FUNDAMENTALS
OF CRISIS
COUNSELING

FUNDAMENTALS OF CRISIS COUNSELING

GERI MILLER

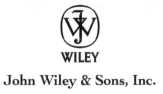

WILEY

John Wiley & Sons, Inc.

Library of Congress Cataloging-in-Publication Data:

    Miller, Geraldine A., 1955–
Fundamentals of crisis counseling / Geri Miller.
      p. ; cm.
Includes bibliographical references and index.
    ISBN 978-0-470-43830-5 (pbk. : alk. paper); 978-1-118-15633-9 (eMobi);
    978-1-118-15634-6 (ePub); 978-1-118-15635-3 (ePDF)
    1. Crisis intervention (Mental health services)   2. Counseling.   I. Title.
    [DNLM: 1. Crisis Intervention.   2. Counseling—methods. WM 401]
RC480.6.M48 2012
362.1'04256—dc23

                                      2011021837

Printed in the United States of America

10 9 8 7 6 5 4 3 2

*This book is dedicated to Ron Hood, my husband and friend, who has survived and shared personal and professional crises with me;
Gale, Abby, and Jason Miller; and
Tom, Laura, Natalie, and Kate Prow—my family;
The many clients I have had the honor of counseling in crisis work;
all of us who have weathered the storms of crisis;
and especially to Lisa Gebo, editor with Wiley, who originally inspired and encouraged this book, who bravely fought for her life, and who finally succumbed to the cancer in 2010.*

Contents

Preface   ix
Acknowledgments   xi

CHAPTER ONE
Introduction/Overview   1

CHAPTER TWO
Crisis Theories, Domains, and Intervention Models   13

CHAPTER THREE
Disaster Mental Health Counseling   27

CHAPTER FOUR
Settings and Commonly Occurring Diagnoses   41

CHAPTER FIVE
Special Populations and Legal/Ethical Issues   73

CHAPTER SIX
Assessment   95

CHAPTER SEVEN
Current Additional Therapies and Concepts   149

CHAPTER EIGHT
Working With Different Cultures   191

CHAPTER NINE
Self-Care   217

References   237
Author Index   259
Subject Index   265

Preface

Fundamentals of Crisis Counseling evolved from my initial national work as a disaster mental health counselor with the American Red Cross in response to the 9/11 tragedy in New York, and then again in 2005 in response to Hurricane Katrina. In 2006, I met Lisa Gebo, Wiley editor, and she encouraged and inspired me to write this book because of my work at local and national levels with the American Red Cross. I would never have taken on this book without her belief in me and her unwavering support. The book is also based on my work in the mental health field since 1976; crisis counseling has always been a part of my work as a counselor under different professional titles.

I have always enjoyed crisis counseling work. Being with clients at their most vulnerable times is an honor, and watching them turn their lives around when they could easily give up is a touching testimony to the power of the human spirit and the loving communities that feed that spirit and keep it alive during adversity. I believe I have watched miracles occur that have inspired me to be a better counselor and person in this world. I have seen counselors committed to the professional field state or demonstrate the same views and feelings I have about this work. I have learned a great deal from my mentors, supervisors, and colleagues, and I hope that I pass on a small amount of this to my own graduate students in counseling.

I wrote this book with my students in mind: what I want them to know of the basics of crisis counseling work. I hope that this book may be helpful to all the readers of the text (students, counselors, etc.) in providing some core information about this important work. This book encourages the application of crisis counseling approaches through the use of case studies, exercises, and questions throughout the book chapters. Also, each chapter provides suggested readings and Web sites; some chapters provide manual, workbook, and videotape/DVD recommendations.

The following is a brief summary of each chapter of the book:

Chapter 1, Introduction/Overview, provides a general overview of crisis counseling and the philosophy of the author toward crisis counseling.

Chapter 2, Crisis Theories, Domains, and Intervention Models, describes crisis theory and general crisis interventions as well as specific crisis intervention models.

Chapter 3, Disaster Mental Health Counseling, summarizes disaster mental health work in terms of its main concepts, techniques, assessment, and treatment.

Chapter 4, Settings and Commonly Occurring Diagnoses, discusses various settings for crisis work (phone, school, agency, private practice) and common diagnoses that can emerge during crisis work (addiction, co-occurring disorders, intimate partner violence, sexual abuse, eating disorders).

Chapter 5, Special Populations and Legal/Ethical Issues, provides an overview of working with specific populations (individual, group, couples/family) with ten practical suggestions for each, as well as a discussion on ethical/legal concerns.

Chapter 6, Assessment, presents an overview on assessment and instrument selection in addition to providing an overview, instruments, case studies, and exercises in each of the following areas: mental health/general trauma, addiction, co-occurring disorders, intimate partner violence, sexual abuse, eating disorders, suicide, and homicide.

Chapter 7, Current Additional Therapies and Concepts, provides the main concepts and techniques of brief therapy, motivational interviewing, stages of change, positive psychology, grief therapy, client resilience, and spirituality.

Chapter 8, Working With Different Cultures, discusses an overall approach to multicultural counseling, multicultural approaches within crisis counseling, and finally, provision of an overview, general approaches, case studies, and exercises with regard to age, gender, sexual orientation, and ethnicity.

Chapter 9, Self-Care, provides an overview, definition, and approaches to self-care as it relates to the counselor, along with case studies and exercises.

Acknowledgments

I have had many great teachers in the counseling field: mentors, supervisors, colleagues, and students of mine. Thank you for all the time and energy you put into teaching me the essentials of counseling and crisis counseling, and for teaching me the power of having compassion for the suffering of others by not only sharing your own stories of suffering but also encouraging me to draw on and learn from the experiences of my own suffering.

In particular, I want to thank the courageous clients I have had the honor of being with in their moments of crisis. To these clients I say: Thank you for trusting me in your sacred space, on your hallowed ground, within your soft spots. You taught me the most important lesson of all: Kindness, a balance of the head and the heart, makes all the difference in life, especially when the volume of life is turned up loud as it is in a crisis. As a result of this lesson, all that is left for me in this world is to practice, to live, to breathe out kindness each day of my life, both personally and professionally. From my work with you, I learned there is nothing more important for me to do in a day than practice kindness. My motto has truly become: If it cannot be done with kindness, then it is not worth doing at all.

Additionally, I want to thank the people at John Wiley & Sons who helped me write this book and supported me on the journey: Lisa Gebo, my first editor, who planted the seed of this book; Isabel Pratt, my second editor, who showed me patience and delighted me with her intellect, humor, and delightful personality; and Marquita Flemming, my third editor, with whom I have had the joy of working on a previous book with Wiley. Marquita's knowledge, precision, enthusiasm, and support never cease to amaze me. I also want to acknowledge the other Wiley employees who worked hard with me on this book and made it an enjoyable experience because of their delightful personalities and intellect: Judi Knott and Heather Dunphy in marketing, Kim Nir in production, and Sherry Wasseeman as editorial assistant.

George Dennis, my computer teacher, again helped me with this book—especially as my computers had crises of their own. George continues to remain a kind, smart, patient, and honest friend of mine. Leila Weinstein, my friend and colleague, assisted me with literature reviews, rewrites, and many miscellaneous details that allowed this book to occur. I especially acknowledge Dr. Betty Gridley, my statistics teacher and mentor, who generously and kindly gave her time and energy to assist me in the development of test questions.

I also thank Susie Greene, Kathleen Kasprick, Alice Krueger, Pat Mitchell, Laurie Percival Oates, Rod and Marilou Steinmetz, and Sue Sweeting, who remained steadfast friends, showing me kindness, compassion, and support and providing me with safe havens on the journey of this book. In addition, I thank my Saturday-morning coffee-drinking buddies, who encouraged me and believed in me and this work.

To Sonny Sweet, former director of the Watauga chapter of the American Red Cross, who encouraged me and others in our work as disaster mental health workers at local, state, and national levels: Thank you.

To the employees of the Paul H. Broyhill Wellness Center—Jodi Cash (director), Paul Moore (assistant director), Michael Darling (personal trainer), and all the rest of my friends who work there and work out there—for encouraging me and supporting me every day with their friendship, laughter, and love: Thank you.

Thank you also to the owners of the Higher Ground Coffee Shop in Boone, North Carolina, Matt and Gloria Scott, who let George and me work on the book for hours in their shop and shared their support and humor with me.

And last on the list, but first in my heart, my husband and best friend, Ron Hood, who continually gave me his love and support by reading every word of every draft of this book and giving up precious evening and weekend time to let me work. My thank you remains the same: "Thank you, Ron, for being with me on this life path. I love you."

CHAPTER ONE

Introduction/Overview

LEARNING OBJECTIVES

1. To learn an overview of the philosophy of crisis counseling.
2. To understand the history of crisis counseling.
3. To develop awareness of areas related to crisis counseling, such as helpful characteristics of counselors and interagency collaboration.

PERSONAL REFLECTIONS ON THE OVERALL BOOK

> Whoever can see through all fear will always be safe.
>
> — *Tao Te Ching*

A few comments regarding this book's philosophy and approach toward crisis counseling need to be presented in this opening chapter. While sometimes this type of information is provided in the preface of a book, it is included in the introductory chapter of this text because of how significantly the underlying philosophy of this book influences each chapter and the general framework of the book.

The motivation for this book stems from my experiences with crisis counseling during 35 years of clinical work. These professional crisis counseling experiences have been augmented recently by my work as a disaster mental health worker with the American Red Cross. This work began in response to the 9/11 attacks in New York and has expanded over the past 10 years to local and state disasters. These combined clinical experiences have resulted in the guiding question used to write this book: "What information is essential to assist mental health professionals in doing crisis work?" This book has evolved from that question and focuses on the goal of the crisis counseling captured in the Tao Te Ching quote at the start of the chapter: to help the client see through the fears of the crisis and feel safe enough in counseling to make the best life-enhancing decisions possible.

In order to assist the client in seeing through the crisis and feeling safe enough to make life-enhancing decisions, the counselor is metaphorically acting as a lighthouse for the client; the client can focus on the guidance of the counselor as the tumultuous waters of the crisis are navigated. As we each think of personal or professional crises we have navigated, we know the power of a caring person simply staying with us through the journey. There is a deep, abiding, sustaining connection offered by the counselor to the client in a crisis situation when the counselor is able to be present with the client and reach out with compassion in response to the client's suffering. The counselor also needs to: (a) help clients proactively respond to the crisis situation, in order to give them a sense of self-control (empowerment); (b) assist clients in getting back into some aspects of their daily routines (activities, rituals), in order to be reassured that the world is a safe place; and (c) provide them with a safe place to vent, where the counselor is listening to the client's storyline (the crisis) but not becoming lost in it to the point of feeling helpless him- or herself or of being drawn to rescue the client and thereby encourage unnecessary dependency of the client on the counselor.

This book, then, is an attempt to provide the reader with practical, hands-on crisis counseling information that will assist clients in crisis and help them heal in their recovery from the crisis. The book can be used as a primer, a handbook presenting an overview of crisis counseling that can be used in clinical work. This can be particularly useful to the reader, because while all clinicians need to be ready to do effective crisis counseling, many of us do not do this work full time. Instead, we have a tendency to integrate this approach into our clinical work when situations arise with clients that require us to have a crisis counseling mindset and crisis counseling skills. Different factors, such as internal client factors (e.g., specific mental health diagnoses that result in the client going in and out of crisis states) or external factors (e.g., life situations such as divorce or natural disasters) may influence the necessary shift to a crisis counseling emphasis in clinical work. To apply effective, timely interventions that operate in the best interests of the client, the reader needs to be prepared to quickly shift to a crisis counseling perspective, often relying solely on his/her clinical judgment under the adage of "the buck stops here."

Because crisis situations require thoughtful clinical decisions that need to be made quickly, the book is designed to expose the reader to an overview of aspects of crisis counseling that one might use infrequently, at best, in clinical work. This approach is intended to help hone the reader's assessment and treatment approach and to enhance the skills that might be required in the crisis counseling situation. The self-reflective aspect of the book (questions, case studies, exercises, etc.) is designed to assist the reader in developing or enhancing his/her crisis counseling mindset by creating an interactive experience between the book and the reader.

This interactive approach is meant to help the reader understand his/her own crisis counseling strengths and weaknesses with the goal of enhancing his/her effectiveness. This self-assessment involves knowledge of critical components, such as: (a) current evidence-based, practical crisis counseling approaches and techniques; (b) operation as an "environmental stress manager" for the client; (c) development of internal and external resources that facilitate client resilience; and (d) self-care approaches that result in the reduction or elimination of burnout.

Finally, the term "counselor" is used throughout the text to describe the mental health professional reader. Readers may identify with different mental health professions and use different labels to describe their work. The term *counselor* has been chosen by the author as a term that represents the application of crisis counseling skills. While it is true that there are emphasis differences in crisis counseling among professionals (due to orientation and training), there are also similar themes and approaches that bridge these differences. While I have attempted to be sensitive to these variances, the reader is asked to acknowledge any limitations of the terminology used in this book and to not allow these limitations to block the potential usefulness of the text.

DEFINITIONS OF CRISIS, CRISIS COUNSELING, AND CRISIS INTERVENTION

There are numerous definitions for crisis (James, 2008). Typically, the crisis is made up of an event that occurs before the crisis, the client's *perception* of the event, and the client's previous coping strategies not being enough in the situation (Roberts, 2005). It is a state of upset-disorganization that is temporary and has the potential for either a "radically positive or negative outcome" (Slaikeu, 1990, p. 15). Essentially, the various definitions state the same components of a crisis: the client's perception or experience of an event/situation as being intolerable and going beyond their resources and coping abilities. There are three components of the crisis: an *event*, the client's *perception*, and the failure of the client's typical *coping methods* (Kanel, 2007). As human beings we are, at least temporarily, unable to find relief in the crisis situation (Hoff, Hallisey, & Hoff, 2009).

When the individual does reach out for assistance, the reaching out can, obviously, include counseling. There are two main components to crisis counseling: first-order intervention (psychological first aid) and second-order intervention (crisis therapy) (Slaikeu, 1990). The first-order intervention of crisis counseling (psychological first aid) has been defined by the National Institute of Mental Health (2002) as making sure clients are safe, stress-related symptoms are reduced, clients have opportunities to rest and recover physically, and clients are connected to the resources and social supports they need to survive and recover from the crisis. The term "psychological first aid" originated in a description of crisis work in response to an Australian railway disaster (Raphael, 1977). It is considered the basic component of crisis intervention (James, 2008).

The goal at this stage of psychological first aid is to break up the behavior cycle that is dysfunctional and help the person return to their previous functioning level. Slaikeu (1990) breaks this stage into five components: psychological contact, problem exploration, solution exploration, concrete action taken, and follow-up. Overall assessment of the client can be done through the BASIC personality profile (Slaikeu, 1990) as described by Miller (2010, p. 100):

1. *Behavioral.* This area focuses on the client's behavior in terms of strengths and weaknesses as well as behavioral antecedents and consequences.
2. *Affective.* The counselor assesses the client's feelings about these behaviors.
3. *Somatic.* The counselor assesses the client's physical health through sensations experienced.
4. *Interpersonal.* This area focuses on examining the quality of various relationships in the client's life.
5. *Cognitive.* The counselor assesses the client's thoughts and self-talk.

When counselors respond, they are intervening in the crisis. In this intervention, counselors are basically assessing the crisis situation at that moment, stabilizing the person, and assisting in the development of a plan to help them move out of the crisis mode. In crisis intervention, the counselor tries to reduce the crisis impact by immersing him- or herself into the client's life and assisting in the development of resources. This involves crisis therapy along a continuum that includes assessment, planning, implementation, and follow-up; the crisis intervention is woven into the context of therapy (Hoff et al., 2009).

Counseling interventions in therapy need to be sensitively timed for the client, because the crisis is both a danger and an opportunity. It is dangerous in that the client may resort to destructive behavior (suicide, homicide), but it is an opportunity because the client may reorganize him/herself and his/her life by reaching out for assistance and thereby developing new knowledge and skills. It is in this development of new knowledge and skills that the counselor can be immeasurably significant in the client's life; this is where therapy can have a long-lasting impact. A well-designed, sensitively timed intervention that is idiosyncratically matched to the individual client and his/her situation can change a life forever.

History of Crisis Intervention

Crisis intervention work has been around since 1942, when the staff of Massachusetts General Hospital responded to the Cocoanut Grove nightclub fire in Boston, where 493 people died (Lindemann, 1944). In their work with survivors and families of the victims, the hospital staff studied their acute and delayed reactions and clinically addressed psychological symptoms (survivors) and the prevention of unresolved grief (family members) (Roberts, 2005). In addition to Lindemann, Gerald Caplan (1961) also worked with these survivors and was a pioneer in defining and developing theory related to crisis (stages). Rapoport (1967) added to Lindemann's and Caplan's work by showing that an event led to a crisis and by describing the nature of the event more precisely, as well as emphasizing the importance of the intervention—particularly in assessment (Roberts, 2005).

This work continued into the 1960s, when suicide prevention (e.g., 24-hour hotlines) and community mental health (e.g., mental health clinics, managing psychiatric patients on medication on an outpatient basis) became popular concerns in the United States. Crisis intervention strategies and research grew out of these concerns (Kanel, 2007). Three major grassroots movements impacted crisis intervention: Alcoholics Anonymous (AA), activism by veterans from the Vietnam War, and the women's movement (James, 2008). The impact came because these three groups of people needed help and were not receiving it. Crisis intervention strategies and research, then, became even more widespread, as there were increased concerns about money and limited resources that could not meet the demands of the population. Since the 1960s, additional crisis management has focused on specific areas, such as domestic violence (hotlines, shelters), child abuse (hotlines, referral networks), and rape crisis programs (Roberts, 2005).

In recent years, crisis intervention has become even more of a core component of the helping professions due to the impact of violent incidents on helping professionals in all areas of the United States because of (a) increased access to information, and (b) violence expressed in terrorist acts in public settings (e.g., the attacks on the Twin Towers, school shootings, etc.). A crisis in one part of the United States can easily set off a secondary trauma in another part of the United States. For example, although the 9/11 terrorist activity took place in New York, Pennsylvania, and Washington, DC, and Hurricane Katrina was physically localized to the southern part of the United States, the impact of these traumas throughout the United States was widespread because of the visual images and information spread through television and the Internet. Additionally, the impact of disasters such as 9/11 and Hurricane Katrina does not remain localized to one specific area, since many individuals needed to relocate themselves in response to the disasters. Finally, shootings such as the ones that occurred at Virginia Tech show that helping professionals are increasingly working with individuals impacted by crises in their communities; the helping professionals need to be prepared to do crisis intervention work at a moment's notice.

The history of crisis intervention work and the current context of this work (increased opportunities for exposure to crisis work) speak again to the focus of this book. This book has an overall goal of providing mental health professionals and students in training in the mental health professions with readily applicable theoretical and practical research-based crisis intervention approaches. Ready access to the essentials of crisis counseling work can assist these individuals in their very important work with the clients in their communities. All counselors will do crisis counseling work, whether it is brief work of a few sessions, working with clients who are in continual crises, and/or working with clients on an ongoing basis who experience a crisis during their therapy.

HELPFUL CHARACTERISTICS OF COUNSELORS

While there may be numerable counselor characteristics that can be helpful in a crisis situation, this section will elaborate on five: life experiences, poise, creativity and flexibility, energy and resiliency, and quick mental reflexes. These are drawn from James's (2008) list of helpful counselor characteristics.

Life experiences means the crisis counselor has emotional maturity that stems from life experiences. Our training as mental health professionals teaches us how to work with clients, whether we have personally experienced their specific crisis or not. Emotional maturity developed through learning from our life experiences can enhance the depth and sensitivity with which we treat our crisis clients. Those of us who have experienced the same type of crisis as our client need to be aware of our countertransference issues that stem from personal and professional biases and "wounds" and work with those issues through consultation with colleagues, mentors, supervisors, and/or personal therapy.

In terms of *poise*, it is important to stay calm, stable, poised, rational, and in control, because in a crisis the client can be out of control and/or might present material that can be shocking and threatening. Here the counselor is acting as the rudder for the client in the storm of the crisis; the client can pick up on the emotional state as well as the physical presence of the counselor. Therefore, the counselor needs to find ways to reassure him/herself in the crisis in order to remain stable for the client. Specific suggestions to the counselor are made in Chapters 3 and 9 of this text with regard to disaster mental health work and self-care. In the overall practice of self-care, the counselor will have the balance and internal resources to be of maximum benefit to the client in the crisis. Or, in terms of the metaphor stated previously, the counselor will be a stable rudder for the client's boat in the storm. Such stability makes an impressive impact on reducing the crisis. In a 9/11 crisis situation, I saw a counselor calmly approach a hostile, belligerent client. In a steady, calming voice and manner, the counselor said, "Friend, I do not think this approach is going to take you far in this situation." Immediately the client calmed down in the situation, making the crisis more manageable.

Creativity and flexibility are major assets and encourage divergent thinking. The more creative and flexible counselors can be in a crisis situation, the more effectively they can meet the needs of the client. If the counselor becomes caught in a formula approach to a crisis situation, then the counselor's response can be an automatic, rigid one that does not meet the unique needs of the client or the possibly changing dynamics of the crisis situation. Rather, if the counselor can approach the crisis with a tentative plan for how to address it, combined with a readiness to let go of that approach if it does not work, then the counselor can be more effective, because a more comfortable intervention fit can evolve for the client through

6

a natural process. For example, a counselor may approach a crisis situation in which the client has been given a terminal illness diagnosis. The counselor may assume the client will want to discuss issues related to death. However, the client may be in a place of denial and may be interested only in discussing how to fight the illness; he or she is unwilling to discuss death at all. The counselor may need to shift the focus of the session to discussing the "battle" first, and then gently but quickly explore the underlying fears related to death.

In terms of *energy and resiliency*, we need to have energy and be organized, direct, and systemic in the actions we take, which means we need to practice self-care to promote our own resiliency. Energy, self-care, and resiliency are discussed more extensively in Chapter 9. To have physical and emotional energy, we need to care for ourselves. The practice of self-care can provide us with resiliency, which is required in the intensity of addressing crises. Clients in crisis will sense when a counselor is balanced, resulting in a helpful contagion effect that may calm the client. When we care for ourselves as mental health professionals, the result is that we are calm and steady in facing the crisis situation, providing the sense that "someone is in charge here." I was told by a mental health worker in a crisis situation where other workers had been having "meltdowns," "Oh, no, you won't have a meltdown—you take care of yourself too well on an ongoing basis."

Quick mental reflexes are critical because the issues in a crisis are steadily emerging and changing. This is very similar to creativity, flexibility, energy, and resiliency. We need to be able to think divergently and be resilient in order to have quick mental reflexes. The nature of the crisis situation calls for us to be able to make quick decisions. This is why I advocate that my students and trainees interested in crisis work have licensure and experience as counselors before doing this type of work, because it is truly work where "the buck stops here." One needs to be comfortable making decisions quickly and often alone in the context of the crisis. There may be time and opportunity for consultation with colleagues, mentors, and supervisors, but we cannot count on it.

This section on characteristics of the counselor is not meant to be discouraging to the reader. No crisis counselor is perfect all the time, nor do any of us handle the crisis perfectly throughout. Rather, we act in the best interest of the client and continually assess the client and the situation for what appears to be the approach that reflects caring for the client's welfare. Rather than focusing on avoiding making a mistake or being flawless, it is more important for us, if and when we make a mistake, to recognize it and recover from it. Most importantly, we need to be human beings with our clients in a crisis situation, for whom everything feels tumultuous. Such humanity can be an umbilical cord of hope for our clients.

INTERAGENCY COLLABORATION

We need to discuss briefly the subject of collaboration with other agencies, because client crises often mean that other agencies will need to be involved somewhere in the process of the intervention—whether it be in terms of referral, assessment, treatment, or follow-up. The same characteristics described above as being helpful with clients are also helpful in working with other agencies: life experiences, poise, creativity and flexibility, energy and resiliency, and quick mental reflexes. Other agency personnel may be almost, or sometimes more, out of balance than the client in the crisis, and through their behavior they may exacerbate the crisis. Or the counselor may approach or interact with the other agency personnel during the crisis in a manner that fuels the crisis.

In crisis situations, emotions tend to run high and just one comment, behavior, intervention, or the like can inflame a crisis through deterioration of a professional relationship. That is why the counselor needs to learn how to remain calm when others are not calm. In Chapter 3, this approach is titled "environmental stress manager." This means that the counselor needs to be able to read his/her own stress levels, those of the client, and those of the surrounding crisis situation, and then intervene on these stressors present in each area—that is, manage the stress. Counselors should not assume that others will pick up on stress indicators and respond to them. Rather, the counselor needs to be cognizant of the skills developed through his/her training to recognize, address, and minimize these indicators. For example, a supervisor at a disaster mental health site had not been caring for herself on a regular basis, but had focused almost exclusively on others. As a result, after a few days on the site, she was very critical and sharp in her dealings with other agencies. Her fellow counselor team members successfully encouraged her to take more breaks, which ended up in her approaching other agencies in a more collaborative manner and reducing the stress in the environment.

SUMMARY

This chapter presented an overview of crisis counseling: philosophy, definition, and history. Finally, it addressed the importance of helpful counselor characteristics and interagency collaboration.

QUESTIONS

1. What is the philosophy of crisis counseling as presented in this book?
2. Describe the history of crisis counseling.
3. What are typical reactions (professional, client) to crisis situations, and what makes interagency collaboration so critical to crisis counseling?

EXERCISE

Write out your philosophy of crisis counseling work in a few sentences. Make sure to address these questions: What is your main focus? How does your current

---

Case Study 1.1

You have a client who requires the assistance of a number of agencies (social services, church, health department, etc.) in dealing with a crisis situation Your client is very distraught, but is willing to contact these agencies to obtain assistance and willing to have you talk with them regarding her situation (she has signed consent forms). You have a history of working with helping professionals at the local health department; you are aware that they do not like to work with clients in crisis mental health situations, and generally, they have not been cooperative with you in the past.

1. How would you approach this situation with the health department?
2. What would you tell your client, if anything, about the history of your experiences in working with the health department?
3. Would you warn your client about some of the barriers she may face in approaching them? If so, what would be your general strategy?

(or anticipated) job/clientele impact your philosophy of crisis counseling? What do you see as your main strengths and weaknesses in this type of work?

SUGGESTED READINGS

Bein, A. W. (2008). *The Zen of helping: Spiritual principles for mindful and open-hearted practice.* Hoboken, NJ: Wiley.

This book has ten chapters that address a mindfulness approach in counseling clients in general.

Briere, J., & Scott, C. (2006). *Principles of trauma therapy.* Thousand Oaks, CA: Sage.

This book is divided into two sections: trauma effects and assessment and clinical interventions.

Greenstone, J. L., & Leviton, S. C. (2002). *Elements of crisis intervention* (3rd ed.). Belmont, CA: Brooks/Cole.

This short book has 11 chapters that briefly cover basic approaches and strategies in crisis work with focused chapters on children, families, hotline workers, loss, legal implications, and disasters.

Hoff, L. A., Hallisey, B. J., & Hoff, M. (2009). *People in crisis: Clinical and diversity perspectives* (6th ed.). New York, NY: Routledge.

This book is an overview of crisis work. It is divided into three sections: understanding crisis intervention, specific crises, and suicide/homicide/catastrophic events.

James, R. K. (2008). *Crisis intervention strategies.* Belmont, CA: Thomson Brooks/Cole.

This book provides an overview of crisis intervention. It has four sections: theory and application, handling specific crises, workplace, and disaster. There is a specific chapter related to addiction.

Kanel, K. (2007). *Crisis intervention* (3rd ed.). Belmont, CA: Thomson Brooks/Cole.

This book has 12 chapters that cover general crisis information (definition, history, ethical/professional issues) as well as chapters on multicultural concerns, the ABC model, and addressing issues related to crisis, such as danger, developmental crises, loss, illness and disabilities, substance abuse, PTSD/community disasters/trauma, and abuse (child, spousal, sexual assault).

Roberts, A. R., & Yeager, K. R. (2009). *Pocket guide to crisis intervention*. New York, NY: Oxford University Press.

This brief book has 33 chapters, each of which, in a few pages, covers major topics of crisis work. It may be thought of as a type of CliffsNotes or a primer of crisis work.

Shea, S. C. (2002). *The practical art of suicide assessment: A guide for mental health professionals and substance abuse counselors*. Hoboken, NJ: Wiley.

This book has three sections: an overview, suicidal ideation, and assessment. It has helpful appendices on assessment documentation, safety contracts, and suicide prevention Web sites.

WEB SITES

Mental health professionals can contact the following Web sites for information on mental health counseling in a crisis context with regard to their professional organizational affiliation.

American Association for Marital and Family Therapy: www.aamft.org
American Counseling Association: www.counseling.org
American Psychiatric Association: www.psych.org
American Psychological Association: www.apa.org
National Association of Social Workers: www.naswdc.org

Co-occurring Disorders

Substance Abuse and Mental Health Services Administration (SAMHSA): www.mentalhealth.samhsa.gov

This Web site provides a variety of information and resources on substance abuse and mental health.

Crisis

Crisis Prevention Institute: www.crisisprevention.com

This Web site provides information on training professionals working with potentially violent people.

National Organization for Victim Assistance: www.trynova.org

This Web site offers information on the rights of victims and services available to them.

General

Department of Health and Human Services (DHHS): www.hhs.gov

This Web site provides information on various aspects of American health concerns. A connecting Web site, www.phe.gov/preparedness, provides information specifically focused on public health emergencies, including crises such as disasters and trauma.

National Institute of Mental Health: www.nimh.nih.gov

This Web site provides information on understanding and treating mental illness and offers helpful publications for the mental health professional.

Suicide

American Association of Suicidology (AAS): www.suicidology.org

One can join this organization. The Web site has facts, warning signs, support groups, crisis centers, a bulletin board (members only), and a bookstore.

American Foundation for Suicide Prevention (AFSP): www.afsp.org

This Web site has statistics and suicide survivor information.

SA/VE: Suicide Awareness Voices of Education: www.save.org

This Web site has suicide prevention education, advocates for suicide survivors, and information on developing a group for suicide survivors.

Suicide Prevention Action Network (SPAN) USA: www.spanusa.org

If You Are Thinking About Suicide . . . Read This First: www.metanoia.org/suicide

This Web site attempts to reduce the stigma around having suicidal thoughts so that the reader is open to receiving help.

CHAPTER TWO

Crisis Theories, Domains, and Intervention Models

LEARNING OBJECTIVES

1. To learn specific theoretical models, domains, and intervention models related to crisis counseling.
2. To apply two general interventions of crisis counseling.
3. To apply these theoretical models, domains, and intervention models to specific crisis situations through the use of case studies and exercises.

> The world is but a resting place.
>
> —*Ancient Proverb*

Counselors need to have a theoretical framework through which to view a client's problem. This is especially important in a crisis counseling situation, in which the counselor often does not have much time to reflect on his/her theoretical views. In such a situation, the counselor needs to almost go into "automatic pilot" regarding a theoretical orientation, because the crisis situation simply needs to be addressed as quickly, thoroughly, and adequately as possible. Such a focused, efficient, yet humane orientation means that the counselor would be well-advised to examine and explore his/her crisis counseling theoretical perspective prior to doing the work of crisis counseling.

While some counselors have jobs that are specifically crisis-focused, and their training for these positions may involve an exploration of theoretical models, domains, and intervention models, many counselors do not have opportunities for such training. At the same time, crisis intervention is seen as a core part of counseling (Hoff, Hallisey, & Hoff, 2009). As a result of these two realities (possibly limited training and required knowledge), this chapter will attempt to assist the counselor in this self-examination process regarding crisis-related theories, domains, and intervention models as a preparation for this type of work.

The theoretical framework (theory, domain, intervention) of the counselor assists the counselor in knowing which factors of the crisis need to be punctuated to adequately address the crisis—which parts of the client's story are drawn into the foreground or dropped into the background. This emphasis guides the counselor through the assessment and treatment aspects of the crisis counseling with regard to the focus on, the priority of, and the intervention on issues; it helps the counselor understand the world of the crisis and attempt to be a part of making the "world as a resting place" for the client. In general, a counselor's theoretical framework acts as his/her rudder. In the navigation of what may be substantial, fragmented, and intense information regarding both the crisis situation and the client's response to it, this rudder is essential. Metaphorically, while a rudder (theoretical framework) is helpful to a boat's balance in the water (general counseling), the sailor (counselor) relies on it even more when the waters are tumultuous (crisis counseling).

Regarding the framework of crisis counseling related areas (theories, domains, and interventions), an overall framework is presented in Figure 2.1 based on James's work (2008). A part of this framework is also based on Janosik's (1984) levels of crisis theory described in James's work (2008).

The framework presented in Figure 2.1 has two main components: crisis theories (which include domains) and crisis intervention models. The theories examine the phenomenon of the crisis, while the intervention models focus on the helping response. The reader is encouraged to choose a core theory, domain, and intervention model from which to view the phenomena of and intervention on the crisis. The reader may also elect to choose one or two adjunctive theories, domains, and intervention models to find a balance between being flexible in applying crisis theory to the crisis situation of the client *and* organizing the fragmentation of the crisis situation to serve the best interests of the client.

Three tables are provided in this chapter to assist the reader in creating a framework that includes theories, domains, and intervention models. Following each table is a case study and exercise(s) to assist in the integration and application of this crisis counseling framework to the reader's overall counseling perspective.

CRISIS THEORIES

A counseling theory is made up of ideas and explanations that require the counselor to prove the theory's fit to the client's situation (Johnson, 2004). The theory

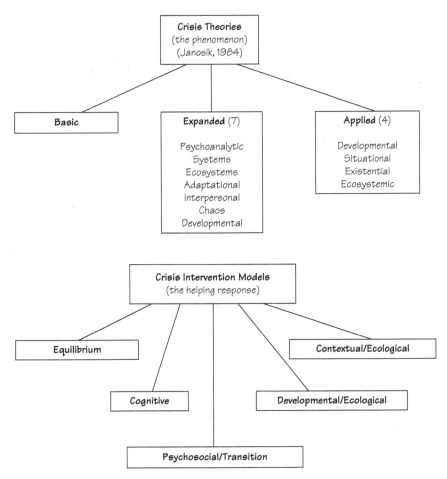

Figure 2.1 Crisis-Related Theories
(James, 2008)

reflects both the personal and professional view of the counselor and is shaped by the populations with whom the counselor has worked and is working currently. In general counseling, no theory explains all counseling problems and required approaches. The same is true for crisis counseling: no one theory explains the phenomenon of crisis adequately. Therefore, the counselor needs to be flexible in drawing upon and applying crisis theory in the same way a counselor would need to be when practicing counseling in general. Such flexibility is very important in crisis counseling so the counselor can readily adapt approaches to fit the uniqueness of the client and the uniqueness of the crisis situation.

The difficulty in choosing a crisis counseling theory may in part be connected to the reality of the numerous crisis counseling theories that exist, as well as the different frameworks developed to organize them. No theoretical discipline can rightfully claim that crisis theory stems solely from it; therefore, crisis counseling theory comes from an "eclectic mixture drawn from psychoanalytic, existential, humanistic, cognitive-behavioral, and general systems theories" (Kanel, 2007, p. 18). To learn more about the overall theories mentioned in this chapter, the reader is referred to general counseling theory textbooks (such as Corey, 2009) and to the resources developed by the respective experts in each of these theoretical orientations. The crisis theories are sorted as *Basic, Expanded,* and *Applied.*

Basic Crisis Theory

As stated in the history of crisis counseling in Chapter 1, Lindemann (1944) and Caplan (1961) helped professionals understand the basic theory and counseling interventions of crisis counseling. Although their work was different in emphasis, both normalized clients' crisis responses and provided short-term intervention techniques that can be used by the counselor. It is this work, discussed both here and in Chapter 1, that makes up basic crisis intervention theory anchored in a psychoanalytic perspective. This psychoanalytic perspective is presented in Table 2.1 in the "Expanded Crisis Theory" section.

Expanded Crisis Theory

Expanded crisis theory evolved because of the limits of basic crisis intervention theory (it did not account enough for the social, environmental, and situational factors that can contribute to a crisis). Thus, crisis counseling expanded from solely *psychoanalytic* theory to the inclusion of six other types of theories: *systems, ecosystems, adaptational, interpersonal, chaos,* and *developmental.* Table 2.1 summarizes each theoretical perspective and its view of the nature, causes, and resolution of crisis.

Table 2.1 Expanded Crisis Theoretical Models

Theory	View of Crisis	Cause of Crisis	Treatment of Crisis
Psychoanalytic (Basic)	Disequilibrium due to unconscious thoughts/ past emotional experiences	Early childhood fixation	Develop client insight into dynamics/causes of behavior
Systems	Interrelationships/ interdependence between people, and between people and events	Interactions between people, and between people and events	Address the interactions

16

Theory	View of Crisis	Cause of Crisis	Treatment of Crisis
Ecosystems	Environmental contexts have an impact on the crisis	Interaction between environmental contexts and the crisis	Examine and address the interrelationships between ecological systems
Adaptational	Maladaptive behaviors, thoughts, defense mechanisms	Interaction of the client's maladaptive behaviors, thoughts, and defense mechanisms	Break the interaction and help the client learn adaptive behaviors, thoughts, and defense mechanisms
Interpersonal	Lack of empowering belief in self, trust in others, confidence in overcoming crisis	External locus of control (self-evaluation based on others)	Assist in shifting locus of control to an internal one (self-evaluation is based on self-view with control and action stemming from that perspective)
Chaos	Presence of a chaotic situation	Chaos that cannot be addressed by known solutions	Understand and cope with the crisis through a trial-and-error process that results in an underlying order
Developmental	Movement through developmental stages has been blocked	Unmet developmental tasks during a life stage	Resolve developmental life tasks

Case Study 2.1

Your client presents with a work situation that has evolved into a crisis because of the current economic problems and politics in the workplace. He is married, has children, and describes himself as a "regular, middle-class, middle-aged guy." He does not know what to do, because his work situation is becoming more abusive due to politics that are hampering the completion of his job responsibilities: for example, people (co-workers, supervisors) are not providing him with necessary information and yet are blaming him and giving him consequences for not meeting his job responsibilities. As a result, he is having to work longer and has less time

(continued)

for his family. This has resulted in problems within his marriage and him being more short-tempered with his children. He wants to leave his career (he has been unhappy with it for a number of years), but does not know how he could find another job in the local area given the current state of the economy. He does not feel suicidal, but he has recently been placed on antidepressants and high blood pressure medication by his general physician. He describes himself as in a crisis and unable to see his way out, which is why he has come for counseling for the first time in his life.

1. Which expanded theory is most complementary to your view of counseling and seems to fit his crisis situation the best?
2. How does this expanded theory explain the cause and resolution of the crisis?
3. How would you approach the assessment and treatment of the client based on your choice of expanded theory?

EXERCISE 2.1

Choose one expanded theory that complements your view of counseling in general and one applied theory that does the same. Write out the pros and cons of the use of this theory in a crisis situation.

Applied Crisis Theory (Domains)

In applied crisis theory, James (2008) discusses the presence of four areas: *developmental, situational, existential, and ecosystemic*. The first three of these areas are based on Brammer's work (1985) and the fourth is a domain added by James (2008). Although theorists will use different domains to understand the crisis (James & Gilliland, 2005), the first two categories (developmental, situational) are most commonly used to understand the domains of the crisis and are typically labeled *maturational/developmental* and *situational/accidental* (Halpern & Tramontin, 2007). The reader may want to explore these two areas (maturational/developmental and situational/accidental) in more depth in Hoff et al.'s (2009) three chapters on life passages, health status and self-image, and occupational and residential security. Table 2.2 summarizes these crisis domains in terms of their views and definitions of crisis.

Case Study 2.2

Using the same case study as in the expanded theory section (p. 17):

1. Which applied theory domain fits this crisis situation?
2. How would you integrate the expanded theory and applied theoretical domain you chose?

Table 2.2 Applied Crisis Theory (Domains)

Domain	View of Crisis	Definition of Crisis
Developmental *"Maturational" commonly used*	Normal	A shift in development that results in abnormal responses (e.g., graduation)
Situational *"accidental"*	"random, sudden, shocking, intense, and often catastrophic" (James, 2008, p. 13).	An uncommon, extraordinary event that an individual cannot predict or control (e.g., rape)
Existential	Inner conflicts/anxieties in relation to basic human existence issues	Confrontation of the void, the emptiness with regard to living (e.g., meaning of life)
Ecosystemic	Disaster results that stem from nature or humans	A consuming disaster in terms of a group of people who are victims of an event (e.g., a flood)

EXERCISE 2.2

Discuss with a colleague how the four applied theoretical domains of crisis counseling can be integrated into your expanded theory of crisis counseling.

EXERCISE 2.3

Write out your experiences with crisis counseling populations in terms of how you would use your expanded crisis theory. Then add in your experiences in working in the four domains and write about how this expanded crisis theory may have assisted in your assessment and treatment of these clinical populations.

GENERAL CRISIS INTERVENTIONS

Before discussing crisis counseling intervention models, we will address a couple of specific interventions, because they can be viewed as overall bridges between theory and application in crisis counseling work. These two interventions are *psychological first aid* and *multimodal therapy*. Each can be used in the various crisis intervention models. As discussed in Chapter 1, Slaikeu (1990) separates them into two main intervention components in crisis counseling: first-order intervention (psychological first aid) and second-order intervention (crisis therapy).

Psychological First Aid (PFA)

This intervention strategy of crisis counseling was discussed in Chapter 1 and will be discussed again in Chapter 3. In Chapter 1, it was discussed in an overview of crisis counseling; in Chapter 3 it will be viewed in the context of disaster mental health counseling specifically with regard to treatment.

Using Slaikeu's (1990) perspective, first-order crisis counseling intervention is psychological first aid (PFA), where the goal is to disrupt the client's dysfunctional behavior and help him/her return to his/her previous functioning level. The term began in a description of crisis work that was done in response to an Australian railway disaster (Raphael, 1977).

PFA has been described as an acute intervention that is one part of a mental health continuum of care (Everly & Flynn, 2006). It is viewed as the basic component of crisis intervention, as it provides physical and psychological support to the client in a manner that is not viewed as invasive. It has been used professionally in different ways that can be confusing; therefore, it may be understood more easily as being like physical first aid: preliminary care ranging from minor care that needs no additional treatment to serious care that can be addressed temporarily until medical professionals arrive on the scene (Jacobs & Meyer, 2006).

PFA has been described as: (a) having five components (psychological contact, problem exploration, solution exploration, concrete action taken, and follow-up; Slaikeu, 1990), (b) defining duty components (problem definition, client safety and support; James, 2008), and (c) being a general approach to assisting clients (safety, stress symptom reduction, physical rest and recovery, connection to resources and social supports; the National Institute of Mental Health [NIMH], 2002). It has also been described as a set of eight core actions that attempt to reduce the initial distress of the trauma by supporting the short- and long-term adaptive functioning of the client (Ruzek, Brymer, Jacobs, Layne, Vernberg, & Watson, 2007):

1. Contact and engage the client
2. Provide safety and comfort
3. Stabilize the client
4. Gather information
5. Provide practical assistance
6. Connect with social supports
7. Provide information on coping supports
8. Connect the client with collaborative services

Finally, PFA can be placed in *Stage 1 (Acute Support)* of a three-stage model of treatment (Housley & Beutler, 2007). In this stage, the counselor's goals with regard to the client are to reduce distress, increase understanding of his/her personal reactions to the crisis, reduce negative coping, and increase knowledge of resources (when needed, how to access). In the provision of acute support, the counselor is establishing rapport with the client, adapting the counseling to fit the client's needs, providing helpful information, supporting the client's positive coping skills, making sure resources are available to meet basic needs, and exploring the existence and use of social networks.

Case Study 2.3

Your client is quite emotional during your first few minutes with him. You are concerned about obtaining accurate information in the assessment because of the extent of the anger being expressed. You are not concerned about violence, but more concerned that you cannot follow your client's train of thought and accurately capture the story of the impact the crisis has had on him.

1. In terms of applying PFA, which aspect(s) of it would you focus on initially?
2. How would you focus on these aspects as a reflection of your view of crisis counseling and your general therapy approach?

All of these perspectives on PFA underscore the importance of using it as a baseline of assistance in crisis counseling work. Although it is technically an intervention strategy, without this strategy, crisis counseling would simply not occur or would be ineffective in its delivery and application. Counselors need to learn how to use PFA as they work with clients in all types of crisis.

EXERCISE 2.4

Find a colleague with whom you can discuss the following questions:

1. Which aspects of PFA do you view as your strengths in crisis counseling?
2. Which aspects of PFA do you believe you need to strengthen?
3. Are these views of your use of PFA based on clinical experiences? If they are, share one of the highlights of both areas with your colleague. If not a part of your clinical experience, share with your colleague what you anticipate to be a strength or a weakness.

Multimodal

One of the developers of the Multimodal therapy approach was Lazarus (1976, 1981). Lazarus (1981) uses the acronym BASIC ID to describe seven modalities of personality: behaviors (B), affective processes (A), sensations (S), images (I), cognitions (C), interpersonal relationships (I), and biological functions–drugs (D).

This BASIC ID framework can be used to both assess and treat the client in crisis therapy. This acronym can be memorized and used by the crisis counselor to ensure that a balanced assessment and treatment approach is done. For example, a client may have a very strong *Affective* orientation during the crisis intake, or a tendency for expressing affect in crisis therapy. The counselor can use the acronym (BASIC ID) as a mental checklist to make sure that the other areas are adequately

---

Case Study 2.4

Your client's physical concerns (Sensations) dominate the counseling session. You believe that it is important to hear the client's story because the physical concerns are core to the crisis. Yet you realize that in order to complete an accurate, overall assessment, you need to address the other areas of the BASIC ID profile (behaviors, affective processes, sensations, images, cognitions, interpersonal relationships, biological functions–drugs). How would you approach the client in a way that would both allow the client the experience of being heard and yet ensure that a complete assessment is done? What would be your concerns about exploring other areas with the client? How would you address those concerns in your approach, whether directly or indirectly, with the client?

---

discussed and explored in the assessment and then expressed in the treatment plan. The use of such an acronym in the assessment and treatment process can assist the counselor in appropriately addressing the client's welfare.

EXERCISE 2.5

Write down your first thoughts to the following questions:

1. What approaches would you use to explore the cognitive domain of a highly affective crisis client? understand feeling / emotion (driven by them) ? why?
2. How would your counseling approach be different if you had a highly cognitive crisis client who was resistant to exploring his/her affective domain in response to the crisis?

CRISIS INTERVENTION MODELS

As stated earlier, no single crisis intervention model captures all crisis intervention approaches. However, as stated in the previous section on crisis theories, the intervention model:

- Reflects the counselor's personal/professional views
- Is shaped by the populations with whom the counselor has worked and with whom he/she is currently working
- Can be flexibly used to fit the unique factors of the client and the crisis

Table 2.3 organizes five crisis intervention models to assist the reader in determining the model or models he/she wants to use in crisis counseling. These five models are: *equilibrium, cognitive, psychosocial* (Belkin, 1984; Leitner, 1974), *developmental-ecological* (Collins & Collins, 2005), and *contextual-ecological* (Myer & Moore, 2006).

Table 2.3 Crisis Intervention Models

Intervention Model	Client Reaction	Counseling Goal	Timing of Use
Equilibrium	Experiences disequilibrium (psychological/emotional) because typical coping mechanisms/problem-solving approaches are inadequate	Help clients obtain pre-crisis equilibrium	Early intervention
Cognitive	Practices faulty thinking about surrounding events or situations of the crisis	Increase client awareness of and change faulty beliefs	After pre-crisis equilibrium is resumed
Psychosocial/ Transition	Reacts out of the combination of biological factors and social learning in response to the environment(s)	Determine internal and external problems that feed the crisis and support in the choice of internal/external alternatives	After pre-crisis equilibrium is resumed
Developmental/ Ecological	Responds to the crisis in terms of resolution of developmental tasks and environmental issues, as well as the interaction between them	Consider the developmental stage of the client at the time of the crisis	No specific time frame
Contextual/ Ecological	Reactions are based on three contextual crisis factors (physical proximity and reactions moderated through perception and attributional meaning; reciprocity between individual and system reactions; impact of time that has passed and special occasions)	Determine the crisis impact by looking at event proximity, event reactions, event relationship, amount of change due to event, and divide by amount of time since the event	Primarily theoretical— no specific interventions

---

Case Study 2.5

Use the same case study as in the expanded theory section (Case Study 2.1, p. 17):

1. Which crisis counseling intervention model most comfortably fits with your general counseling approach and this crisis situation?
2. How would you integrate this model into the expanded theory and applied theoretical domain you chose?

EXERCISE 2.6

Rank order the five crisis counseling intervention models in terms of your comfort level using them. Discuss the order of your rankings with a colleague in terms of the factors that shaped your rankings (e.g., client population, timing of crisis intervention work, theoretical counseling framework).

SUMMARY

This chapter focused on specific theoretical models, domains, and intervention models related to crisis counseling. In an attempt to enhance the reader's capacity to go into "automatic pilot" in the application of one's theoretical orientation in a crisis counseling situation, a figure and three tables related to the core crisis theories and crisis intervention models were provided. The text, visual images, case studies, and exercises were provided to assist the reader in choosing and applying these frameworks and interventions to crisis situations.

QUESTIONS

1. What are specific theoretical models, domains, and intervention models related to crisis counseling?
2. What are some general interventions of crisis counseling?
3. How might these theoretical models and interventions be applied in clinical settings of the reader?

SUGGESTED READINGS

Overall (Psychological First Aid, Multimodal Therapy, Theory)

Slaikeu, K. A. (1990). *Crisis intervention: A handbook for practice and research* (2nd ed.). Needham Heights, MA: Allyn & Bacon.
This 519-page book has 21 chapters divided into four sections: theoretical considerations, intervention strategies, service delivery systems, and training and

research. In addition, it has three appendices: crisis therapy groups, crisis question-naire, and glossary of crisis therapy techniques.

Psychological First Aid

Halpern, J., & Tramontin, M. (2007). *Disaster mental health: Theory and practice.* Belmont, CA: Thompson Brooks/Cole.

This 366-page book provides a thorough overview of disaster mental health coun-seling. It has two main sections (disaster mental health theory and disaster mental health practice), which are each divided into twelve chapters (six per section). The first section provides an overview, disaster characteristics, and a history of this approach, as well as a discussion of risk factors, both typical and extreme reactions, and vulnerable populations. The second section covers challenges, psychological first aid, early interventions, debriefing, long-term treatment, and new directions. It has five appendices: sample common reactions document, Internet resources for children, group therapy (air disaster), articles, and a resource list for disaster men-tal health workers.

Housley, J., & Beutler, L. E. (2007). *Treating victims of mass disaster and terrorism.* Cambridge, MA: Hogrefe & Huber.

This 72-page book can be viewed as a "CliffsNotes" version of disaster mental health work. It has four chapters (description of diagnoses, theories and treat-ment models, diagnosis and treatment indications, and treatment using the three-stage model of principle-driven treatment for early intervention following mass casualty events), a chapter on case vignettes, recommended reading, and an appendix of tools and resources (coping tools handout, helpful information hand-out, potential psychoeducation topics, overview of tools associated with each stage).

Multimodal Therapy

Lazarus, A. A. (1989). *The practice of multimodal therapy: Systematic, comprehensive, and effective psychotherapy.* Baltimore, MD: The Johns Hopkins University Press.

This 272-page book contains 11 chapters that explain the rationale, concepts, and application of multimodal therapy. It has three appendices: a multimodal life history questionnaire, a glossary of principal techniques, and a marital satisfaction questionnaire.

Theory

Hoff, L. A., Hallisey, B. J., & Hoff, M. (2009). *People in crisis: Clinical and diversity perspectives* (6th ed.). New York, NY: Routledge.

This book is an overview of crisis work. It is divided into three sections: understanding crisis intervention; specific crises; and suicide, homicide, or catastrophic events.

James, R. K. (2008). *Crisis intervention strategies.* Belmont, CA: Thomson Brooks/Cole.

This book provides an overview of crisis intervention. It has four sections: theory and application, handling specific crises, workplace, and disaster. There is a specific chapter related to addiction.

Kanel, K. (2007). *Crisis intervention* (3rd ed.). Belmont, CA: Thomson Brooks/Cole.

This book has 11 chapters that cover general crisis information (definition, history, ethical/professional issues) as well as chapters on multicultural concerns, the ABC model, and addressing issues related to crisis such as danger, developmental crises, loss, AIDS/HIV, substance abuse, PTSD/community disasters/trauma, and abuse (child, spousal, sexual assault).

VIDEOTAPES

Multimodal Therapy

Allyn & Bacon (Producer). (1998). *Psychotherapy with the experts: Multimodal therapy with Dr. Arnold Lazarus* [Video]. Available from www.abacon.com. ISBN 0-205-28187-7.

This video is a part of a video series on counseling approaches. It has an opening section in which the therapist, Dr. Lazarus, is interviewed about the approach. This section is followed by a counseling session with Dr. Lazarus, and finally, the third section is a follow-up to the session, in which Dr. Lazarus is interviewed again.

WEB SITES

National Institutes of Mental Health. www.nimh.nih.gov

This Web site provides information on understanding and treating mental illness.

CHAPTER THREE

Disaster Mental Health Counseling

LEARNING OBJECTIVES

1. To learn an overview of disaster mental health counseling.
2. To apply disaster mental health counseling in the context of crisis counseling.
3. To use main concepts and techniques from disaster mental health counseling as they apply to crisis counseling.

> Small service is true service . . . The daisy, by the shadow that it casts,
> protects the lingering dewdrop from the sun.
>
> *—William Wordsworth*

The reader may wonder about the importance of including a chapter on disaster mental health counseling in a book on crisis counseling. Such a focused chapter is included because of two factors—a tendency for counselors to do this work as an adjunct to their typical clinical load and the uniqueness of disaster mental health counseling. Often those of us who practice disaster mental health counseling do so outside of our typical counseling framework. We may not see ourselves as experts *per se* in this line of work, but rather as therapists who do this work on a part-time or as-needed basis. This type of work classifies as crisis counseling because it happens in relation to a crisis situation, such as a natural disaster. However, disaster mental health counseling is distinct from general counseling and crisis counseling in important ways that need to be discussed and explored. This chapter, then, will examine disaster mental health counseling and its underlying philosophy as it expresses itself through main concepts and techniques that can be used in crisis counseling situations.

MAIN CONCEPT

There is a distinction between crises and disasters. A crisis is a critical point where a person's resources and coping mechanisms are stretched too far. There are two types of crises: *developmental* (key issues are related to a certain life point) and *situational* (unexpected events) (Halpern & Tramontin, 2007). Situational crises and natural or human-caused catastrophes will be the underlying focus of this chapter. While all crises are not disasters, disasters may be crises.

Disaster is: "Natural or human-caused catastrophe that causes destruction, frequently including loss of life, with permanent changes to an environment and a community" (Halpern & Tramontin, 2007, p. 3). Often there is little or no warning with a disaster, but they can cause significant death and destruction (Dass-Brailsford, 2010). Keep in mind, though, that types of crises are not mutually exclusive: clients may be facing developmental crises at the same time as a situational one that is a catastrophe for them. For example, a client who has recently retired (developmental crisis) may have had his home destroyed and lost his wife in a hurricane disaster (situational crisis/disaster).

In terms of disasters, there are seven stages/phases of disasters (Kafrissen, Heffron, & Zusman, 1975; Raphael, 1986 as described in Halpern & Tramontin, 2007):

1. Warning (alarm): first awareness of the potential disaster.
2. Threat: imminent danger time frame.
3. Impact: when the disaster hits (acute trauma phase).
4. Inventory: examination and categorization of damage done by disaster.
5. Rescue: efforts are organized.
6. Remedy: relief efforts are present.
7. Recovery: some initial stability occurs.

Disaster mental health counseling attempts to support individuals and communities as they experience, survive, and respond to disasters in these phases. This chapter looks at disaster mental health counseling primarily, although not exclusively, in phases 5 through 7.

The guiding question regarding disaster mental health counseling for this chapter is: "What makes disaster mental health counseling different from regular counseling? From crisis counseling?" Halpern and Tramontin (2007) provide an overview of disaster mental health counseling that is summarized as follows.

Disaster mental health counseling is a distinct, new, and developing field that has a history; involves professional organizations; has its own publications, theory, research methodology/measurement, and intervention technology; and plays a role in impacting public policy and the judicial system. Disaster mental health counseling became common in disaster responses in the early 1990s; three factors that contributed to its development were recognition of trauma as having an impact on mental health (last 25 years); awareness in the 1980s that disasters could be used to understand trauma; and increased prevalence of technology (resulting in an increase of problems when it is impacted).

The American Red Cross (ARC) has played the largest role in the development of disaster mental health work: It was the first agency to acknowledge the need for that type of mental health care in the United States and the first one to develop standards for provision and training. In the late 1980s, following two major disasters, ARC workers were dissatisfied and resigning at high rates because they were overworked and not receiving enough support (Weaver, Dingman, Morgan, Hong, & North, 2000). A task force formed in 1990 resulted in the ARC Mental Health Services (MHS) to reduce/eliminate post-disaster stress responses in survivors and workers. In 1991, systemic training for mental health professionals began. The work of the ARC has been a baseboard for disaster mental health counseling in the United States. Note that Web sites for different mental health professional organizations are listed at the end of this chapter and, if interested, the reader is encouraged to contact them regarding information on how to become a disaster mental health worker with their chosen professional organization.

There are differences between traditional clinical work and disaster mental health counseling work. In traditional clinical work, counselors are typically viewed as experts by their clients; they meet with their clients at prescribed times and locations; and they typically have more than one session with their client. In contrast, disaster mental health counseling may involve counseling overwhelmed, resistant clients who vary significantly in their relationship to the disaster (survivors, their loved ones, other site workers, etc.); involve frequent, sudden changes in terms of counseling routine, location, and clients; occur in various settings that can be noisy, chaotic, public, unpleasant, and dangerous; and be short and infrequent in terms of sessions.

Regarding the earlier question ("What makes disaster mental health counseling different from regular counseling? From crisis counseling?"): Disaster mental health counseling is not an entirely different sort of counseling, but it does have different emphases. For example, a counselor needs to have the capacity to develop relationships with others as well as a capacity for flexibility. Both of these abilities are emphasized and required in disaster mental health work. The counselor working in a disaster setting needs to be able to establish rapport with a client quickly and also be quite flexible in adapting to the client's needs within the context of the situation. I will provide an example of disaster mental health counseling I have done that exemplifies the necessity of these traits.

I had the honor and opportunity to work as a disaster mental health counselor with the ARC in response to the 9/11 attack in New York City. I found that *rapport* needed to be established quickly with clients as they waited for services, during which time they could be called at any moment by various workers with the ARC or other disaster service organizations. The counseling connection needed to be inviting, not pushy, and needed to focus on the individual client's needs at that moment. I developed a client approach while engaging in two 2-week volunteer responses to the disaster where I would extend a friendly greeting accompanied by the underlying (if not explicitly stated) question, "How can I be helpful to you right now?" The *flexibility* required of a disaster mental health counselor was apparent in numerous ways: the length of time of contact, the setting (often public), the focus that the client wanted for the "session," etc. I needed to be willing to shift on a moment's notice to any one of these areas. Some "sessions" were cut short because a client's name was called for services, and, while there were areas that were more private than others, often "sessions" needed to occur in lines or seated areas where people were waiting for services. In terms of "session" focus, some clients wanted to talk about their 9/11 experiences at length while others simply wanted assistance with having their needs for food and shelter met.

One strong example of a combination of *rapport-building* and *flexibility* was an experience I had with a client who was waiting to meet someone for housing services. The client did not want to talk about his 9/11 experiences, but did respond to an offer of coffee and thereby a connection was made upon which a counseling contact could be developed. After bringing the client coffee and having a brief conversation with the client, the housing services worker appeared and the counseling "session" ended. In this example, I recognized, acknowledged, and responded to our shared humanness, thereby making a counseling connection and then recognizing the need to let go of the session in terms of both focus and length. This example shows the necessity in disaster mental health work to be both quick and flexible in rapport-building.

TECHNIQUES

Prior to discussing some of the techniques in disaster mental health counseling, it is necessary to present some of the hazards in this type of work (Miller & Hood, 2005, 2009). First, the counselor needs to manage countertransference by viewing disaster sites as places of daily living where the volume is turned up. What this means is that even in a disaster, there is a range of human behaviors that occur. Clients may try to be conning others or the system or simply may be more difficult in a disaster situation than at other times in their lives. As one client once said of himself to me in frustration at a 9/11 disaster site after struggling with a copying machine, "I'm not always this difficult." A second danger for the disaster mental health counselor is becoming caught up in the intensity of the situation. Disaster situations may fluctuate in emotional intensity from high to low (and vice versa) quite suddenly, and the worker needs to be able to adjust to such intensity. Third, the mental health professional needs to check his/her ego at the door. This means that the professional needs to work collaboratively with others and approach the disaster with the underlying question, "How can *i* be helpful here?" rather than, "How can *I* be helpful here?" Finally, this type of work can be draining, relentless, and may appear futile in the face of the disaster. However, the disaster mental health counselor needs to remember the adage, "Be responsible for the effort, not the outcome." This means the counselor is responsible for giving 100 percent in effort, but at the same time must be aware that there may not be a difference made in the client's life; if there is a difference made, the counselor may not have the privilege of being aware of it, given the nature of disaster mental health work— follow-up and ongoing appointments may not be possible. The disaster mental health worker needs to remember that his/her job is simply to put forth his/her best possible effort in the disaster situation.

Overall, in the disaster setting, the mental health worker needs to know him/ herself, practice the client-centered approach (genuineness, respect, empathy), establish relationships quickly, provide assistance that is therapeutic, and be able to remain calm (Halpern & Tramontin, 2007). The worker can help manage the stress of the environment for everyone by using his/her trained eye to scan situations for stressors and by responding in ways that reduce the environmental stress for the wide continuum of clients. For example, at the 9/11 site, I noted there were empty body bags lying on the floor near the family reception area. Worried that family members who had lost a loved one in the disaster may inadvertently walk by and see them, I informed my supervisor of the situation. My supervisor, who had already seen them, had contacted someone to have them removed quickly from that site location. Such an intervention reduced the potential environmental stress for all the clients (workers, survivors, family members, etc.).

ASSESSMENT

Assessment in general crisis counseling is discussed in Chapter 6. Also in that chapter are summaries of assessment with regard to mental health/general trauma work, addiction, co-occurring disorders, intimate partner violence, sexual abuse, eating disorders, suicide, and homicide. The reader is encouraged to use that chapter as a reference for disaster mental health assessment.

Specifically, in disaster mental health work, assessments generally need to be done quite quickly. There are numerous checklists for responses to a disaster (emotional, cognitive, behavioral, physical) that can be accessed through various books (e.g., Halpern & Tramontin, 2007; Weaver, 1995) and through the professional Web sites listed at the end of this chapter. Such checklists can assist the disaster mental health worker in reassuring clients that they are having normal reactions to the disaster, in educating them about possible problems they can watch for in themselves and/or others impacted by the disaster, and in referring clients for additional assistance.

In addition to the seven stages/phases of disasters discussed earlier in this chapter, the disaster mental health counselor may find it helpful to learn the four time frames describing the period after a disaster (DeWolfe, 2000):

1. *The Heroic Phase*: In this phase are responses in which great, noble efforts are made to help those who have been impacted.
2. *The Honeymoon Phase*: In this stage, compassion and relief are expressed to the impacted.
3. *The Disillusionment Phase*: This phase is an anticlimactic experience where resources and attention are diminished.
4. *The Reconstruction Phase*: This phase can last a long time, and can possibly always be present.

Knowledge of these phases can be helpful in the mental health professional's assessment process in two ways. First, the survivors of the disaster will generally have emotions that match the phase, which can then be used to guide the clinician's choice of intervention. For example, during the heroic phase (also the impact stage of the disaster), clients may experience shock, yet may be in a high state of arousal. In this phase, the disaster mental health counselor may encourage the client to pace him/herself in responding to the disaster situations that present themselves, rather than having a fever-pitch response to all situations. Second, knowledge of the phases can assist the disaster mental health counselor in educating the community about how reactions to the disaster will generally change over time and about how this is a normal and natural process—not necessarily a negative one. For example, during the disillusionment phase, it does not mean that people do not care; it simply means that the community is adjusting naturally to the disaster over a period of time and attempting to go back to "normal."

When assessing the client's reaction to disaster, as stated previously, it is necessary to assess what is a normal reaction and what is atypical. It is also impor- tant to look for common diagnoses present in relation to a disaster, such as acute stress disorder (ASD), posttraumatic stress disorder (PTSD), complicated grief, depression, and substance use/abuse/dependence (Halpern & Tramontin, 2007; Housley & Beutler, 2007).

TREATMENT

Chapter 7 discusses different forms of therapy (brief therapy, motivational inter- viewing, positive psychology, grief therapy) and related techniques. Also discussed in that chapter are the concepts of stages of change, resilience, and the integration of spirituality into counseling, which can be used in disaster mental health work to help the client regain a sense of balance and safety in the context of the disaster. The reader is encouraged to read that chapter for specific techniques related to these therapies and concepts that can be used in counseling in a disaster situation.

Disaster mental health counseling applies crisis intervention strategies in the field. This form of counseling requires a focus on practical concerns and includes interventions that have psychoeducational components and stress management techniques. The following is a list of general techniques that can be used by mental health workers in responding at a disaster site (Miller & Hood, 2005, 2009):

1. Find out what you do well in disaster settings and look for opportunities to do those things.
2. Be present for people.
3. Avoid placating or pathologizing people.
4. Treat everybody as a unique person.
5. Use common-sense responses and problem-solving approaches.
6. Respect the confidences of everyone (survivors, family members, workers, etc.).
7. Remember that disasters are hard on marginalized people.

Some specific counseling techniques will be housed in a discussion of the three stages of disaster treatment (Housley & Beutler, 2007).

In *Stage 1 (Acute Support)*, the goal is to reduce the distress of the client, increase the client's understanding of his/her reactions, reduce negative coping, and increase the client's knowledge of when additional resources may be needed and how they can be accessed. Psychological first aid (PFA) is included for use in this stage. In the past, PFA has included critical incident stress debriefing (CISD), but has been more recently used to describe manualized techniques that do not include CISD (National Child Traumatic Stress Network and National Center for PTSD, 2005). CISD is discussed at the end of this section. As discussed in Chapter 2, acute support, then, includes making sure basic needs are met; developing rapport; encouraging social networks; shaping the approach to the survivor's needs; obtaining/providing information that may help the survivor; and encouraging positive coping skills.

In *Stage 2 (Intermediate Support)*, the therapeutic relationship is critical and the focus is on assisting the client in coping with the daily stressors experienced from the disaster. In this stage, repeated visits (three to five) are needed. Techniques include psychoeducational information, cognitive-behavioral approaches (thought identification, restructuring, homework), and anxiety management.

During *Stage 3 (Ongoing Treatment)*, the interventions are shaped to fit the individual client and his/her problems, such as anxiety disorders (cognitive-behavioral interventions), chemical abuse/dependency (consideration of impairment level and client resistance), and depression and comorbidity (consideration of impairment level, client resistance, and coping styles). As stated in the assessment section of this chapter, common diagnoses in relation to a disaster include acute stress disorder (ASD), posttraumatic stress disorder (PTSD), complicated grief, depression, and substance use/abuse/dependence. Each of these diagnoses can be treated based on the clinical expertise and theoretical orientation of the mental health professional and there are specific approaches typically used in response to each of these areas. For example, in trauma counseling, some recent and trauma-specific treatment techniques that can be used are dialectical behavior therapy (DBT) and Seeking Safety. Resources for these two treatment approaches are included at the end of this chapter.

CISD is the most widely used debriefing model that is a part of critical incident stress management. Debriefing simply means that clients are able to talk about what happened to them during an event—they have a chance to process the experience. It has been used as a specific, delineated technique with emergency service workers to help them manage stress and was developed by Mitchell in the early 1980s. The approach is mentioned here because often disaster mental health workers may have been exposed to the model or are asked in their work to provide such an approach to workers (Mitchell, 1983). There are some cautions with regard to this approach: (a) it has not demonstrated effectiveness in clinical trials and (b) no one should be "pressured or ordered to participate in critical incident stress debriefing" (Harvard Mental Health Letter, 2006, p. 2).

In practicing any of the above techniques with clients, the disaster mental health worker also needs to be simultaneously practicing self-care. There are some specific challenges to counselors working at a disaster site: having a lack of structure and resources, experiencing changing leadership, being direct victims in the disaster, experiencing a lack of rewards while having personal challenges (Dass-Brailsford, 2010). As discussed in Chapter 9 of this book, self-care can make a significant difference in the quality of the counseling the mental health professional can provide to clients. By caring for ourselves, we can care more effectively for our clients. Disaster mental health counselors can reduce stress during their preparation to volunteer by talking with family and employers about the work; preparing a bag that includes the necessary professional materials (credential documentation, business cards, handouts, notebooks/writing utensils, contacts, etc.) and personal materials (calling card, water bottle, snacks, etc.); and attending ongoing education and training that may include mentors and disaster drills (Housley & Beutler, 2007).

Disaster mental health counselors can also practice self-care during and after the disaster through self-observation where negative coping reactions (increased substance use, isolation/withdrawal, and high-risk/self-destructive behaviors) are prevented or replaced by positive coping reactions that include intentionally practicing healthy eating/drinking/exercise habits, obtaining support from colleagues and family, following shift schedules, taking time off, and breathing deeply

(Halpern & Tramontin, 2007). Miller and Hood (2005) also make the following specific self-care suggestions to disaster mental health workers:

- Take things with you that reassure you (pictures, jewelry, reading materials, etc.).
- Build in reassuring rituals daily.
- Watch out for heroic tendencies in responding to the "ocean of need," and pace yourself instead.
- Listen to your body and remember HALT: Avoid getting too Hungry, Angry, Lonely, or Tired.
- Take breaks and encourage other workers to take breaks.
- Watch for appropriate use of humor (humorous moments and people with a sense of humor) to assist in breaking the tension and stress.
- Find ways to feed your spirit by appreciating life, remembering what is important, and living within your values.
- Be willing to "pass the baton" to the next mental health counselor when it is time for you to leave the disaster site.

Finally, when the counselor and the client share the traumatic reality (e.g., a hurricane hits the area where they both live), counselors need to be aware that their internal and external boundaries may be blurred by the experience; in such circumstances, we need to work carefully and thoughtfully with these experiences with an awareness of countertransference issues, using supervision, and practicing self-care (Baum, 2010).

The disaster mental health counselor who practices self-care can work more effectively professionally. As counselors, by practicing self-care, we can more easily integrate this type of work into our professional and personal lives.

SUMMARY

This chapter provided an overview of disaster mental health counseling in terms of philosophy, approaches, and techniques. It specifically focused on using this approach from a crisis counseling perspective to:

1. Learn an overview of disaster mental health counseling.
2. Apply disaster mental health counseling in the context of crisis counseling.
3. Use therapeutic concepts and techniques from disaster mental health counseling as they apply to crisis counseling.

QUESTIONS

1. Define disaster mental health counseling.
2. What are some of the main concepts of disaster mental health counseling?
3. What are some core techniques of disaster mental health counseling?

Case Study 3.1

Your client is a woman with two children who has just had her home destroyed by a flood. You are visiting with her in a crowded shelter as she sits in a chair with her sleeping toddler in her arms and a child about age 6 sitting quietly at her feet. She is saying very little in response to your light, conversational comments. She is looking down and away from you as you speak. Periodically, during your five-minute conversation she has wiped a tear from her eye. In terms of rapport-building:

1. What might you do to extend an invitation to engage her in a dialogue?
2. What might you do to show flexibility in terms of discussing the topic?

EXERCISES

Exercise 3.1

What are ways that you welcome (or anticipate welcoming) clients into sessions? Jot down these thoughts quickly and then share these thoughts with a colleague, mentor, or supervisor. Additionally, tell that person how you might avoid using these welcoming strategies in a disaster setting, or how you might adapt such approaches to a disaster mental health setting.

Exercise 3.2

Imagine that you are counseling someone at a disaster site. What types of natural or human-caused disasters do you anticipate being difficult for you? How would you work with these difficulties? Discuss your answers with a colleague, mentor, or supervisor.

Exercise 3.3

Take a sheet of paper and draw three columns. In the first column, list all the disasters (natural, human-caused) you have personally experienced in life. In the second column, list the internal resources you had that helped you cope with the accompanying disaster. In the third column, list the external resources you used that helped you cope with the disaster. Now process, with a colleague, mentor, or supervisor, those internal and external resources that you believe may be generally helpful to clients in disaster situations.

SUGGESTED READINGS

Disaster Mental Health Counseling

Dass-Brailsford, P. (Ed.) (2010). *Crisis and disaster counseling: Lessons learned from Hurricane Katrina and other disasters*. Los Angeles, CA: Sage.

This 258-page book has 15 chapters that provide an overview of disaster and crisis counseling, specific disasters, interventions, and populations impacted by disasters (families, children, older adults, rural and diverse communities) as well as the impact on workers and specific topics (spirituality, federal government involvement).

Halpern, J., & Tramontin, M. (2007). *Disaster mental health: Theory and practice.* Belmont, CA: Thompson Brooks/Cole.

This 366-page book provides a thorough overview of disaster mental health counseling. It has two main sections (disaster mental health theory and disaster mental health practice) that are divided into twelve chapters (six per section). The first section provides an overview, disaster characteristics, and a history of this approach, as well as a discussion of risk factors, both typical and extreme reactions, and vulnerable populations. The second section covers challenges, psychological first aid, early interventions, debriefing, long-term treatment, and new directions. It has five appendices: sample common reactions document, Internet resources for children, group therapy (air disaster), articles, and a resource list for disaster mental health workers.

Housley, J., & Beutler, L. E. (2007). *Treating victims of mass disaster and terrorism.* Cambridge, MA: Hogrefe & Huber.

This 72-page book can be viewed as a "CliffsNote" version of disaster mental health work. It has four chapters (description of diagnoses, theories and treatment models, diagnosis and treatment indications, and treatment using the three-stage model of principle-driven treatment for early intervention following mass casualty events), a chapter on case vignettes, recommended reading, and an appendix of tools and resources (coping tools handout, helpful information handout, potential psychoeducation topics, overview of tools associated with each stage).

Weaver, J. D. (1995). *Disasters: Mental health interventions.* Sarasota, FL: Professional Resource Press/Professional Resource Exchange.

This 204-page book has 16 chapters that describe crisis/disaster and mental health aspects of disaster impact. It provides practical suggestions for mental health professionals regarding the application of clinical work to a disaster setting as well as chapters on loss, self-awareness, stress management, and working with the media.

Trauma Counseling

Dialectical Behavior Therapy (DBT) Readings

Dimeff, L. A., Comtois, K. A., & Linehan, M. M. (2009). Co-occurring addiction and borderline personality disorder. In R. K. Ries, D. A. Fiellin, S. C. Miller, & R. Saitz (Eds.), *Principles of addiction medicine*, 4th ed. (pp. 1227–1237). Philadelphia: Wolters Kluwer/Lippincott Williams & Wilkins.

This chapter provides a concise overview of DBT as applied to a substance-abusing borderline population.

Dimeff, L. A., & Linehan, M. M. (2008). Dialectical behavior therapy for substance abusers. *Addiction Science & Clinical Practice, 4,* 39–47.

This article provides a concise overview of DBT as applied to a substance-abusing borderline population.

Goldstein, E. G. (2004). Substance abusers with borderline disorders. In S. L. A. Straussner (Ed.) *Clinical work with substance-abusing clients*, 2nd ed. (pp. 370–391). New York, NY: Guilford.

This chapter discusses characteristics and causes of borderline personality disorders as well as assessment and treatment strategies.

Linehan, M. M. (1993a). *Cognitive-behavioral treatment of borderline personality disorder*. New York, NY: Guilford.

This book comprehensively describes this treatment approach.

DBT and Seeking Safety Manuals/Workbooks

Linehan, M. M. (1993b). *Skills training manual for treating borderline personality disorder*. New York, NY: Guilford.

This book comprehensively describes this treatment approach in terms of skills, teaching strategies, and discussion topics in groups.

Linehan, M. M. (in press). *Skills training manual for disordered emotional regulation*. New York, NY: Guilford.

Marra, T. (2004). *Depressed & anxious: The dialectical behavior therapy workbook for overcoming depression & anxiety*. Oakland, CA: New Harbinger.

Najavits, L. M. (2002). *Seeking safety: A treatment manual for PTSD and substance abuse*. New York, NY: Guilford.

The manual has a chapter that provides an overview of PTSD and substance abuse and a chapter that discusses how to conduct the treatment. The remainder of the manual focuses on treatment topics. This book has nine chapters, the first of which is an overview of DBT. The remaining eight are meant for the client to use as exercises (dialectics of anxiety and depression, feelings, "there must be something wrong with me," meaning making, mindfulness skills, emotional regulation, distress tolerance skills, and strategic behavioral skills).

VIDEOTAPES/DVDS

Disasters

American Psychological Association (Producer). (2002). *Reclaiming hope in a changed world (Broadcast version)*. [Videotape]. Available from www.apa.org/pubs/videos

This 56-minute video includes interviews with professionals about how people can regain their balance and hope in response to 9/11. Interspersed in the video are sections on spirituality.

American Psychological Association (Producer). (2002). *Reclaiming hope in a changed world (Classroom/Community version)*. [Videotape]. Available from www.apa.org/pubs/videos

This 18-minute video includes interviews with professionals about how people (especially children) can regain their balance and hope in response to 9/11. There are specific cues adults are told to look for in terms of difficulties, as well as suggestions on how to help children cope.

American Psychological Association (Producer). (2002). *Reclaiming hope in a changed world (for kids)*. [Videotape]. Available from www.apa.org/pubs/videos
This 18-minute video, meant for children in response to 9/11, discusses the concept of RICH (Respect, Information, Connection, Hope) as elements of relationships. There is also a section where children discuss their spirituality.

Spirituality

HBO Home Video (Producer). (1996). *How do you spell God?* Available from Amazon.com or other vendors for VHS films.
This 32-minute film has children from different religions (Christianity, Judaism, Buddhism, Islam) talk about their views of God. It is interspersed with three animated stories used to elaborate on different perspectives.

PBS & HBO Home Video (Producer). (2002). *Frontline: Faith & doubt at Ground Zero*. Available from Amazon.com or other vendors for videos/DVDs.
This 120-minute film looks at the spiritual lives of believers and non-believers in response to questions regarding good and evil following the 9/11 attacks.

WEB SITES

Mental health professionals can contact the following Web sites for information on disaster mental health counseling with regard to their professional organizational affiliation.

Professional Organization Web Sites (Disaster Mental Health Counseling)

American Association for Marital and Family Therapy. www.aamft.org
American Counseling Association. www.counseling.org
American Psychiatric Association. www.psych.org
American Psychological Association. www.apa.org
National Association of Social Workers. www.naswdc.org

National Organization Web Sites (Disaster Mental Health Counseling)

American Red Cross. www.redcross.org
This Web site provides information on trainings and opportunities on how to be generally involved with the American Red Cross. By accessing this site, one can find out information on one's local chapter and then contact that chapter regarding

involvement with the American Red Cross Disaster Mental Health Counseling division.

There are excellent publications for both mental health professionals and clients at this Web site. For example, two helpful publications for clients are coloring books for children (*After a Fire; After the Flood*).

National Institute of Mental Health. www.nimh.nih.gov

This Web site offers helpful publications for the mental health professional. For example, there is one titled *Helping Children and Adolescents Cope with Violence and Disasters (For Teachers, Clergy, and Other Adults in the Community): What Community Members Can Do* — NIH Publication No. 08-3519.

Substance Abuse and Mental Health Services Administration (SAMHSA). www.samhsa.gov

This site has disaster health information in general and has a link to *Mental Health Response for Mass Violence and Terrorism: A Field Guide* as well as excellent publications such as *Psychosocial Issues for Children and Adolescents in Disasters* (DHHS Publication No. ADM 86-1070R), *Psychosocial Issues for Older Adults in Disasters* (DHHS Publication No. ESDRB SMA 99-3323), and *Responding to the Needs of People with Serious and Persistent Mental Illness in Times of Major Disaster* (DHHS Publication No. SMA 96-3077).

Trauma Counseling

Seeking Safety. www.seekingsafety.org

This Web site provides general information about the Seeking Safety approach. It includes article and training information on the topic.

CHAPTER FOUR

Settings and Commonly Occurring Diagnoses

LEARNING OBJECTIVES

1. To learn typical crises/issues and helpful responses in specific crisis counseling settings.
2. To learn common diagnoses that occur in crisis counseling work.
3. To practice applying helpful crisis counseling approaches to these common diagnoses through case studies and exercises.

> When you come to the edge of all that you know, you must believe in one of two things: there will be earth upon which to stand, or you will be given wings.
>
> —*Author unknown*

Both counselor and client in crisis situations can experience a sense of letting go of the "known" and trusting the "unknown" with a sense of hope for the future, as described in this quote. This chapter is an attempt to encourage the reader's sense of confidence and hope in dealing with crisis situations in specific settings and with specific diagnoses.

This chapter is intended to provide an overview of typical crises/issues and helpful responses that can occur in specific crisis counseling settings: phone, school, agency, and private practice. This overview will focus on only a few of the typical crises/issues in each area. The reader can use these crises and suggested responses as guidelines for other crises that occur in the specific setting discussed. Again, the reader is encouraged to use the information that is helpful as a guide.

Crises may occur across many settings, and the settings may shape the assessment, treatment, and aftercare process. For example, the issue of intimate partner violence can occur in a phone, school, agency, or private practice setting, but may express itself differently in these different settings. Over the phone, the client may be a survivor (adult, child) calling a hotline for assistance as the intimate violence is occurring. In a school setting, a child may be telling a teacher about the intimate partner violence occurring at home. At an agency, the perpetrator may be showing signs of intimate partner violence in the assessment phase, alerting the counselor that the survivor is in danger because of him. In private practice, the counselor may be working with a couple and pick up on the issues of intimate partner violence that are contributing to the marital crisis they are experiencing. The same issue, intimate partner violence, can express itself in terms of client, information, and aftercare in the assessment, treatment, and aftercare process. That is why there is no one typical crisis that adheres itself to one setting; instead, there may be typical issues faced by the counselor in a particular setting.

The reader should note that the four settings presented above (phone, school, agency, private setting) may not be pertinent at this point in time for his/her work, but they may be considered a future resource should the reader work in this area. Particularly now in the counseling field, counselors need to be very flexible in the job market. For example, a school counselor may be laid off from his/her position and find him/herself opening a private practice. Beyond the basic need to be aware of the different types of crises that can arise in a setting, as well as how the setting can shape the crisis, this chapter has the intention of helping the counselor learn how to shape crisis responses to adapt to various settings. An excellent resource for counselor stories in different settings is the book *Days in the Lives of Counselors*, which is described more thoroughly in the resource section at the end of this chapter (Dingman & Weaver, 2003). In this book, counselors in different settings describe their personal experiences as counselors, with three of the stories focused on crisis counseling experiences.

The second main purpose of this chapter is to assist the reader in developing a sensitivity to certain problems that are often at the core of the crisis or are fueling the crisis at hand. The diagnoses examined here are: addiction, co-occurring disorders, intimate partner violence, sexual abuse, and eating disorders. Once again, there are other diagnoses that may be at the crisis core or fueling the crisis, but these five are ones I have chosen based on clinical experience in doing crisis counseling work. These five areas are presented in this text in Chapter 6, which discusses assessment. In Chapter 6, an overview is provided of each area and a review of the assessment process with appropriate instruments is provided. This section of this chapter is a preparation for Chapter 6 in that it describes each of the five areas in terms of a general overview but specifically addresses the application of information in each of these areas to the crisis counseling context.

SETTINGS

Telephone

Typical Crises/Issues

In the 1960s and 1970s, suicide prevention became a focus of 24-hour crisis lines, and phones are the most used crisis counseling medium. There are "warm lines," which focus on non-life-threatening topics (e.g., support for latchkey kids) and "hotlines," which address critical, life-threatening situations such as suicide (James, 2008). This text will focus on the crisis or "hotlines," where assessment and management of the problem is prompt, the caller is anonymous, and a wide range of issues can be addressed (suicide, depression, addiction, intimate partner violence, rape, and crime victimization; Roberts, 2005).

Crisis lines are convenient, inexpensive forms of assistance where the client can start and stop the contact and avoid dependency on the counselor. The counselor can readily provide information on services and consult with others, as well as reach numerous clients and clients who are isolated. The counselor in this context is practicing crisis counseling by making a therapeutic connection, an assessment, a plan, and a referral. Issues counselors face in this setting include variation in clientele, an unpredictable workload, unrealistic expectations of themselves (e.g., needing to be an expert, needing to defend themselves), and difficult clients (manipulative, unlikeable, regular/disturbed/abusive) (MacKinnon, 1998; James, 2008).

Helpful Responses

These issues can be addressed through practicing self-care, being flexible, realistically addressing counselor expectations of themselves, and accepting the reality of the clients with whom they work. For example, there are specific suggestions for working with regular callers, disturbed callers, and abusive callers (James, 2008). For the *regular callers* the counselor needs to be aware of the caller's agenda. For the *disturbed callers*, the counselor needs to slow his/her own emotional reactions, and in addition to being a professional (establishing boundaries, having realistic expectations, avoiding placating), the counselor needs to avoid joining with the hallucinations or delusions, determine the medication being used, and assess lethality.

For *problem callers*, the counselor needs to use open-ended questions, set time limits, terminate the abuse, switch counselors, use covert modeling (use mental imagery to extinguish a behavior), and form administrative rules.

Some additional suggestions are as follows. When specific populations are focused on, comprehensive training needs to be given to workers to ensure they have enough knowledge about callers and their problems (Bryant & Harvey, 2000). Suicide risk assessments and strategies to improve referral follow-up are needed (Kalafat, Gould, Munfakh, & Kleinman, 2007). There needs to be quality assurance, standardized practices, and research examining the relationship between interventions and outcomes (Mishara, et al., 2007). Finally, outreach needs to be done to adolescents to encourage their use of this resource (Gould, Greenberg, Munfakh, Kleinman, & Lubell, 2006).

School

Typical Crises/Issues

The new school system is like a penitentiary, in that it is increasingly designed to enhance security and safety; it also has a social structure and community of its own that can influence a crisis (James, 2008). Violent crises that erupt in this set-ting are due to numerous factors (parenting issues, disenfranchised individuals, weapons access, gangs, drugs, physical abuse, lack of positive role models, pres-ence of negative role modeling, etc.). Lethality shows up in ". . . assaults, threats, intimidation, property destruction, bullying, and physical injury [which] occur fairly often" (James, 2008, p. 404). Violence in school has been separated into two forms—bullying through homicide and "catastrophic outbursts" against others— both requiring professional intervention (Stewart & MacNeil, 2005). The violence emerges out of a complex interaction between individual, relationship, and family/ community factors (Stewart & MacNeil, 2005).

Schools are often able to handle the *developmental* crises of students, but do not handle *situational* crises, especially unexpected and violent ones, as well (James, 2008). In all fairness to schools, they are designed for educational goals and, as a result, do not necessarily have plans developed and/or implemented for address-ing student and staff psychological and emotional needs in a crisis (Newgass & Schonfeld, 2005). Common crises include ". . . gang activities, school shootings, physical assault, suicides, natural disasters, terrorist assaults, drug abuse, physical and sexual abuse, medical emergencies, and classmate, parent, and teacher deaths . . ." (James, 2008, p. 406).

Helpful Responses

Planning allows schools to address a crisis in a ". . . thoughtful, broad, and long term view of the needs of students and staff" (p. 502) (Klingman, 1988, as refer-enced in Newgass & Schonfeld, 2005). Schools need a crisis plan that involves a crisis response planning committee and a school crisis response team (SCRT), and in order to implement the crisis plan, the following need to be taken into account: physical needs (i.e., counseling space), logistics, and responding to the crisis (obtaining facts, assessing, providing psychological first aid, screening for fur-ther issues, briefing/debriefing, demobilizing) (James, 2008). Both individual and group work can be of benefit to the school community. In the resource section at the end of this chapter, specific texts are described that provide guidelines for crisis interventions within the school system.

In response to community trauma, schools are encouraged to connect children with their parents/caretakers as soon as possible (Cohen, Mannarino, Gibson, Cozza, Brymer, & Murray, 2006). In the short term (one month), schools need to provide trauma assessment for the children and educate the school personnel about common reactions and effects of trauma on children. Beyond one month, the authors recommend ongoing screening for trauma as well as making individual counseling (referrals) and group interventions available for the children, in addition to psychoeducational training and therapy for the parents.

Agency

Typical Crises/Issues

The Community Mental Health Centers Act of 1963 was legislation that directed all states to provide crisis mental health treatment. These community mental health centers originally focused on psychiatric services to meet the needs of the chronically ill mental patients who had been deinstitutionalized. However, over time, counselors in these centers began to see clients that were healthier and less dysfunctional.

There is little written on agency work *per se* as a part of crisis counseling. While agency counselors have clients in crisis in the assessment, treatment, or aftercare process, their clinical issues with clients may be more similar to counselors in private practice, although they have the additional burden of the agency bureaucracy. Currently, much of agency counseling work that addresses crises specifically focuses on a crisis intervention team that works in coordination and collaboration with three groups: the client, the community mental health agency, and the community at large. Issues related to this setting of crisis counseling are often connecting to resources available for the client to use, matching those resources with client need, and coordinating the implementation of such resources between the individual, agency, and community. All three (client, agency, community) can have different motivations, values, and agendas, which can be further complicated by politics and personality clashes within the systems or between the systems.

To further complicate this crisis work, the influence of the current economy has impacted crisis counseling done in these settings. Increasingly, as mentioned in other places in this text, counselors are asked to do more with less. As community and agency resources for clients become increasingly scarce (e.g., psychiatric hospital beds), and as counseling positions are cut in agencies, clients and counselors find that these realities can fuel the crisis situation. Increasingly, clients seen in a crisis context are more dysfunctional and have longer, more complicated histories of mental health problems. It is as though the system is returning to the state of the client and the service delivery model as originally designed by The Community Mental Health Centers Act of 1963, with shrinking services and resources available. Shrinking services and resources can encourage crises, because by the time clients enter the system and/or are eligible for assistance from the system, their problems have evolved into a crisis or a more extreme form of crisis. For example, because of issues such as health insurance, clients may have to "'invent' a life-threatening crisis as a ticket to hospital admission" (Hoff, Hallisey, & Hoff, 2009, p. 72). Also, there are communities that do not even have comprehensive crisis programs, and if they do, they are "far from ideal," with political and fiscal policies playing parts in this situation (Hoff, Hallisey, & Hoff, 2009, p. 14).

Helpful Responses

When reading such bleak news about the current state of the mental health delivery system and the stresses on both the client and the counselor that can exacerbate the crisis, the reader is encouraged not to give up hope. As I tell my students, there is an ebb and a flow to the funding of counseling, and a counselor needs to remember this during the ebb times.

Because crisis service need is growing and supports are declining, community programs need to create and implement services that are a good match to the community's needs (Ligon, 2005). In the past, crises may have been addressed by taking clients to emergency facilities, but because fewer of these facilities exist, and because of the influence of managed care, the practical reality is that communities are increasingly forced to address client crises within their own community resources, such as agencies (Ligon, 2005). One example of effectively meeting the needs of the community through agency crisis counseling work is the Mobile Crisis Unit. The units involve trained professionals who typically deliver services in the home of the client. They have advantages that include: accessible services, assessment of the client's natural environment, prompt intervention, and avoidance of arrests/hospitalizations (Zealberg, Santos, & Fisher, 1993, as referenced in Ligon, 2005).

Specifically, counselors working in these settings can do a number of things to address the issues related to crisis counseling work in these settings:

1. Advocate in conjunction with professional organizations for increased resources for clients in counseling.
2. Work closely with community agencies to develop resources that complement agency resources to deal with the crisis.
3. Work on a team, formally or informally, that is supportive to crisis counseling work and understands and respects the importance of that work.
4. If an agency team is not available formally or informally, develop a relationship with an outside supervisor or mentor who is encouraging and supportive.
5. If personality clashes occur in the system delivery of crisis client services, carefully examine how to reduce such personality conflicts (e.g., addressing the conflict directly or indirectly through dialogue or systemic intervention).
6. Determine whether systemic interventions can be made to decrease the crisis. For example, are there ways that the needs of less dysfunctional individuals can be met by the agency?
7. Develop Mobile Crisis Units that intervene at the local level (i.e., the client's home).
8. Practice self-care, as discussed in Chapter 9 of this text, and encourage clients in crisis to practice self-care within the realistic limits of time, energy, and money.

Private Practice

Typical Crises/Issues

This setting of crisis counseling, the private practice, has the least written on it. What has been written are excellent texts that address crisis counseling in general (Roberts, 2005) or specific aspects of crisis counseling work, such as disaster mental health (Dingman and Weaver, 2003; Webber, Bass, & Yep, 2005), divorce counseling (Granvold, 2005), or the development of a crisis component aspect in one's practice (Wise, 2000).

The private practice counselor can be a generalist, a specialist, or both in terms of various counseling issues. As a result, the crisis issues faced by the counselor are unique to his/her practice. However, in spite of this uniqueness, there are some general aspects to a crisis.

The issues faced by the private practice counselor are those discussed in Chapters 1, 2, and 6 of this book. These include, respectively: (a) personal characteristics that may inhibit crisis counseling, (b) the lack of a strong theoretical framework that quickly facilitates the counseling relationship, and (c) an inability to assess the crisis and its influencing factors as quickly as possible.

Helpful Responses

Overall, the private practice counselor needs to be able to address the emergence of a crisis at any given moment within the context of the counseling. The counselor also needs to have a known, reliable, and easily accessible form of crisis support available to clients in the event a crisis emerges outside the counseling setting. These responses are standard in terms of keeping the client's welfare the focus of counseling.

In addition, the counselor needs to (as all crisis counselors need to do in whatever setting they work): (a) examine his/her characteristics that are conducive to crisis counseling; (b) form a strong theoretical framework that facilitates the development of the counseling relationship; and (c) assess the crisis situation as quickly as possible. Characteristics that are particularly helpful in the development of the therapeutic relationship are: poise, creativity/flexibility, energy/resilience, quick mental reflexes, and an ability to collaborate with agencies. Finally, there may be times where the private practitioner needs to carefully consider screening for crisis potential—times when perhaps other community resources (e.g., mobile crisis teams) could more efficiently respond to the crisis or a potential pattern of crises.

COMMONLY OCCURRING DIAGNOSES

Addiction

Because many Americans use alcohol and drugs (129 million Americans drink alcohol and 20.1 million used an illicit drug the month before their Substance Abuse and Mental Health Services Administration [SAMHSA] interview; SAMHSA, 2008b), all counselors need to be aware that they may be seeing a client who has an alcohol and/or drug problem. Crisis counselors need to keep this at the forefront of the crisis assessment, treatment, and aftercare, because of the strong influence an alcohol and/or drug problem can have on the crisis counseling process. Essentially, all the crisis counseling work may be ineffectual if there is an active alcohol or drug problem.

In Chapter 6, on assessment, the reader is encouraged to ask the client about his/her alcohol and drug usage in an open, direct, and respectful manner with an awareness that the client may deny or minimize usage. The counselor is also encouraged to examine his/her personal and professional reactions to alcohol/drug use in clients, as well as his/her own usage. This examination process can assist the counselor in reducing countertransference during the crisis counseling process. Finally, the counselor is encouraged to use a broad assessment instrument to assess for a problem that may be contributing to the crisis situation.

EXERCISE 4.1 ADDICTION

Find a colleague, supervisor, or mentor to process this exercise. Ask yourself the following questions:

1. What do I believe causes addiction?
2. Where did I obtain this information?
3. How do my views on addiction impact the work I see myself doing as a crisis counselor (e.g., how much emphasis do I view myself putting on addiction in a crisis situation; what biases—negative or positive—might I be bringing to the crisis situation with regard to addiction)?

Case Study 4.1 Addiction

Your client recently experienced a disaster related to a terrorist attack. All you know about your client is that he is male, addicted (you do not know if he has been formally diagnosed as such, has been treated for it, is in active addiction, or is in recovery), and he has "lost everything." You have been contacted as a counselor to assist in this situation.

1. Which setting (phone, school, agency, private practice) might increase or decrease the likelihood you would be contacted as a counselor to assist in the situation?
2. In each setting, how might you handle this situation generally?
3. What would be your first priority in terms of the welfare of your client?

Co-Occurring Disorders

When alcohol and drugs are involved in a client's situation, often it is common for another disorder to be present. This is called a co-occurring disorder (COD). SAMHSA (2007) estimates that 5 million Americans have COD. Because of the frequency of alcohol/drug use problems and accompanying mental health issues, the crisis counselor, again, needs to be sensitive to these issues.

As stated in Chapter 6, the crisis counselor is advised to assess for additional mental health problems not being discussed in the crisis situation and consider that alcohol/ drug problems might be present. Also, the counselor needs to note that the client may be using alcohol or drugs to medicate his/her mental health problems. This reality means that the crisis counselor needs to be aware that in addition to the crisis being presented, the client may, like a Russian doll, have additional inner layers of substance abuse and undiscussed mental health issues that are a part of the crisis situation and that require further examination and inclusion in the crisis intervention plan.

EXERCISE 4.2 CO-OCCURRING DISORDERS

Write a brief list of at least three mental health diagnoses you are comfortable addressing in a general counseling setting. Next to this list, write a list of three mental health diagnoses you are comfortable addressing in a crisis counseling situation. Repeat this process with three mental health diagnoses you are uncomfortable addressing in both general and crisis counseling contexts. Finally, note what actions you may take to enhance your comfort level with addressing these diagnoses in a crisis counseling context.

Intimate Partner Violence

SAMHSA (1997) defines intimate partner violence (IPV), which has been historically named "domestic violence," as force that is verbal, psychological, or physical

---

Case Study 4.2 Co-Occurring Disorders

Your client is elderly and is part of a racial/ethnic minority. She needs to be assessed for a guardianship because of her living problems. The crisis is that her living situation has come under the auspices of the Department of Social Services. You have been contacted as a counselor to assist in this situation.

1. Which setting (phone, school, agency, private practice) might increase or decrease the likelihood you would be contacted as a counselor to assist in the situation?
2. In each setting, how might you handle this situation generally?
3. What would be your first priority in terms of the welfare of your client?

in nature used by one family member toward another family member. It is violence used to control the other person. Again, alcohol or drugs may be used by the perpetrator (Bureau of Justice, 2005) and this may be used to explain their violence or their lack of impulse control (Jacobson & Gottman, 1998). Alcohol or drugs might also be used by survivors who have substance abuse problems (Erbele, 1982) or who use alcohol/drugs to self-medicate (Gomberg & Nirenberg, 1991). Again with regard to the Russian doll metaphor, the crisis counselor may need to look for another layer of the crisis problem (intimate partner violence) if alcohol and drugs are involved in the crisis.

EXERCISE 4.3 INTIMATE PARTNER VIOLENCE

As with any counseling issue, IPV can be a stressful area in which to work as a crisis counselor. Some dynamics of violence, such as life-and-death situations or innocent individuals being hurt, can be especially difficult for some of us to work with in a crisis counseling context. Write out a holistic self-care plan (physical, cognitive, emotional, and spiritual) that addresses specific actions you will take in order to care for yourself when the crisis counseling you do in your current or anticipated work setting involves an IPV component.

Sexual Abuse

Childhood sexual abuse and rape may overlap with problems of substance abuse and mental health issues. As stated in Chapter 6, the best predictor of female alcohol dependence is childhood sexual abuse (Van Wormer & Davis, 2008). Rape survivors have shown an increase in alcohol use (McMullin & White, 2006) or prescription drugs (Sturza & Campbell, 2005), and survivors may experience posttraumatic

---

Case Study 4.3 Intimate Partner Violence

Your client is a child whose parents are in an intimate partner violence crisis. All you know is that your client, who is in kindergarten, has told his teacher that his parents fight a lot and the police were contacted over the weekend by neighbors who were worried about the fighting. The child is crying uncontrollably in the classroom and the teacher does not know how to handle the situation. You have been contacted as a counselor to assist in this situation.

1. Which setting (phone, school, agency, private practice) might increase or decrease the likelihood you would be contacted as a counselor to assist in the situation?
2. In each setting, how might you handle this situation generally?
3. What would be your first priority in terms of the welfare of your client?

---

stress disorder (PTSD) (Sturza & Campbell, 2005). Sexual abuse offenders may use alcohol/drugs to overcome their abuse inhibitions (Finkelhor, 1986), and may use the alcohol or drugs as an excuse for why they offended. Because these areas overlap, SAMHSA (2000a) recommends that counselors screen for trauma if PTSD, major depression, or mood disorders are present. Crisis counselors need to be aware of these overlapping areas of sexual abuse, mental health issues, and substance abuse issues in terms of their relationship with the crisis situation.

EXERCISE 4.4 SEXUAL ABUSE

Allow yourself to free associate in this exercise. Imagine yourself in your current or anticipated work setting in a common crisis situation. Although sexual abuse is not a core aspect of the crisis, it is one of the contributing factors to the crisis. What action would you take as a counselor to prevent or minimize the impact of the sexual abuse on the crisis situation? How might the context of the setting in which you work and/or the type of crisis impact the type and amount of intervention you can make?

Eating Disorders

Because Chapter 6 defines three eating disorders according to the *DSM-IV-TR* criteria (anorexia nervosa, bulimia nervosa, and eating disorder not otherwise specified [NOS]), those definitions will not be repeated in this section. However, what will be emphasized in this chapter is, again, the fact that many issues can overlap. Eating disorders and sexual abuse show an overlap (K. MacDonald, Lambie, & Simmonds, 1995). Also, eating disorders have components that are similar to other addictive behaviors—compulsiveness, powerlessness, preoccupation, avoidance of feeling,

---

Case Study 4.4 Sexual Abuse

Your client is gay and is talking about sexual abuse issues from his childhood. He has never talked with anyone about them before. He states he is afraid to trust counselors because he has heard that they "put ideas in your head" about sexual abuse, meaning that they encourage false memories. He states that he is so angry he feels like he is about to explode with violence. You have been contacted as a counselor to assist in this situation.

1. Which setting (phone, school, agency, private practice) might increase or decrease the likelihood you would be contacted as a counselor to assist in the situation?
2. In each setting, how might you handle this situation generally?
3. What would be your first priority in terms of the welfare of your client?

Case Study 4.5 Eating Disorders

Your client is a recovering alcoholic who has recently admitted to her Alcoholics Anonymous (AA) sponsor that while she has remained sober for two years, she has been bingeing and purging during that entire time. She has a lot of shame about her eating disorder, and when she approached her AA sponsor, who had been very kind, supportive, and reliable for two years, her sponsor was very critical and judgmental of her, making statements such as "This is not a big problem." "You need to simply eat differently and use the 12 Steps to help you with this issue." Your client is having trouble talking because she is crying so hard and because of the shame she is experiencing following her contact with her sponsor. You have been contacted as a counselor to assist in this situation.

1. Which setting (phone, school, agency, private practice) might increase or decrease the likelihood you would be contacted as a counselor to assist in the situation?
2. In each setting, how might you handle this situation generally?
3. What would be your first priority in terms of the welfare of your client?

---

relief by substance abuse — with the dissimilarity that food cannot be totally avoided. Finally, women in the United States make up 90%–95% of the clients diagnosed as having this disorder (APA, 1996). Crisis counselors need to: (a) be aware of the overlapping issues, (b) know there are similarities with other addictive behaviors, and (c) be sensitive to the high number of women diagnosed with these disorders.

EXERCISE 4.5 EATING DISORDERS

In this reflective exercise, examine the amount of knowledge and experience you have in working with eating disorders. Further examine this knowledge and experience in terms of crisis situations. What are the gaps (information, experience) you have in general in these areas? What are your concerns about applying your knowledge and experience in this area in a crisis situation? What can you do to address these concerns?

SUMMARY

This chapter presented typical crises and issues that occur in crisis counseling work. Also, helpful responses to these typical crises/issues were highlighted. In addition, common diagnoses that occur in this work were discussed with case studies and exercises provided to assist in the application of crisis counseling approaches.

QUESTIONS

1. What are some typical crises/issues in crisis counseling settings (phone, school, agency, private practice)?
2. How might I respond in a helpful way to such typical crises/issues?
3. What are some common diagnoses that occur in crisis counseling work? Which ones do I feel strongest in addressing? Which ones do I feel weakest in addressing? What can I do in settings to "play" to my strong areas and minimize my weak ones?

SUGGESTED READINGS

Settings

Telephone

James, R. K. (2008). *Crisis intervention strategies* (6th ed.). Belmont, CA: Thomson Brooks/Cole.

The author provides an entire chapter on telephone crisis counseling, and includes suggestions on handling specific issues that might arise for workers.

Roberts, A. R. (2005). Bridging the past and present to the future of crisis intervention and crisis management. In A. R. Roberts (Ed.), *Crisis intervention handbook* (3rd ed., pp. 3–34). New York, NY: Oxford University Press.

This chapter provides an overview of crisis counseling in terms of intervention and management and has sections on crisis lines.

Roberts, A. R., & Yeager, K. R. (2009). *Pocket guide to crisis intervention*. New York, NY: Oxford University Press.

This brief book has 33 chapters. Each of them covers, in a few pages, the major topics of crisis work. It may be thought of as a "CliffsNotes" or a primer of crisis work. It has a specific, concise chapter on "do's and don'ts."

School

James, R. K. (2008). *Crisis intervention strategies* (6th ed.). Belmont, CA: Thomson Brooks/Cole.

The author provides an entire chapter on crises in the schools with a particular emphasis on specific crises (gangs, bereavement, suicide) and suggestions on a framework for schools on how to handle different crises.

Juhnke, G. A., Granello, D. H., & Granello, P. F. (Eds.) (2011). *Suicide, self-injury, and violence in the schools*. Hoboken, NJ: Wiley.

This book provides an excellent overview of assessment, prevention, and intervention strategies within the school system. It has 11 chapters that are separated into three sections: suicide and self-injurious behaviors (five chapters), violence assessment, response, and postvention (four chapters), and legal issues and preparation (two chapters).

Newgass, S., & Schonfeld, D. J. (2005). School crisis intervention, crisis prevention, and crisis response. In A. R. Roberts (Ed.), *Crisis intervention handbook* (3rd ed., pp. 499–518). New York, NY: Oxford University Press.

This chapter outlines the components of a school crisis response initiative, with guidelines for specific components such as support rooms and classroom interventions.

Stewart, C., & MacNeil, G. (2005). Crisis intervention with chronic school violence and volatile situations. In A. R. Roberts (Ed.), *Crisis intervention handbook* (3rd ed., pp. 519–540). New York, NY: Oxford University Press.

This chapter describes a specific crisis intervention model of cognitive therapy.

Agency

Dingman, R. L., & Weaver, J. D. (2003). *Days in the lives of counselors*. Boston, MA: Allyn & Bacon.

In this book, counselors in different settings describe their experiences, with three of the 33 chapters (stories) focusing on crisis counseling. Two of the three stories are specifically related to agency work. One story is based on a crisis counselor who works with the chronically mentally ill, and another is from a counselor at a psychiatric facility.

Ligon, J. (2005). Mobile crisis units: Frontline community mental health services. In A. R. Roberts (Ed.), *Crisis intervention handbook* (3rd ed., pp. 602–618). New York, NY: Oxford University Press.

In this chapter, the author provides an overview of community crisis services with a special emphasis on mobile crisis units.

Private Practice

Dingman, R. L., & Weaver, J. D. (2003). *Days in the lives of counselors*. Boston, MA: Allyn & Bacon.

In this book, counselors in different settings describe their experiences, with three of the 33 chapters (stories) focusing on crisis counseling. One of these three stories addresses disaster mental health work with the American Red Cross.

Granvold, D. K. (2005). The crisis of divorce: Cognitive-behavioral and constructivist assessment and treatment. In A. R. Roberts (Ed.), *Crisis intervention handbook* (3rd ed., pp. 650–681). New York, NY: Oxford University Press.

This chapter focuses on working with the crisis of divorce from both cognitive-behavioral and constructivist approaches. Divorce crisis, psychosocial needs, risk assessment, client strengths, and interventions are examined.

Webber, J., Bass, D. D., & Yep, R. (Eds.) (2005). *Terrorism, trauma, and tragedies: A counselor's guide to preparing and responding* (2nd ed.). Alexandria, VA: American Counseling Association.

This book provides practical suggestions for counselors in various settings, including private practice, on how to effectively approach traumatic events.

Wise, E. A. (2000). Mental health intensive outpatient programming: An outcome and satisfaction evaluation of a private practice model. *Professional Psychology: Research and practice, 31*, 412–417.

This article describes the development of an intensive outpatient program in a private practice that uses crisis intervention and group therapy approaches.

General Crisis

Greenstone, J. L., & Leviton, S. C. (2002). *Elements of crisis intervention* (3rd ed.). Belmont, CA: Brooks/Cole.

This short book has 11 chapters that briefly cover basic approaches and strategies in crisis work with chapters focused on children, families, hotline workers, loss, legal implications, and disasters.

Hoff, L. A., Hallisey, B. J., & Hoff, M. (2009). *People in crisis: Clinical and diversity perspectives* (6th ed.). New York, NY: Routledge.

This book, an overview of crisis work, is divided into three sections: understanding crisis intervention; specific crises; and suicide, homicide, and catastrophic events.

James, R. K. (2008). *Crisis intervention strategies*. Belmont, CA: Thomson Brooks/Cole.

This book provides an overview of crisis intervention. It has four sections: theory and application, handling specific crises, workplace, and disaster. There is a specific chapter related to addiction.

Roberts, A. R., & Yeager, K. R. (2009). *Pocket guide to crisis intervention*. New York, NY: Oxford University Press.

This brief book has 33 chapters. Each of them covers, in a few pages, the major topics of crisis work. It may be thought of as a "CliffsNotes" or a primer of crisis work. It has a specific, concise chapter on "do's and don'ts."

General Mental Health/General Trauma

Briere, J., & Scott, C. (2006). *Principles of trauma therapy*. Thousand Oaks, CA: Sage.

This book is divided into two sections: trauma effects and assessment and clinical interventions.

Foa, E. B., Keane, T. M., Friedman, M. J., & Cohen, J. A. (2009). *Effective treatments for PTSD: Practice guidelines from the International Society for Traumatic Stress Studies* (2nd ed.). New York, NY: Guilford.

This book is divided into five sections: assessment and diagnosis (two chapters); early interventions (three chapters); treatment for chronic PTSD (15 chapters, children/adolescents/adults, various treatment approaches); treatment guidelines (18 sections); and conclusions.

Hien, D., Litt, L. C., Cohen, L. R., Miele, G. M., & Campbell, A. (2009). *Trauma services for women in substance abuse treatment*. Washington, DC: American Psychological Association.

This book has three sections about: the relationship between trauma and substance abuse; the impact of trauma on functioning; and strategies for implementation.

Ogden, P., Minton, K., & Pain, C. (2006). *Trauma and the body: A sensorimotor approach to psychotherapy*. New York, NY: Norton.

This book is divided into two sections: theory and treatment. The theoretical section has seven chapters that look at thoughts, feelings, and sensorimotor reactions to trauma. The treatment section has five chapters that provide the counselor with information on how to apply the theory to clinical practice with trauma survivors.

Rothschild, B. (2000). *The body remembers*. New York, NY: Norton.

This book is divided into two sections: theory and practice. The theoretical portion of the book describes the main impacts of trauma on the mind and body. The practice section provides the counselor with practical suggestions on working with trauma survivors.

Addiction

Dimeff, L. A., Comtois, K. A., & Linehan, M. M. (2009). Co-occurring addiction and borderline personality disorder. In R. K. Ries, D. A. Fiellin, S. C. Miller, & R. Saitz (Eds.), *Principles of addiction medicine* (4th ed., pp. 1227–1237). Philadelphia, PA: Wolters Kluwer/Lippincott Williams & Wilkins.

This chapter provides a concise overview of DBT as applied to a substance-abusing borderline population.

Dimeff, L. A., & Linehan, M. M. (2008). Dialectical behavior therapy for substance abusers. *Addiction Science & Clinical Practice, 4*, 39–47.

This article provides a concise overview of DBT as applied to a substance-abusing borderline population.

Goldstein, E. G. (2004). Substance abusers with borderline disorders. In S. L. A. Straussner (Ed.), *Clinical work with substance-abusing clients* (2nd ed., pp. 370–391). New York, NY: Guilford.

This chapter discusses characteristics and causes of borderline personality disorders as well as assessment and treatment strategies.

Harvard Health Publications (2008a). *Alcohol use and abuse*. Boston, MA: Harvard University.

This booklet provides a concise overview of the continuum of alcohol use (use, abuse, addiction) as well as sections on women, adolescents, and the elderly.

Harvard Health Publications (2008b). *Overcoming addiction*. Boston, MA: Harvard University.

This booklet gives a summary of the causes of addiction, how people recover from addiction, and different types of addiction.

Margolis, R. D., & Zweben, J. E. (1998). *Treating patients with alcohol and other drug problems: An integrated approach*. Washington, DC: American Psychological Association.

This 358-page book has an excellent section on techniques a counselor can use to encourage abstinence.

Miller, G. A. (2010). *Learning the language of addiction counseling* (3rd ed.). Hoboken, NJ: Wiley.

This book provides a summary of addiction counseling. It has 14 chapters (introduction, theories, assessment of addiction, assessment of co-occurring disorders, treatment, treatment-related issues, relapse prevention, self-help groups, current and evolving therapies, culturally sensitive counseling, spirituality, chronic pain, personal and professional development, preparation of certification and licensure). The text has numerous case studies and exercises to facilitate application of the material.

Schenker, M. D. (2009). *A clinician's guide to 12 step recovery: Integrating 12 step programs into psychotherapy*. New York, NY: Norton.

This book has 12 chapters that are designed to educate the clinician about the core components of 12-step recovery programs and how to integrate them into a clinical practice. Chapters address topics such as the history of AA, what happens in meetings, common treatment issues as they relate to AA, and critiques and challenges.

Shaw, B. F., Ritvo, P., & Irvine, J. (2005). *Addiction & recovery for dummies*. Hoboken, NJ: Wiley.

This book has 20 chapters divided into five sections: the detection of addiction, taking initial steps, treatment approaches, a recovery life, and 10 ways to help a loved one and self-help resources. It is written for a layperson.

Co-Occurring Disorders

Center for Substance Abuse Treatment (CSAT) (2005). *Substance abuse treatment for persons with co-occurring disorders*. Treatment Improvement Protocol (TIP) Series, No. 42. DHHS Publication No. (SMA) 05-3922. Rockville, MD: Substance Abuse and Mental Health Services Administration.

The manual provides a general overview of treatment for these disorders.

Center for Substance Abuse Treatment (CSAT) (2008). *Managing depressive symptoms in substance abuse clients during early recovery*. Treatment Improvement Protocol (TIP) Series, No. 48. DHHS Publication No. (SMA) 05-3922. Rockville, MD: Substance Abuse and Mental Health Services Administration.

This manual is the first TIP manual using a new format that describes working with this population in three parts for substance abuse counselors (part 1: counseling methods and frameworks), program administrators (part 2: provision of administrative support for part 1 to be integrated), and clinical supervisors (part 3: online literature review that is updated every six months for five years and can be accessed at www.kap.samhsa.gov).

Daley, D. C., & Moss, H. B. (2002). *Dual disorders: Counseling clients with chemical dependency and mental illness* (3rd ed.). Center City, MN: Hazelden.

This book has 15 chapters that provide an overview of dual disorders and the treatment (including group treatment) and recovery process (including relapse

prevention) as well as chapters that focus on the family, specific disorders (personality, antisocial, borderline, depression, bipolar, anxiety, schizophrenia, cognitive),
and specific program development issues.

Evans, K., & Sullivan, J. M. (2001). *Dual diagnosis: Counseling the mentally ill substance abuser* (2nd ed.). New York, NY: Guilford Press.
This book provides suggestions for working with a dually diagnosed population.

Hamilton, T., & Samples, P. (1994). *The twelve steps and dual disorders*. Center City,
MN: Hazelden.
This book describes how the 12 steps can be effectively used with this population.

Hazelden (1993). *The dual disorders recovery book*. Center City, MN: Hazelden.
This book focuses on the 12-step program for dual disorders (Dual Recovery
Anonymous), using the stories of individuals.

L'Abate, L. L., Farrar, J. E., & Serritella, D. A. (1992). *Handbook of differential treatments for addictions*. Boston, MA: Allyn & Bacon.
This book provides information on a variety of addictions that the authors describe as
socially destructive (alcohol, substance abuse, tobacco, domestic violence, sexual abuses
and offenses), socially unacceptable (interpersonal/love, eating disorders), or socially
acceptable (gambling, workaholism, exercise, spending, religion, codependency).

McGovern, M. (2009). *Living with co-occurring addiction and mental health disorders*.
Center City, MN: Hazelden.
This book is written to the person struggling with these disorders. It has
14 chapters that explain basic concepts of dual diagnosis and its treatment.

Mueser, K. T., Noordsy, D. L., Drake, R. E., & Fox, L. (2003). *Integrated treatment
for dual disorders*. New York, NY: Guilford Press.
This is an excellent workbook that generally describes co-occurring diagnosis and
then provides information on working with this population in the assessment and
treatment process—including individual, group, and family therapy. Its appendix
contains 16 educational handouts and 20 assessment and treatment forms.

National Institute on Drug Abuse (NIDA) (2008a). Comorbidity: Addiction and
other mental illnesses. *Research Report Series*. Rockville, MD: NIDA.
This 11-page publication provides an excellent summary of comorbidity.

Smith, T. (2008). *A balanced life: 9 strategies for coping with the mental health problems of a
loved one*. Center City, MN: Hazelden.
This book is written for the family and friends of a loved one who struggles with
mental illness. It provides nine strategies to help the individual cope with the daily realities of this situation within a balanced lifestyle. It incorporates a Higher Power concept.

Solomon, J., Zimberg, S., & Shollar, E. (Eds.) (1993). *Dual diagnosis: Evaluation,
treatment, training, and program development*. New York, NY: Plenum Press.
This book covers theory, research, and practice concerning co-occurring diagnosis. Specific suggestions are made regarding assessment and treatment of the
dually diagnosed.

Substance Abuse and Mental Health Services Administration (SAMHSA) (1994). *Assessment and treatment of patients with coexisting mental illness and alcohol and other drug abuse* (DHHS Publication No. 94-2078). Rockville, MD: Author.

This publication has nine chapters that provide basic information on co-occurring diagnosis and treatment (issues, collaboration, medication), and a separate chapter on specific diagnoses (mood disorders, anxiety disorders, personality disorders, psychotic disorders).

Substance Abuse and Mental Health Services Administration (SAMHSA) (2002). *Report to Congress on the prevention and treatment of co-occurring substance abuse disorders and mental disorders* (www.samhsa.gov). Rockville, MD: Author.

This report is divided into five chapters: characteristics/needs, impact of federal block grants, prevention, evidence-based practices, and a five-year action blueprint.

Watkins, T. R., Lewellen, A., & Barrett, M. C. (2001). *Dual diagnosis: An integrated approach to treatment.* Thousand Oaks, CA: Sage.

This book covers general issues related to co-occurring diagnosis and then provides separate chapters on assessment and treatment for specific disorders in relation to substance abuse (schizophrenia, depression, bipolar, personality disorders, anxiety disorders).

Intimate Partner Violence

Professional

Domestic Abuse Intervention Project (2002). *A guide for conducting domestic violence assessments.* Duluth, MN: Author.

This manual has four sections (using the assessment guide, assessing social risks of battered women, preparing for the assessment, assessment interview format) and 10 appendices. It provides a domestic violence matrix and a risk assessment for women that focuses on the woman's safety.

Edelson, J. L., & Tolman, R. M. (1992). *Intervention for men who batter: An ecological approach.* Newbury Park, CA: Sage.

This manual is designed to provide practical suggestions to the counselor who wants to counsel batterers.

Goodman, M. S., & Fallon, B. C. (1995). *Pattern changing for abused women.* Thousand Oaks, CA: Sage.

This text provides an overview of domestic violence counseling theory and approaches. The accompanying workbook has helpful exercises that a counselor can use in working with this population; one especially helpful handout is "Your Bill of Rights."

Graham-Bermann, S. A., & Edleson, J. L. (Eds.) (2001). *Domestic violence in the lives of children.* Washington, DC: American Psychological Association.

This book is divided into three sections: understanding children's exposure to intimate partner violence, the role of families and social support, and preventive intervention initiatives and evaluations.

Hilton, N. Z., Harris, G. T., & Rice, M. E. (2010). *Risk assessment for domestically violent men*. Washington, DC: American Psychological Association.

This book provides information on the Ontario Domestic Assault Risk Assessment (ODARA) and the Domestic Violence Risk Appraisal Guide (DVRAG), which can be used to predict recidivism in male domestic violence offenders. It has seven chapters that provide an overview and six appendices on the instruments, including one specifically on scoring criteria for the ODARA and one for the DVRAG.

Hines, D. A., & Malley-Morrison, K. M. (2005). *Family violence in the United States*. Thousand Oaks, CA: Sage.

This book has 12 chapters that address: definition issues, cultural contexts, religious contexts, child physical abuse, child sexual abuse, child neglect, wife abuse, husband abuse, GLBT abuse, elder abuse, hidden types of abuse, and effective responses.

Holden, G. W., Geffner, R., & Jouriles, E. N. (Eds.) (1998). *Children exposed to marital violence*. Washington, DC: American Psychological Association.

This book covers theoretical and conceptual issues, research, and applied issues.

Knapp, S. J., & VandeCreek, L. (1997). *Treating patients with memories of abuse: Legal risk management*. Washington, DC: American Psychological Association.

This book presents suggestions on how to treat clients who have been abused from a risk management perspective. It provides helpful guidelines for practice in working with this population.

Leventhal, B., & Lundy, S. E. (1999). *Same-sex domestic violence*. Thousand Oaks, CA: Sage.

This book is divided into four sections: personal stories, legal perspectives, organizing coalitions/building communities, and providing services.

Miller, G., Clark, C., & Herman, J. (2007). Domestic violence in a rural setting. *Journal of Rural Mental Health, 31*, 28–42.

This journal article provides a summary of barriers that face intimate partner violence survivors in a rural setting, along with specific counseling examples. Recommendations are made to rural health care professionals.

Minnesota Coalition for Battered Women (1992). *Safety first: A guide for battered women*. St. Paul, MN: Author.

This is a useful book for survivors of intimate partner violence because it provides both theoretical and practical information and suggestions.

Schechter, S. (1987). *Guidelines for mental health practitioners in domestic violence cases*. Washington, DC: National Coalition Against Domestic Violence.

This booklet has basic information on intimate partner violence (definition, misconceptions, indicators) as well as clinical suggestions on working with this population.

Substance Abuse and Mental Health Services Administration (SAMHSA) (1997). *Substance abuse treatment and domestic violence*. Rockville, MD: Author.

This manual summarizes the knowledge base of intimate partner violence (male batterers to female survivors), the relationship between substance abuse and intimate partner violence, and how to screen for it in treatment. It also provides instruments that can be used for assessment.

Substance Abuse and Mental Health Services Administration (2002). *Domestic violence and the new Americans: Directory of programs and resources for battered refugee women* (CMHS-SVP-0061). Rockville, MD: Author.

This book provides information about services and programs available by state.

Trickett, P. K., & Schellenbach, C. J. (1998). *Violence against children in the family and the community*. Washington, DC: American Psychological Association.

This book has five sections: developmental consequences, causes of different forms of violence, effective interventions, prevention, and effectiveness of interventions.

Personal

NiCarthy, G. (1987). *The ones who got away: Women who left abusive partners*. Seattle, WA: Seal Press.

This book has 33 stories of women from different walks of life who left their abusers. There is also a chapter on the lessons the women who leave provide and a chapter on why they left and how they were able to stay away.

NiCarthy, G. (1997). *Getting free: You can end abuse and take back your life*. Seattle, WA: Seal Press.

This book provides general information on intimate partner violence with exercises to facilitate the survivor's awareness. There are chapters on teen abuse, lesbian abuse, and emotional abuse.

White, E. C. (1994). *Chain, chain, change: For black women in abusive relationships*. Seattle, WA: Seal Press.

This book has nine chapters that attempt to provide information to the reader to assess whether she is in a violent relationship and explore actions she may choose to take. The book includes a chapter on lesbians and abuse.

Sexual Abuse

Professional

Cunningham, C., & MacFarlane, K. (1991). *When children molest children: Group treatment strategies for young sexual abusers*. Orwell, VT: The Safer Society Press.

This book contains simple activities for children ages 4 to 12, which counselors can use in addressing sexual offender behaviors in young children. It has three sections (interventions, skills/competencies, progress measures) with accompanying exercises the counselor can use in group counseling.

Finkelhor, D. (1986). *A sourcebook on child sexual abuse*. Beverly Hills, CA: Sage.

This book provides an excellent general overview on sexual abuse.

Gonsiorek, J. C., Bera, W. H., & LeTourneau, D. (1994). *Male sexual abuse.* Thousand Oaks, CA: Sage.

This book covers basic information on male sexual abuse with specific counseling suggestions.

Schwartz, M. F., & Cohn, L. (Eds.) (1996). *Sexual abuse and eating disorders.* New York: Brunner/Mazel.

This book provides an excellent overview of the overlap of the issues between sexual abuse and eating disorders.

Substance Abuse and Mental Health Services Administration (2000b). *Substance abuse treatment for persons with child abuse and neglect issues.* Rockville, MD: Author.

The seven chapters in this manual cover areas that include working with these issues: screening, assessment, treatment, therapeutic issues, breaking the cycle, and legal concerns.

Personal

Bass, E. (Ed.) (1983). *I never told anyone: Writings by women survivors of child sexual abuse.* New York, NY: Harper Perennial.

This book has 33 stories of survivors of sexual abuse, organized by perpetrator type (fathers, relatives, friends/acquaintances, strangers).

Bass, E., & Davis, L. (1988). *The courage to heal.* New York, NY: Harper & Row.

This book was written for female survivors. It has five sections (taking stock, the healing process, changing patterns, survivor supporters, and courageous women) that provide information as well as questions and exercises to assist the survivor in the healing process.

Lew, M. (1988). *Victims no longer: Men recovering from incest and other sexual child abuse.* New York, NY: Harper & Row.

This book has five sections (general information, information about men, survival, recovery, and other people/resources). Each section provides information and the story of a survivor.

Lew, M. (2004). *Victims no longer: The classic guide for men recovering from sexual child abuse.* New York, NY: Harper Paperbacks.

This book describes how culture inhibits men's ability to see abuse and obtain treatment for it.

Mendel, M. P. (1995). *The male survivor.* Thousand Oaks, CA: Sage.

This book has eight chapters that each provide information on male sexual abuse and are accompanied by a survivor's story. The final chapter discusses the male survivor in general.

Eating Disorders

Schwartz, M. F., & Cohn, L. (Eds.) (1996). *Sexual abuse and eating disorders*. New York, NY: Brunner/Mazel.

This book provides an excellent overview of the overlap of the issues between sexual abuse and eating disorders.

Stromberg, G., & Merrill, J. (2006). *Feeding the fame*. Center City, MN: Hazelden.

This book tells the stories of 17 celebrities who struggled with eating disorders and are in the process of recovery. It does an excellent job of personalizing and demystifying the struggle with eating disorders. The celebrities come from all types of careers (political, journalistic, acting, writing, modeling, religious, entertaining, sports, paranormalistic).

Thompson, J. K., Heinberg, L. J., Altable, M., & Tantleff-Dunn, S. (1999). *Exacting beauty: Theory, assessment, and treatment of body image disturbance*. Washington, DC: American Psychological Association.

This book provides an excellent overview of theoretical approaches (societal/ social, interpersonal, feminist, behavioral, cognitive, and integrative) that explain eating disorder prevalence. It has 36 scales, surveys, and questionnaires that can be used with this population.

Manuals/Workbooks

General Mental Health/General Trauma

Linehan, M. M. (1993a). *Cognitive-behavioral treatment of borderline personality disorder*. New York, NY: Guilford.

This book comprehensively describes this treatment approach.

Linehan, M. M. (1993b). *Skills training manual for treating borderline personality disorder*. New York, NY: Guilford.

This book comprehensively describes this treatment approach in terms of skills, teaching strategies, and discussion topics in groups.

Linehan, M. M. (in press). *Skills training manual for disordered emotional regulation*. New York, NY: Guilford.

Marra, T. (2004). *Depressed & anxious: The dialectical behavior therapy workbook for overcoming depression & anxiety*. Oakland, CA: New Harbinger.

This book has nine chapters. The first is an overview of DBT. The remaining eight are meant for the client to use as exercises (dialectics of anxiety and depression, feelings, "there must be something wrong with me," meaning making, mindfulness skills, emotional regulation, distress tolerance skills, and strategic behavioral skills).

Najavits, L. M. (2002). *Seeking safety: A treatment manual for PTSD and substance abuse*. New York, NY: Guilford.

The manual has a chapter that provides an overview of PTSD and substance abuse and a chapter that discusses how to conduct the treatment. The remainder of the manual focuses on treatment topics.

Rosenbloom, D., & Williams, M. B. (1999). *Life after trauma: A workbook for healing*. New York, NY: Guilford.

This workbook is meant for trauma survivors in general. It has eight sections that have accompanying exercises to facilitate awareness in trauma survivors. It also has a prologue with suggestions on how to use the book and an epilogue on long-term healing. Finally, it has appendices on recommended readings, the psychotherapy process, and suggestions to counselors on how to use the book.

Williams, M. B., & Poijula, S. (2002). *The PTSD workbook*. Oakland, CA: New Harbinger.

This book has 15 chapters. Each chapter has exercises that facilitate awareness about the impact of the trauma on the survivor and ways to heal from the trauma.

Addiction

Documentation Resources

Berghuis, D. J., & Jongsma, A. E. (2002). *The addiction progress notes planner*. Hoboken, NJ: Wiley.

This book is a guide to documenting the therapeutic process and can assist in determining eligibility for reimbursable treatment. It complements *The Addiction Treatment Planner, Second Edition* (2001), also published by Wiley.

Finley, J. R., & Lenz, B. S. (1999a). *The chemical dependence treatment documentation sourcebook*. Hoboken, NJ: Wiley.

This book has more than 80 forms that cover the continuum of addiction treatment and can be readily copied. It also has a disk of the forms.

Finley, J. R., & Lenz, B. S. (1999b). *Chemical dependence treatment homework planner*. Hoboken, NJ: Wiley.

This 302-page book has 53 homework assignments that can be readily copied. It also has a disk of the assignments.

Finley, J. R., & Lenz, B. S. (2003). *Addiction treatment homework planner* (2nd ed.). Hoboken, NJ: Wiley.

This book has 78 homework assignments for chemical and nonchemical addiction treatment issues. The book contains a CD with all the forms.

Jongsma, A. E., & Peterson, L. M. (2003). *The complete adult psychotherapy treatment planner*. Hoboken, NJ: Wiley.

This book covers numerous diagnoses and has two sections specifically on chemical dependency: chemical dependence and chemical dependence-relapse. For each one, it provides behavioral definitions, long-term goals, short-term objectives/ therapeutic interventions, and diagnostic suggestions. It provides a section on how to write a treatment plan as well as two sample treatment plans.

Perkinson, R. R., & Jongsma, A. E. (1998). *The chemical dependence treatment planner*. New York, NY: Wiley.

This 248-page book provides guidelines for writing treatment plans as well as specific goals and objectives that can be used in treatment plan writing.

Resources (Workbooks)

Hazelden (2005a). *Client recovery workbook*. Center City, MN: Author.

This 143-page workbook has five sections: getting started, you and your team, 12-step and other group meetings, AA/NA/CA recovery basics, and getting ready to go off probation/parole or leaving the safety of the drug court. It has 52 exercises, each of which has an introduction and a set of questions.

Hazelden (2005b). *Client cognitive skills workbook*. Center City, MN: Author.

This 148-page workbook has eight parts: mapmaking, criminal and addiction history, becoming aware of your inner maps, learning to think about your thinking, learning to think about your behaviors, socialization, what works/what doesn't, and how do I change. It has 45 exercises designed to facilitate self-exploration.

Hazelden (2005c). *Client life skills workbook*. Center City, MN: Author.

This 100-page workbook has four parts: have a plan, plan the work, the many parts of the plan, and work the plan. There is a good, simple explanation of the Stages of Change model on page 11. It looks at recovery in a holistic way. There are 52 exercises designed to facilitate the client's self-exploration.

Substance Abuse and Mental Health Services Administration (1996). *Counselor's manual for relapse prevention with chemically dependent criminal offenders* (Technical Assistance Publication Series 19; DHHS Publication No. SMA 96-3115). Rockville, MD: Author.

This 181-page booklet provides general information on addiction, relapse prevention treatment, a guide to professionals on how to use the workbook, and an appendix workbook on relapse prevention that has 27 exercises.

Co-Occurring Disorders

Center for Substance Abuse Treatment (CSAT) (2003). *Co-occurring disorders: Integrated dual disorders treatment: Implementation resource kit*. Rockville, MD.

Intimate Partner Violence

Fall, K. A., & Howard, S. (2004). *Alternatives to domestic violence* (2nd ed.). New York, NY: Brunner/Routledge.

This is a homework manual for participants in a battering intervention group. It has 12 chapters that include exercises meant to facilitate self-awareness.

Goodman, M. S., & Fallon, B. C. (1995). *Pattern changing for abused women*. Thousand Oaks, CA: Sage.

This text provides an overview of intimate partner violence counseling theory and approaches. The accompanying workbook has helpful exercises that a counselor can use in working with this population; one especially helpful handout is "Your Bill of Rights."

Minnesota Coalition for Battered Women (1992). *Safety first: A guide for counselors and advocates*. St. Paul, MN: Author.

This workbook provides very helpful guidelines on working with survivors of domestic violence.

Rosenbloom, D., & Williams, M. B. (1999). *Life after trauma: A workbook for healing*. New York, NY: Guilford.

This workbook is meant for trauma survivors in general. It has eight sections that have accompanying exercises to facilitate awareness in trauma survivors. It also has a prologue with suggestions on how to use the book and an epilogue on long-term healing. Finally, it has appendices on recommended readings, the psychotherapy process, and suggestions to counselors on how to use the book.

Sexual Abuse

Carter, W. L. (2002). *It happened to me: A teen's guide to overcoming sexual abuse*. Oakland, CA: New Harbinger.

This book has five sections with exercises in each section meant to help teenagers become aware of their reactions to the sexual abuse they have experienced.

Davis, L. (1990). *The courage to heal workbook*. New York: Harper & Row.

This workbook is designed for women and men who have survived sexual abuse. It has three sections (healing survival skills, taking stock, and healing aspects). Each section has subsections with specific exercises meant to help the survivor learn about self and heal from the sexual abuse.

Rosenbloom, D., & Williams, M. B. (1999). *Life after trauma: A workbook for healing*. New York, NY: Guilford.

This workbook is meant for trauma survivors in general. It has eight sections that have accompanying exercises to facilitate awareness in trauma survivors. It also has a prologue with suggestions on how to use the book and an epilogue on long-term healing. Finally, it has appendices on recommended readings, the psychotherapy process, and suggestions to counselors on how to use the book.

VIDEOTAPES/DVDS

General Mental Health/General Trauma

Cavalcade Productions (Producer) (1998a). *Trauma and substance abuse I: Therapeutic approaches* [video]. Available from www.cavalcadeproductions.com

This 46-minute video discusses ways to work with substance abuse trauma survivors.

Cavalcade Productions (Producer) (1998b). *Trauma and substance abuse II: Special treatment issues* [video]. Available from www.calvacadeproductions
This 40-minute video discusses the issues of countertransference, codependency, crisis, and relapse.

Cavalcade Productions (Producer) (2005). *Numbing the Pain: Substance abuse and psychological trauma* [video]. Available from www.calvacadeproductions.com
This 30-minute video examines how substance abuse has assisted survivors in their lives and the ways therapy can provide challenges and benefits to the survivor.

CNS Productions (Producer) (2008). *In & out of control* [video]. Available from www.cnsproductions.com
This 38-minute video provides general information about emotional, physical, and sexual violence.

Addiction

A&E (Producer). Investigative reports: Inside Alcoholics Anonymous [DVD]. Available from www.aetn.com
This 50-minute DVD provides an overview of Alcoholics Anonymous.

Films for the Humanities & Sciences (Producer) (2004). Understanding addiction [DVD]. Available from www.films.com
This 24-minute DVD provides overall information about addiction with one individual's story of recovery highlighted.

Hazelden (Producer) (2004). The Hazelden Step Series for Adults [3 DVDs]. Available from www.hazelden.org
These three DVDs are each 12 minutes in length and each covers one of the first three steps of Alcoholics Anonymous.

HBO Documentary Films (Producer) (2007). Addiction [4 DVDs]. Available from www.hbo.com/documentaries
This four-set DVD is divided into: (a) 1 & 2 (90 minutes), which focus on "What is Addiction?"; "Understanding Relapse"; "The Search for Treatment: A Challenging Journey"; and "The Adolescent Addict"; and (b) 3 & 4 (270 minutes), which have four interviews with addiction professionals, three sections on treatment, one section on drug court, and one about a mother.

Co-Occurring Disorders

See General Mental Health section, above.

Intimate Partner Violence

Domestic Abuse Intervention Project (Producer). (2011a). *Power & control: A woman's perspective* [video]. Available from www.theduluthmodel.org
This one-hour video discusses power and control issues from a woman's perspective through interviews with survivors.

Domestic Abuse Intervention Project (Producer) (2011b). *Power & control: The tactics of men who batter* [video]. Available from www.theduluthmodel.org
This 40-minute video discusses power and control issues from a man's perspective through interviews with perpetrators.

New Day Films (Producer). *To have and to hold* [video]. Available from www.new day.com
This 20-minute film interviews men who have assaulted their wives.

Sexual Abuse

KB Films (Producer). *The healing years* [DVD]. Available by e-mailing: kbfilms@ compuserv.com
This 52-minute DVD has a summary of different women's stories of sexual abuse and incest. A former Miss America tells her story.

WEB SITES

General Mental Health/General Trauma

Behavioral Tech. www.behavioraltech.org
This Web site provides information on workshops, training (intensive, online), and educational products related to DBT.

Seeking Safety. www.seekingsafety.org
This Web site provides general information about the Seeking Safety approach. It includes article and training information on the topic.

Addiction

National Association of Drug Court Professionals (NADCP). www.nadcp.org
NADCP provides general information about their organization at this Web site.

National Drug Court Institute. www.ndci.org
The National Drug Court Institute provides education, research, and scholarship for drug court intervention programs. This Web site provides information on how to access these resources.

Restorative Justice. www.restorativejustice.org
This Web site provides resources such as crime victim support. The focus of this group is to repair the harm done by crime.

The National Institute on Alcohol Abuse and Alcoholism (NIAAA). www.niaaa .nih.gov
The NIAAA Web site provides general information on alcohol use as well as resources helpful to the counselor.

National Institute on Drug Abuse (NIDA). www.nida.nih.gov
The NIDA Web site provides general information about drug abuse as well as numerous resources.

Substance Abuse and Mental Health Services Administration (SAMHSA). www.samhsa.gov
The SAMHSA Web site assists in treatment location and services as well as providing resources (publications, etc.) on substance abuse.

Co-Occurring Disorders

National Institute on Drug Abuse. www.drugabuse.gov
This Web site provides general information on drug abuse and addiction.

National Institute of Mental Health. www.nimh.nih.gov
This Web site provides information on understanding and treating mental illness.

Substance Abuse and Mental Health Services Administration (SAMHSA). www.samhsa.gov
This Web site provides a variety of information and resources on substance abuse and mental health.

Treatment Improvement Exchange (TIE) (SAMHSA-funded). www.treatment.org
This Web site provides information on the treatment of addiction, with a special topics section that addresses concerns such as co-occurring disorders, gambling, and homelessness.

Intimate Partner Violence

The Domestic Violence Initiative for Women with Disabilities. www.dviforwomen.org
This Web site provides information regarding domestic violence within the disabled population of women.

The Domestic Abuse Intervention Project. www.theduluthmodel.org
This Web site provides overall information on intimate partner violence.

National Latino Alliance for the Elimination of Domestic Violence. www.dvalianza.org
This Web site provides information on intimate partner violence in the Latino population.

The Institute on Domestic Violence in the African-American Community. www.dvinstitute.org
This Web site provides information on family violence in the African-American community and provides an avenue where individuals can state their perspectives.

Jewish Women International. www.jwi.org
This Web site provides information on programs, education, and advocacy within the Jewish population.

Minnesota Coalition for Battered Women. www.mcbw.org

This organization provides general information, books, stickers, pins, posters, referrals, trainings, research, networking, and legislative lobbying.

Mending the Sacred Hoop: Technical Assistance Project. www.msh-ta.org

This Web site provides training and technical assistance to American Indians and Alaskan Natives in the effort of eliminating intimate partner violence in this population.

National Coalition Against Domestic Violence. www.ncadv.org

This Web site provides information helpful at the regional, state, and national levels. Information includes safe homes/shelters, policy development and legislation, public education, and technical assistance.

Sacred Circle: National Resource Center to End Violence against Native Women. www.sacred-circle.com

This Web site provides information on intimate partner violence in American Indian and Alaskan Native tribal communities.

Sexual Abuse

Posttraumatic Stress Disorder Alliance. www.ptsdalliance.org

This Web site has general information on PTSD as well as articles and support group information.

Rape, Abuse, & Incest National Network (RAINN). E-mail: info@rainn.org; Web site: www.rainn.org

This Web site provides information about services, education, and advocacy regarding rape, abuse, and incest

Sacred Circle: National Resource Center to End Violence against Native Women. www.sacred-circle.com

This Web site provides information on sexual assault in American Indian and Alaskan Native tribal communities.

Substance Abuse and Mental Health Services Administration (SAMHSA). www .samhsa.gov

This Web site provides the TIP series and their related products. Two helpful, free brochures are called *Helping Yourself Heal*. One is written for recovering men (DHHS Publication No. SMA 04-3969) who have been abused as children, and one is written for recovering women (DHHS Publication No. SMA 06-4132).

S. E. S. A. M. E. (Stop Educator Sexual Abuse, Misconduct, and Exploitation). E-mail: Babe4justice@aol.com; Web site: www.sesamenet.org

This Web site is for the group S. E. S. A. M. E. (Stop Educator Sexual Abuse, Misconduct, and Exploitation), whose goal is to be a national voice for preventing sexual exploitation, abuse, and harassment of students by teachers and school staff.

Survivorship. E-mail: info@survivorship.org; Web site: www.survivorship.org

This Web site provides resources for survivors of ritualistic abuse, mind control, and torture.

Special Populations and Legal/Ethical Issues

LEARNING OBJECTIVES

1. To learn an overview of individual, group, and couples/family counseling as well as overall legal and ethical issues as they relate to crisis counseling.
2. To understand 10 practical suggestions that can be used in these different counseling special populations (individual, group, couples/family).
3. To practice applying the overview and the related suggestions through exercises and a case study.

> You can cut all the flowers, but you can't keep spring from coming.
>
> —*Pablo Neruda*

This chapter is a transitional chapter. Up to this point, the book has focused on general crisis counseling, theoretical orientation, types of disasters, and common crisis counseling contexts and issues. This chapter begins the specific application of crisis counseling as it relates to special populations (group, couples/family) and how individual assessments are applicable to special populations.

In crisis counseling, no matter what the population context, we, as counselors, attempt to provide clients with a sense of hope—a sense that while all the flowers have been cut in one's life, spring will still come. We attempt to do this in a variety of ways, but basically we are trying to assist the individual(s) in regaining their balance and sense of hope by normalizing their routine and by treating them as normally as possible. What this means in practice is that when one has had his/her world turned upside down through a crisis, he/she is encouraged to return as much as possible to a daily routine that helps them feel safe and reassured in the world. When we are treated normally by others, we tend to behave more normally, and this leads to others treating us normally, and so on. This cycle of normalcy helps calm the client in a holistic manner (mentally, physically, emotionally, spiritually), inviting the client to survive a crisis that seems insurmountable and overwhelming and return to a more balanced state of coping with life—inviting spring to return.

A brief review of the information leading us to this chapter on special populations in crisis work is necessary. Chapter 1 described the client's subjective reaction to the crisis in terms of perceiving him/herself as unable to cope due to the event, perception, and coping abilities. The counselor's role in the crisis is to assess, stabilize, and develop a plan that includes resources. Specific counselor characteristics (life experiences, poise, creativity and flexibility, energy and resilience, and quick mental reflexes) are discussed in this chapter. The client's reactions, the counselor's role, and the specific characteristics of the counselor all play important, interactive parts in the process of inviting spring back into the client's life.

Chapter 2 built on this base by encouraging the reader to examine his/her theoretical orientation so that it is focused, efficient, and humane and is on "automatic pilot," which it needs to be in a crisis situation. An examination of theory, domain, and interventions in terms of expanded crisis theoretical models (psychoanalytic, systems, ecosystems, adaptational, interpersonal, chaos, developmental) and applied crisis models (developmental, situational, existential, ecosystemic), as well as some specific techniques (psychological first aid, multimodal therapy), are provided. The theoretical orientation allows the counselor to operate more effectively in the crisis, because it guides the counselor toward what is most important to focus on with the client and also provides the counselor with a secure home base on which to stand when addressing the crisis.

Chapter 3 provided information on developmental and situational disasters, where once again specific counselor characteristics, such as rapport and flexibility, are important. Also, the counselor was encouraged to know him/herself, practice core counseling skills (genuineness, empathy, respect), provide assistance, remain calm, assess quickly, and help the client understand what is normal, as well as to educate and provide assistance to the client.

Chapter 4 addressed common counseling contexts and issues in crisis counseling. These first four chapters provided the baseline upon which this chapter is built. The overall view of crisis, theoretical orientation, counselor characteristics, and specific contexts of crisis counseling will assist the reader in working with special populations. The special populations have been chosen because these areas are not affiliated with any specific theoretical orientation or grouping of clients. Rather, it is the context in which the counselor is treating the client. The crisis emerges within the boundaries of the special population context, which influences the crisis interventions. The exercises and case study focus on the special populations to assist the reader in learning the unique aspects of each of the contexts and the contrasts between them.

The special populations of individual, group, couples/family, and community could each be the topic of a textbook in their own right. Rather than overwhelm the reader with the wealth of information available on treatment in these contexts, the information provided will be an overview of basic principles and orientation in general and then specifically as they apply in a crisis counseling situation. Resources mentioned at the end of the chapter are provided to assist in managing the wealth of available information. The goal in this chapter is to leave the reader with the "flavor" of each of these special populations, which might encourage the reader to further explore crisis counseling work within these contexts.

INDIVIDUAL

Overview

Information about individual interventions is presented, as they also apply to special populations. Individual counseling in general needs to be a safe place where the client can sort out sensitive, personal problems (Johnson, 2004). The counselor needs to be an anchor for the client while assisting the client in personalizing information about the changes that need to be made. How does a counselor accomplish such a task, especially in a crisis situation where this invitation to trust and collaborate needs to be done in a quick, almost automatic manner by the counselor?

As stated previously in this chapter, the counselor needs to be genuine, direct, and honest with the client. In addition, the counselor needs to be firm, supportive, calm, and clear in communication, while providing an honest encounter and honest feedback to the client. The counselor needs to slow down the client's reaction to the crisis to better facilitate the client's ability to hear the information being given and to allow the client to make the most empowering choice possible out of their collaborative interactions.

In the relationship with the client, the counselor is, overall, trying to help the client through the crisis period by providing support (Roberts, 2005). Also, because a crisis is an isolating experience where one feels very alone, the counselor is trying to draw the client back into the human community beginning with individual counseling. The individual counseling relationship is one in which the client can begin to trust again and feel less isolated and alone; the client can build on this relationship in the recovery process from the crisis.

Different authors provide suggestions on specific techniques that can be helpful to individual clients in crisis situations. Some of these are as follows:

- Chemical dependency: inpatient/outpatient treatment (James, 2008)
- Posttraumatic stress disorder (PTSD): multimodal therapy emphasizing behavioral and cognitive-behavioral therapy (James, 2008)

- Burnout: BASIC ID (Lazarus, 1976 as cited in James, 2008)
- Childhood trauma: trauma-focused cognitive-behavioral treatment (Cohen, Berliner, & Mannarino, 2010)
- Traumatized children: expressive arts (Malchiodi, 2008).

Techniques to facilitate the crisis counseling relationship are discussed throughout this book. The specific approaches of motivational interviewing (MI) and the stages of change model that will be discussed in Chapter 7 are briefly reviewed here because of the excellent fit to and readiness for use in an individual crisis counseling situation. They are discussed in this section on individual counseling because the individual client is a part of each population context (group, couples/family, community).

MI (W. R. Miller & Rollnick, 2002) encourages an empowering approach that stems from its collaborative nature. In this approach, the counselor provides empathy, points out discrepancies, avoids arguments, rolls with the client's resistance, and supports the client's self-efficacy (perception of ability to persist) in developing the counseling relationship and facilitating the willingness to make a change(s). Regarding burnout, the client may make change by deciding to take direct action (dealing with the environmental stress through group therapy) or palliative action (reducing cognitive and emotional disturbances through exercise) (James, 2008). Using the MI approach can help the client more readily trust the counselor and then be open to making changes necessary due to the crisis situation.

The stages of change model can help the counselor assess the level of the client's readiness to change and thereby assist in determining the most effective treatment approach. The stages are *precontemplation, contemplation, preparation, action, maintenance*, and *termination* (Prochaska, DiClemente, & Norcross, 1992). The stages refer to exactly what they sound like they are describing. Respectively, the client: has not thought about change, is thinking about making a change, is preparing to make a change, is taking action to change, is maintaining the change, and has integrated the change deeply into their lives.

In general, clients come to counseling with various levels of motivation to change. In crisis counseling, clients often present themselves as very willing to receive assistance because of the level of psychic pain they are experiencing—they want to experience relief. Yet, once presented with options for reducing the pain, the client may naturally resist because the treatment sounds as bad as or worse than the current crisis situation. Metaphorically, we can compare it to going to a physician's office because we do not feel well and wanting to feel better—wanting to do anything to get out of the discomfort. Yet once the doctor brings up options for how we can feel better, we may lose our motivation to change. For example, the doctor may suggest that we will feel better if we make changes in our diet; if we let go of our comfort foods, we would lose weight. The resistance we might feel toward this may be the same experience the crisis client might have.

Counselors need to remember, then, that the presenting motivation and actual motivation to change may be quite different for the crisis client. Even when clients may present themselves as ready to change, clients are in actuality most likely to be at the *precontemplation, contemplation*, or *preparation* stages with regard to actually making the change. Because the crisis is recent, the exact change level may not be apparent until the counselor begins to make recommendations of resources or options for change.

This situation is why the combination of MI and the stages of change model can be so helpful in a crisis situation. The counselor can use MI strategies to assist in the development of rapport, and then, while assessing the client and making recommendations of options, the counselor can determine the *actual* level of readiness for change. The counselor can do a "dance" between them by using client resistance as a marker to go back and build up rapport and then resume realistic work at the client's actual stage of change. Interventions that are carefully arranged can both help clients survive the stress and develop coping skills (Dattilio & Freeman, 2007). Note that specific processes to assist the client in moving from one stage to another are presented in Chapter 7.

Regarding counseling perspectives, counselors need to avoid becoming caught in the biomedical model perspective, in which the focus is on the individual as the source of the problem. Instead, take a more public health perspective, in which social, cultural, and environmental factors are considered as contributing or mitigating in the crisis situation (Hoff, Hallisey, & Hoff, 2009). This is why the other special populations are examined for the remainder of this chapter: they (group, couples/family) can be resources for therapy and emotional growth (Dziegielewski & Sumner, 2005).

Top 10 Practical Suggestions

1. Provide a safe, confidential space to process the crisis.
2. Assist the client in personalizing information about the crisis.
3. Be genuine, honest, direct, and firm in clear communications with the client.
4. Collaborate with the client to enhance choice (empowerment).
5. Be an anchor of support.
6. Draw the client out of isolation and into the human community by establishing a therapeutic relationship that can be generalized to other relationships.
7. Determine with the client direct actions and palliative actions that can be taken.
8. Determine how much the client is willing to change.
9. Examine social, cultural, and environmental factors that can be impacting the crisis.
10. Determine resources (supports, strategies) needed for therapy and emotional growth (group, couples/family, community).

EXERCISE 5.1 INDIVIDUAL

Either in writing or in dialogue with another (fellow student, colleague, supervisor, mentor), react to the following questions:

1. Which suggestions are you already committed to use in your counseling work?
2. How do you incorporate or plan to incorporate these suggestions into your work?
3. Which suggestions are new ones or ones you want to enhance in your practice?
4. What is your plan for incorporating these new suggestions into your practice?
5. How do these suggestions shift for you when you compare how you apply or plan to apply them in your general counseling and then when you think of applying them to crisis counseling?
6. Choose the top three suggestions you believe are most important for you in crisis counseling work in this population context.

GROUP

Overview

Group counseling began after World War II because of the ratio of clients who needed counseling to the number of counselors available; in order to provide help to those who needed it, group counseling was used (Hoff et al., 2009). Group therapy is a re-creation of one's family of origin (Yalom, 1985). This means that in group settings, clients will naturally project onto the group their experiences in the families in which they grew up. It is also a microcosm of the real world (Yalom, 1985). In a group it is very difficult to maintain a "front" that will not be seen through by at least one group member; we cannot help but be in a group as we are in the real world. We get caught "being ourselves" in groups. Finally, groups can help clients with a sense of isolation, because they are focused on forming and maintaining relationships. It is important for the counselor to remember, then, that groups, which by their very nature reflect family, the real world, and a sense of community, can be both powerfully healing and powerfully destructive. They can encourage people to rebuild themselves or destroy themselves.

Crisis can appear in at least two basic forms in terms of group counseling. First, the crisis may occur as a part of the group counseling process. Clients may be coming to group counseling for help and may experience a crisis as a part of the group or have a personal crisis outside the group that they bring in as a group issue. Second, a group counseling framework may be formed around a specific crisis. There are numerous examples of these types of groups (e.g., disaster-related, specific issues such as trauma, etc.). One such example is group counseling with children in response to 9/11 (Haen, 2005). This section will focus on both types of groups.

Crisis Within a Group Counseling Context

Prior to discussing how to handle these types of group crises, some general comments on group work need to be made. First, counselors need specific training on group counseling that assists them in looking at the pragmatics of group (type of group they want to create, size of the group, group norms) as well as the developmental structure of the group in terms of group stages (issues, leadership functions, etc.). Some overall suggestions for group work are made:

- If possible, have at least a 15- to 20-minute interview with a client to determine whether they are appropriate, hear the client needs, educate about the group's purpose and norms, and meet the leader (counselor) of the group.
- Encourage the client during the interview to "do it differently"—to practice different behaviors in the group than they normally practice in life (e.g., if the client is quiet, he/she should talk more).
- If an interview is not possible, make some type of individual connection with the new group member prior to the group or right away during their first group (e.g., shake hands).
- Practice the integration of the healing aspects of group, such as installation of hope and universality (common existential factors for all humans) (Yalom, 1985).
- Encourage honesty and respect among members in order to create a healing atmosphere in group.
- Work with emotional reactivity and poor impulse control that may act as destructive influences on the group.

When developing a group, decide on a general framework (alone or with a co-leader) on how to handle crises that occur in group. These may be crises that occur as a part of the group sessions or crises that occur outside the sessions that members need to process as a part of the group. Planning ahead on how to generally handle such crises can be of long-term benefit to the leader and to the group members by protecting the members' trust in the group process and keeping a strong sense of community in the group. Two areas of prime concern are: (1) group members feeling punished/ostracized and (2) secret-keeping. There are times that a member may evidence behavior that indicates they are a poor match for the group (motivation to change, problem intensity, etc.). In this case, the group member may need to leave the group for the overall benefit of the group. Such a decision should not be made lightly and needs, ideally, to be made in consultation with another professional (colleague, supervisor, mentor). With such a decision, the group leader needs to make sure that the action taken does not make the member feel punished/ostracized for his or her behavior and/or that the other members view it that way. In addition, while group members do not need to be told all the information about how the situation was handled (e.g., specific confrontation in an individual session about group behavior), there needs to be avoidance of any secrets because of the destructive, trust-eroding dynamics this can set up in a group.

Lastly, crises may happen in groups because of the developmental stage of the group. Corey (1995) presents four group stages: Initial Stage—Orientation and Exploration (Stage 1), Transition Stage—Dealing with Resistance (Stage 2), Working Stage—Cohesion and Productivity (Stage 3), and Final Stage—Consolidation and Termination (Stage 4). Each stage has different developmental tasks and leadership functions. An effective group leader needs to understand the dynamics of each stage and how to assist the group in meeting that stage's tasks in order to move on to the next stage. This is why specific training in group development is needed by the leader in order to ensure that the welfare of the group is met and that healing dynamics occur for all group members. An understanding of leadership functions required at these stages can reduce or contain crises that occur in the group process.

Specific Crisis Counseling Groups

These groups are focused on helping the client resolve the crisis through the process of group; clients focus on the crisis and are restricted as to how much individual history and feelings they express. These groups can help clients figure out the coping mechanisms they lack through group interaction; feel confident and in control; reduce the isolation they feel in the crisis; and be beneficial to as many clients as possible if there are a limited number of counselors available to assist in the crisis (Hoff et al., 2009). They help clients express feelings, understand the crisis, explore resources/solutions, and determine strategies that may reduce future risks. Specific suggestions regarding the establishment of these groups are to limit the number of sessions (some experts say six sessions, others recommend considering each individual's coping abilities and external resources in terms of number of sessions) and have clients attend one or two times a week for one and a half to two hours for a maximum of ten sessions (Hoff et al., 2009).

When working with these types of groups, especially those involving critical incident stress debriefing (CISD) (Mitchell & Everly, 1999) and critical incident stress management (CISM)—an integrated, multifaceted approach (Mitchell & Everly, 1999; Mitchell & Everly, 2001)—there are some additional cautions and suggestions (Everly, Lating, & Mitchell, 2005). First, group members might be exposed to traumatogenetic material they might not otherwise be exposed to, so the leader needs to make sure the groups are naturally formed or that the members have been exposed to similar levels of trauma. Second, the leader needs to give out empowering educational crisis-related information to prevent highly suggestible group members from developing crisis-related signs and symptoms they learn

---

Top 10 Practical Suggestions

General

1. Admit clients who need a decreased sense of isolation.
2. Admit clients who may benefit from a group viewing them as confident and in control.
3. Remember that groups can powerfully heal or hurt members.

Crisis within a Group Counseling Context

4. Develop a framework for handling crises in group.
5. Avoid action that punishes members or encourages secret-keeping.

Specific Crisis Counseling Groups

6. Focus on the crisis.
7. Form groups naturally or at similar levels of trauma experience.
8. Give information that empowers people.
9. Assess group members for fragility.
10. Avoid specific techniques (deep probing, interpretation, paradoxical intentions).

---

about educationally in the group. Third, cathartic ventilation might simply be too much for some members, so counselors need to assess for fragility in clients and avoid techniques that can stir up an overwhelming amount of emotion for clients (deep probing, interpretation, paradoxical intentions).

EXERCISE 5.2 GROUP

Either in writing or in dialogue with another fellow student, colleague, supervisor, mentor), react to the following questions:

1. Which suggestions are you already committed to use in your counseling work?
2. How do you incorporate or plan to incorporate these suggestions in your work?
3. Which suggestions are new ones or ones you want to enhance in your practice?
4. What is your plan for incorporating these new suggestions into your practice?

5. How do these suggestions shift for you when you compare how you apply or plan to apply them in your general counseling and then when you think of applying them to crisis counseling?

6. Choose the top three suggestions you believe are most important for you in crisis counseling work in this population context.

COUPLE/FAMILY

Overview

Couples/families can experience crises like individuals (Hoff et al., 2009). As in group counseling, a couple or family may come to counseling due to a crisis, or a crisis may evolve while they are in the process of counseling. The reader may want to note that individuals in crisis tend to receive help more quickly than groups or families (Roberts, 2005). This section will examine couple/family crises, beginning with a brief overview of the systemic perspective of couple/family counseling, and then will examine some specific factors related to couple and family work.

Individuals as a part of a couple or a family are in constant interaction with one another and, therefore, influence one another. The "couple" and the "family" systems develop a life-force of their own; they are more than the individuals that make them up because of the influencing interactions between them. The counselor working in this area, then, needs to be sensitive to the interactions between members and treat the interaction, rather than the individual members. Problems are viewed from the overall system and interactions within the system (Stanton & Heath, 1997). This is especially important as couples and families may present themselves in counseling through the behavior of the identified patient, the symptom-bearer of the family (Hoff et al., 2009). The client presented as the "problem" to the counselor in actuality lives in the couple's relationship, or in the family relationships—where individuals are mutually influencing one another and shaping the relationship in an ongoing fashion. The actual client is the couple/family relationship within the symptoms presented, maintaining the functioning of the couple/family.

In terms of the systemic perspective, each person lives in the context of the relationships in his/her life. From this perspective, the counselor is attempting to understand how each individual contributes to the crisis that has presented itself. The focus is on *how* the couple or the family functions, rather than on *why* there is a problem: *How* do the relationships within the system keep the problem alive? Therefore, counseling is an attempt to understand the subjective, interactional view of each of the individuals involved in the crisis situation, rather than to find an objective, causal reality of the problem. The behavior of the individual is examined within the context of the relationship(s), with an emphasis on the exploration of the patterns of behavior of both the individual and the couple/family as they impact the crisis (Winek, 2009).

Regarding how couples in crisis come into therapy, often there are events that have overwhelmed one or both of the individuals in terms of their abilities to cope (Halford, 2001). Many times, they are major events such as death, financial problems, life-threatening illness, extreme conflict (intimate partner violence), or an affair. There are other concerns that may present themselves, such as problems with communication, conflict, intimacy, etc. Couples who come in with crises often have poor relationship skills or extreme defensive posturing that prevents intimacy (Snyder & Mitchell, 2008).

An assessment in counseling needs to be done to determine whether the partners still have positive feelings for each other; then, focus on what immediately needs to be done; delay long-term decisions until the impact of the crisis is under more control; resolve the immediate crisis; and then decide if ongoing couple's therapy is needed (Halford, 2001). A problem-solving approach with an emphasis on quick cognitive-behavioral strategies that assist with the restructuring of the couple's thoughts and perceptions is needed to prevent further deterioration of the couple's functioning (Dattilio & van Hout, 2006; Schlesinger & Epstein, 2007). Williams, Edwards, Patterson, and Chamow (2011) present the "Eight Cs for Couple Functioning and Assessment: Communication, Conflict resolution, Commitment, Contract, Caring and cohesion, Character, Culture, and Children" as a framework for couples' assessment.

Regarding family, families can be a source of support or a source of extreme distress (Hoff et al., 2009). Stress experienced by a family depends on the resources both within and outside the family, as well as how the family defines the traumatic event. Some families have multiple problems that are quite complex, interactive, and caused by different factors (Lawrence & Sovik-Johnston, 2010). Family crises are "short term, overwhelming, and understandably stressful" (Patterson, Williams, Grauf-Grounds, & Chamow, 2009, p. 117). They can be unexpected external events or developmental or maturational events. Whatever type of crisis it is, there is at its core a disruption in the functioning of the family.

The high-functioning family looks at a problem as resulting from different factors and tends to respond to the situation in a pragmatic manner, while poorly functioning families tend to focus on one explanation of the problem, lock into a single cause of the problem, and blame and scapegoat someone for the problem (Walsh, 2006). Counselors need to assess: (a) how the family defines and frames the problem and (b) who the family blames for the problem. The counselor then needs to use techniques that help the family reflect on the cause of the problem. Counselors need to be aware of family system dynamics, dysfunctional patterns within a family, and power and communication problems within a family (NIDA, 2003). Some presentations of various family crises and how to treat them as presented are available on alcoholism (James, 2008) and separation/divorce (Granvold, 2005; James, 2008). Crisis interventions that are unique from the systemic view include (Patterson et al., 2009):

- Altering the hierarchy
- Boundary-making

- Enactment (have the family reenact the event)
- Exploring exceptions to presenting problems
- Externalizing problems (i.e., give the problem a name and work on the relationship between the client and the name)
- Genogram development (look for family themes and patterns)
- Identifying and interrupting negative interactional patterns
- Identifying family strengths
- Inviting absent family members to sessions
- Timeline development (look at family problems in a context)

EXERCISE 5.3 COUPLE

Either in writing or in dialogue with another (fellow student, colleague, supervisor, mentor), react to the following questions:

1. Which suggestions are you already committed to using in your counseling work?
2. How do you incorporate or plan to incorporate these suggestions in your work?

Top 10 Practical Suggestions

General

1. Remember the client is the couple or the family, not an individual member (the identified patient).
2. Examine how the system is keeping the problem alive in terms of interactions.

Couples

3. Focus on what needs to be done immediately.
4. Delay long-term decisions until the crisis is under control.
5. Have a problem-solving approach.

Family

6. Assess how the family defines and frames the problem(s) and who is viewed as to blame for it.
7. Be aware of the family system dynamics.
8. Examine dysfunctional patterns in the family.
9. Look at power and communication problems in the family.
10. Use systemic crisis interventions.

---

3. Which suggestions are new ones or ones you want to enhance in your practice?
4. What is your plan for incorporating these new suggestions in your practice?
5. How do these suggestions shift for you when you compare how you apply or plan to apply them in your general counseling and then when you think of applying them to crisis counseling?
6. Choose the top three suggestions you believe are most important for you in crisis counseling work in this population context.

Exercise 5.4 Family

Either in writing or in dialogue with another (fellow student, colleague, supervisor, mentor), react to the same questions in Exercise 5.3.

Ethical/Legal

Overview

These two areas are combined here because of the overlap that can occur between them in areas such as confidentiality, documentation, and consultation. While these three areas can involve extensive overlap, other areas of counseling may or may not have much crossover. They are combined in this section to remind the reader that there may be crossover. However, ethical and legal concerns are dealt with separately in this section because of the variation that can occur in a crisis counseling context due to the counselor's role, client population, and the like. The reader may want to refer to additional readings in the ethical and legal areas related to telephone and Internet counseling and school crises (James, 2008), and intimate partner violence and stalking, as well as working with adolescents in suicide and psychiatric emergencies (Roberts, 2005).

To facilitate the reader's application of this information, this section will not have an exercise or a box of ten practical suggestions, but will be included as a part of the case study that comes at the end of this section. While reading the following section, counselors need to remember that they may be sued or have professional board ethic complaints against them for the work they do professionally. It is probably best to protect oneself from this reality by only practicing common practices of counseling in one's area of competence, consulting with other professionals when necessary (and documenting that consultation), and having good malpractice insurance for both legal action and board complaints. Having an attorney as a legal consultant is also recommended.

Each of these areas, ethical/legal, needs to be defined prior to a discussion of the issues that can emerge in crisis counseling. *Ethical principles* of one's professional orientation act as a rudder guiding counselor behavior, and *laws* as the formal version of a culture's moral decisions. *Moral decisions* are "the concrete decisions counselors make in a situation based on the values (beliefs, attitudes, and behaviors) that have important personal meaning to them." (Miller, 2010, p. 359). We need to remember that no counselor is morally free, and one's morals can influence counseling.

Ethical

Counselors need to have a heightened sensitivity for ethics because of the vulnerability of clients in the unstable, off-balance state in which they come to counseling. Their intense negative emotionality, especially fear, can cause them to grasp intensely at what appears to be a solution to their problems or a comfort to reassure them; as human beings, we are very vulnerable, highly suggestible, and not at our best in terms of our thoughts, feelings, and behaviors when we are afraid. This is why it is important for counselors to be self-aware and work with their countertransference issues in order to avoid taking advantage of clients and to act at all times in their clients' best interest (Kanel, 2007).

Ethics can parallel the law because they guide our professional conduct principles. One area of ethical concern is *dual relationships*. Dual relationships are defined here as more than the counseling relationship: an additional relationship that may be personal or professional (Moleski & Kiselica, 2005). Ideally, the crisis counselor needs to not have another relationship with the client in crisis except for the relationship related to the crisis (Kanel, 2007). However, as with informed consent, this may shift depending on the context of the crisis counseling. For example, the same private practice counselor may be able to have only the counseling relationship with the client, but if that counselor practices in a rural setting, the counselor may have no choice but to have some type of dual relationship—for example, if the client is the only one who performs a specific type of surgery that the counselor needs. Also, the counselor may inherently have a dual relationship with the client in responding as a mental health worker in a local or state disaster. These relationships inherently occur when one practices as a counselor in a rural community or in a "small-town clientele context in a larger community" (e.g., being a gay therapist with GLBT clients) (Coombs, 2005, as cited in Miller, 2010, p. 363). Possibly the best approach for the crisis counselor is to follow the guidelines of one's professional organization regarding dual relationships, and to follow the motto of "The fewer the roles, the better."

Another major area of concern for crisis counselors is the area of *confidentiality*. There is a distinction that needs to be made here between confidentiality and disclosure:

Confidentiality means that the information obtained in a counseling session is not shared with others unless written permission has been given by the client. *Privileged communication* is legal protection for the benefit of the client in working with certain professionals under state law, which prohibits information being given without the client's consent. Therefore, while a counselor has a professional, ethical commitment to confidentiality, this commitment may or may not be held up under privileged communication laws in the state where the counselor works (Miller, 2010, p. 360).

Certain special populations of counseling bring up confidentiality issues in unique ways. In group counseling, for example, the counselor needs to inform group members that he/she will keep information confidential and can encourage that within the group by having people sign forms or make a verbal commitment to confidentiality, but the counselor is not able to enforce such a commitment. Confidentiality in a family counseling context is complex in a similar way, in that counselors may need to talk with clients about what they discuss with others outside the family session (Winek, 2009). Counselors need to be clear with their clients from the beginning in written guidelines as to the limits of confidentiality, since counselors may vary in terms of how they structure counseling (e.g., individual sessions alongside family sessions), their philosophy of family counseling (no secrets), and practices regarding providing the family with a fair warning (Patterson et al., 2009). This same importance exists for stating the limits of confidentiality with couples (Halford, 2001).

Confidentiality of counseling brings up an exception to privilege in terms of _informed consent_. There are three aspects to informed consent: (a) knowing that clients • can make rational decisions and, if not, making sure a parent or guardian can give consent; (b) providing clear information about the risks and benefits of counseling; and (c) making sure clients have freely consented to treatment (Kanel, 2007). As a part of informed consent, exceptions to confidentiality need to be outlined clearly. One of these exceptions involves the need and extent of a disclosure regarding issues such as videotaping, supervision, consultation with others, and the like. Counselors need to check their professional organizations for ethical guidelines regarding informed consent. Some examples of thoughtful professional discussions on ethical issues related to crisis counseling are discussed by American Psychological Association (Campbell, Vasquez, Behnke, & Kinscherff, 2010) and American Counseling Association (Sommers-Flanagan & Sommers-Flanagan, 2008). Counselors also need to consider how aspects such as setting may shape the need for and type of informed consent. For example, an informed consent for counseling may be required for a private practice counselor, but not for a disaster mental health worker.

Two other exceptions to privilege, _duty to report_ and _duty to warn_, are critical for the counselor to take into account. Keep in mind that there may be variations in these duties from state to state so the counselor needs to know the requirements of the state in which he/she practices (Haley, 2008). If there is a conflict between state and federal guidelines, the federal guidelines take precedent (Myers & Salt, 2007). "_Duty to report_ means that the counselor has an ethical obligation to break confidentiality by contacting authorities when the client or a third person can be harmed" • (Miller, 2010, p. 360). Counselors need to report suspected child abuse and adult abuse to authorities. A report of child abuse is a crisis for both parent and child; remember that the parent might be overlooked in this process. An outline of crisis intervention work with the parents when making such a report is in Hoff and others' book, Chapter 11, "The Crisis of Victimization by Violence." The counselor needs to view such a report as a possible turning point for the parent, who may experience a lot of guilt and fear in relation to the report. The use of *compassionate accountability* can be applied to these parents: Parents are held accountable for their behavior (given consequences) within an atmosphere of compassion for their suffering (they have made grievous errors out of their pain and fear).

"*Duty to warn* means that the counselor needs to determine whether the client is seriously dangerous and, in some states, that the potential victim can be identified" (Miller, 2010, p. 260). In this situation, the counselor may want to consult with another professional, a legal representative, make a referral(s), contact the police, and contact the victim (B. S. Anderson, 1996). In addition to consulting professionals about how to handle this situation and keeping notes on the consultation, crisis counselors should develop a plan for handling violent crisis situations ahead of time by consulting with experts on violence (James, 2008). Regarding specific issues, such as HIV/AIDS, crisis counselors need to stay current on professional and legal guidelines in dealing with these situations.

Case Study 5.1 Individual, Group, Couple/Family

The following case study is the most involved one in this book and asks the reader to explore a number of aspects that include special populations and related factors. The reader is encouraged to not be overwhelmed by the case study, but to explore those aspects that seem appropriate and then process this exploration through writing or dialogue. The complications in this case study are meant to encourage the reader to look at the same crisis situation from different angles and to be aware of any shifts within him- or herself when viewing the same situation from a different perspective.

Your client is a 56-year-old male who has talked with you over the phone prior to your session in order to set up an appointment with you. On the phone, he struck you as suspicious and seemed to be interviewing you with cautiousness, thoroughness, and a sense of mistrust. These were the underlying emotional themes you picked up in the 5-minute conversation. He also described his situation as urgent in terms of a relationship ending that means a lot to him. You respond to his urgency by scheduling him for an appointment later in the day, since one of your appointments had canceled and he could come in at that time. Now do the following either in writing or in dialogue with another (fellow student, colleague, supervisor, mentor): First, develop an overall, tentative plan for your session based on what you picked up over the phone in combination with both your personal and professional approach to counseling. Second, review this plan from different angles by taking into account the contexts and information you obtain in the session that could reshape the plan. Third, apply any of the 10 practical

---

---

suggestions for the different areas that seem appropriate for this plan as you review it from different angles.

Special Populations

Individual

Your client has definite problems trusting others and is quite defensive, as evidenced in the counseling session. You also found out that he has a history of posttraumatic stress disorder (PTSD) that has been basically untreated, and you believe this history is being stirred up by his potential relationship breakup and is enhancing his sense of mistrust and defensiveness, which is reaching almost a paranoid level.

Group

You have your client join the group you have that evening, based on your brief intake for the group you did earlier in the day. Your client seems appropriate for the group, which is focused on the loss of relationships. In the mixed-gender group he begins to cry almost uncontrollably as other members discuss their losses in relationships. He is having difficulty sharing words with the group because of his mistrust of others and his history of PTSD, which he briefly discloses to the group.

Couples/Family

Your client unexpectedly brings his partner to your intake session. They discuss how their breakup appears to be necessary and imminent. You have never interacted with your client's partner until this moment. While they both appear to be sad and angry about the breakup, your client is almost hysterical when discussing it and your client's partner is the more verbal of the two. During the discussion, your client shares a small piece of information about his history of PTSD, and you believe that that history is impacting his difficulty sharing and trusting in the session and is also affecting the impact of the relationship ending. You also become aware that though the couple has been together a few years, your client's partner's family of origin has never liked your client and they have been indirectly unkind and mean-spirited toward your client in hopes the relationship would break up.

Related Factors

Finally, with regard to this case study, ask yourself the following questions in response to these different special populations:

1. Are there any legal or ethical issues involved? For example, are there confidentiality issues of concern when shifting the intake to a couples/family context when you believed it was going to be individual? Do you need to assess for suicidal/homicidal tendencies?

2. How would you address any of these ethical/legal issues?

3. How would any of the factors discussed in Chapter 8 (age, gender, sexual orientation, ethnicity), as relating to your clients, possibly impact your approach in this crisis?

4. How would any of the factors discussed in Chapter 8 (age, gender, sexual orientation, ethnicity), *as they apply to you*, possibly impact your approach in this crisis? Particularly focus on those factors that are differences between you and your client(s) and those that are strong personal and/or professional values for you.

SUMMARY

This chapter provided an overview of individual, group, couple/family, and community counseling, with practical suggestions associated with each. Additionally, an overview of legal and ethical issues was discussed. Reader application was facilitated through the use of exercises to accompany each of the population areas (individual, group, couple/family). Finally, a case study was given that examined a crisis counseling approach through these different client special populations and ethical/legal issues.

QUESTIONS

1. What are the five common special populations of crisis counseling work discussed in this chapter?

2. What are 10 practical suggestions that can be used with the different special populations of crisis counseling (individual, group, couple/family)?

3. What are some legal and ethical issues commonly involved in crisis counseling work?

SUGGESTED READINGS

General

Hoff, L. A., Hallisey, B. J., & Hoff, M. (2009). *People in crisis: Clinical and diversity perspectives* (6th ed.). New York, NY: Routledge.

This book is an overview of crisis work. It is divided into three sections: understanding crisis intervention; specific crises; and suicide, homicide, or catastrophic events.

James, R. K. (2008). *Crisis intervention strategies*. Belmont, CA: Thomson Brooks/ Cole.

This book provides an overview of crisis intervention. It has four sections: theory and application, handling specific crises, workplace, and disaster. There is a specific chapter related to addiction.

Kanel, K. (2007). *A guide to crisis intervention* (3rd ed.). Belmont, CA: Thomson Brooks/Cole.

This book has 11 chapters that cover general crisis information (definition, history, ethical/professional issues). It also has chapters on multicultural concerns, the ABC model, and addressing issues related to crisis, such as danger, developmental crises, loss, HIV/AIDS, substance abuse, PTSD/community disasters/trauma, and abuse (child, spousal, sexual assault).

Miller, G. A. (2010). *Learning the language of addiction counseling* (3rd ed.). Hoboken, NJ: Wiley.

This book provides a summary of addiction counseling. It has 14 chapters (introduction, theories, assessment of addiction, assessment of co-occurring disorders, treatment, treatment-related issues, relapse prevention, self-help groups, current and evolving therapies, culturally sensitive counseling, spirituality, chronic pain, personal and professional development, preparation of certification and licensure). The text has numerous case studies and exercises to facilitate application of the material.

Roberts, A. R. (Ed.) (2005). *Crisis intervention handbook* (3rd ed.). New York, NY: Oxford University Press.

This book has 32 chapters divided into six sections: Overview, Disaster Mental Health and Crisis Intervention and Trauma Treatment, Crisis Assessment and Intervention Models with Children and Youth, Crisis Intervention and Crisis Prevention with Victims of Violence, Crisis Assessment and Crisis Intervention in Health-Related and Mental Health-Related Crises, and Evidence-Based Practice and Research.

Group

Connors, G. J., Donovan, D. M., & DiClemente, C. C. (2001). *Substance abuse treatment and the stages of change.* New York, NY: Guilford Press.

This 274-page book has a section on group treatment that discusses "resolution-enhancing" exercises that can assist clients in addressing their ambivalence about their alcohol and drug use (good or less good things about use, decisional balance, looking back/looking forward, exploring goals, the "miracle question").

Corey, G. (2004). *Theory and practice of group counseling: Student manual* (6th ed.). Belmont, CA: Brooks/Cole.

This 217-page book has five chapters on general group concerns (leadership, ethics, stages), 10 chapters on specific theoretical approaches to group work (psychoanalytic, Adlerian, psychodrama, existential, person-centered, Gestalt, transactional analysis, behavioral, rational emotive behavior therapy, reality therapy), and two chapters comparing the different theories and looking at group from an integrated perspective. It has excellent sections in the general group concerns area on proposal development of a group and opening and closing comments for group sessions.

Corey, G., Corey, M. S., Callanan, P., & Russell, J. M. (2004). *Group techniques* (3rd ed.). Pacific Grove, CA: Brooks/Cole.

This 199-page book has two chapters on general and ethical issues related to techniques and five chapters of techniques, each specific to a group stage (forming, initial, transition, working, final).

Ingersoll, K. S., Wagner, C. C., & Gharib, S. (2002). *Motivational groups for community substance abuse programs*. Richmond, VA: Mid-Atlantic ATTC (804-828-9910). E-mail: mid-attc@mindspring.com

This work addresses the application of motivational interviewing (MI) to group therapy with substance abusers.

Kelin, R. H., & Schermer, V. L. (Eds.) (2000). *Group psychotherapy for psychological trauma*. New York, NY: Guilford.

This book focuses specifically on trauma in terms of group work.

Malekoff, A. (2004). *Group work with adolescents: Principles and practice* (2nd ed.). New York, NY: Guilford.

This book has 17 chapters on group work with the adolescent population. Chapter 9 has an appendix that provides information on group manuals specifically designed for this age-group.

Metcalf, L. (1998). *Solution focused group therapy*. New York, NY: Free Press.

This book addresses the application of solution-focused therapy to a group setting. It has an excellent admission interview form and forms for notes for the client and therapist to complete after each session to monitor clinical work from a solution-focused perspective.

Rogers, C. (1970). *Carl Rogers on encounter groups*. New York, NY: Perennial.

This book provides an overview on encounter groups.

Velasquez, M. M., Maurer, G. G., Crouch, V., & DiClemente, C. C. (2001). *Group treatment for substance abuse: A stages-of-change therapy manual*. New York, NY: Guilford.

This 222-page book has three sections: The first section provides an overview of the stages of change model, and the next two sections cover the five stages, providing thorough outlines for each session.

White, J. R., & Freeman, A. S. (2000). *Cognitive-behavioral group therapy for specific problems and populations*. Washington, DC: American Psychological Association.

This book provides a cognitive-behavioral focus.

Yalom, I. D. (1985). *The theory and practice of group psychotherapy* (4th ed.). New York, NY: Basic Books.

This book provides an in-depth look at group counseling.

Couples/Family

Williams, L., Edwards, T.M., Patterson, J., & Chamow, L. (2011). *Essential assessment skills for couple and family therapists*. New York, NY: Guilford.

This book has 13 chapters that address assessment, interviews, and treatment with regard to children, adolescents, adults, couples, and families.

Patterson, J., Williams, L., Grauf-Grounds, C., & Chamow, L. (2009). *Essential skills in family therapy* (2nd ed.). New York, NY: Guilford.

This book has 11 chapters that describe the interview, assessment, treatment, and termination process with families. It has separate chapters on working with families with children, couples, and a family with a mentally ill member.

Winek, J. (2009). *Systemic family therapy: From theory to practice.* Thousand Oaks, CA: Sage.

This book is divided into five sections: history and development, first-generation models, systemic models, postmodern models, and processes and outcomes. It provides an overview of family therapy with brief summaries on effectiveness research on adolescent substance abuse, and alcohol abuse.

Ethical/Legal

Anderson, B. S. (1996). *The counselor and the law* (4th ed.). Alexandria, VA: American Counseling Association.

This 149-page book has six chapters: the counseling profession, overview of law and ethics, the counseling relationship, protecting client confidence, avoiding liability, and managing your counseling practice. It also provides a section on suggested readings.

Brooks, M. K. (1997). Ethical and legal aspects of confidentiality. In J. H. Lowinson, P. Ruiz, & T. P. Remley (Eds.). *Substance abuse*: *A comprehensive textbook* (3rd ed.), pp. 884–899. Baltimore, MD: Williams & Wilkins.

This chapter provides an overview of confidentiality issues.

Remley, T. P. (1993). *The ACA Legal Series* (vols. 1–12). Alexandria, VA: American Counseling Association.

This series covers a number of legal issues counselors typically face. Particularly relevant to issues in this chapter are volumes 6 (*Confidentiality and Privileged Communication*) and 8 (*The Danger-to-Self-or-Others Exception to Confidentiality*).

MANUALS/WORKBOOKS

For Motivational Interviewing and Stages of Change resources, see Chapter 7.

VIDEOTAPES/DVDs

For Motivational Interviewing and Stages of Change resources, see Chapter 7.

Couples/Family

American Psychological Association (Producer) (2007). *Couples therapy for extra-marital affairs: Don-David Lusterman, Ph.D.* (APA Psychotherapy Videotape Series II). Available from www.apa.org/pubs/videos

WEB SITES

Professional Organizations

The reader is encouraged to check with the national professional organization with which he/she is affiliated in order to obtain current information, guidelines, and resources related to the practice of crisis counseling within specific special populations.

American Association for Marital and Family Therapy. www.aamft.org
American Counseling Association. www.counseling.org
American Psychiatric Association. www.psych.org
American Psychological Association. www.apa.org
National Association of Social Workers. www.naswdc.org

CHAPTER SIX

Assessment

LEARNING OBJECTIVES

1. To learn diagnoses common in crisis counseling work.
2. To develop a familiarity with assessment instruments related to some of these diagnoses that may be used in crisis counseling situations.
3. To practice applying these diagnoses and use of the instruments to case studies and exercises.

> To work in the world lovingly means that we are defining what we
> will be for, rather than reacting to what we are against.
>
> —*Christina Baldwin*

This chapter addresses diagnoses that are common to crisis counseling work. In addition to crises being different in type, as discussed in Chapter 2, they also occur in different settings, and counselors may operate under different titles and from different theoretical orientations. Diagnostic assessment in crisis situations, then, can vary among counselors substantially because of these influencing factors.

The reader may ask, "Why have a chapter on assessment in a crisis counseling book? A counselor does not need to assess different diagnoses in a crisis—a counselor simply needs to assess the crisis situation in the moment, stabilize the person, and move on." There may have been a time when that was the case—and counselors do still continue to work in settings and have roles that reflect that philosophy. In those contexts, assessment can be done in the moment of the crisis and can rely on the judgment of the counselor without the support of additional, instrument-based assessment. However, there are some exceptions to this, and there have been some shifts in the counseling field that merit a chapter on assessment.

First, there are clients who have so-called "patterns of crisis"—they go in and out of crises in their lives due to various mental health disorders. A counselor working with this type of client needs to consider doing an overall assessment within the context of the crisis in order to be truly helpful to the client.

Second, referral sources for crisis counseling have been changing. Some sources now ask for information about diagnoses (in addition to information about the crisis presented) as well as documented support of clinical information provided by the counselor. In such situations, the counselor and client are well served to have the additional information provided by a more extensive assessment, possibly supported by psychometric instrument data.

This chapter provides information on some brief assessment scales a clinician may use in the crisis context. A counselor may want to have such assessments available to make differential diagnoses that may assist the client in crisis in receiving the best services available. However, some settings prohibit the use of instruments (e.g., a natural disaster site). In such settings, the counselor may find it helpful to operate from a theoretical/philosophical orientation that can be useful in the assessment and intervention of a crisis within this context. Information derived from psychometric instruments or a theoretical/philosophical perspective that can be used in an interview may deepen or expand the information the counselor is already gathering in the crisis and thereby enhance the welfare of the client. The use of assessment instruments can facilitate the development of crisis treatment planning and long-term treatment goals.

While the crisis assessment is the primary focus of the assessment process done by the counselor, assessment of other issues is also pertinent at times because of these issues' potential to influence the crisis assessment and intervention. For example, a client who has returned from deployment and is struggling substantially with reintegration because of posttraumatic stress disorder (PTSD) issues that are causing marital and family problems may also be having difficulties with alcohol and drugs that are contributing to the crisis situation. The counselor, who is aware of the possible connection between coping with PTSD and alcohol/drug use, may decide to use a broad screening measure of alcohol and drug use to determine whether the substance use is an additional problem related to the crisis and whether it also needs to be addressed.

In this chapter, psychometric instruments or a philosophical perspective are centered on eight common diagnostic areas in crisis counseling: mental health/general trauma, addiction, co-occurring disorders, intimate partner violence, sexual abuse, eating disorders, suicide, and homicide. Within each topic, a brief overview is provided. The brief overview of each of the eight areas is followed by a summary of an instrument (or instruments) that can be used for assessment of the diagnosis, or a theoretical/philosophical approach that can be used in the assessment process. The instruments or theoretical/philosophical approaches presented here are broad in nature, because counselors may vary in specialization and therefore in their exposure to or training in each of the eight common diagnostic areas. Limitations regarding expertise in a particular area of specialty may lead the counselor to make a placement or referral to a specialist for further assessment.

The reader is also cautioned that: (a) the instruments summarized are not inclusive and at best provide an example or examples of a broad type of instrument that can be used in this area, and (b) instrument selection hinges both on the training and comfort level of the counselor using the instrument and the appropriateness of the use of the instrument, given specific crisis factors such as type, context, and location. In spite of these limitations, the types of instruments are included so that the reader has an example of at least one instrument or theoretical/philosophical orientation that might be helpful in the assessment of the specific diagnosis in the context of a crisis. It is important for the reader to note that few instruments have been chosen for review. The limited number chosen is due to the length of instruments available (which makes such a choice practically prohibitive), as well as the focus of the instrument for a specific population. Simply stated, I found few brief, general instruments that could be effectively and practically used in a crisis counseling situation.

This chapter begins with a general overview of assessment and assessment instrument guidelines that can be used by the reader in the selection of instruments. Once an instrument is selected by the counselor, the counselor may decide to incorporate the assessment instrument as a standard part of crisis assessment work and/or have copies of the instrument readily available to access in a crisis assessment situation that calls for additional assessment of the area. Ready access to the instrument may facilitate both the ease and quality of the assessment, and possibly, the placement and referral process.

Overview of Assessment

During psychological first aid, according to Slaikeu's model (1990) discussed in Chapter 1, the counselor makes the assessment of the crisis situation. Other authors (James, 2008) have stated that assessment needs to be done throughout the crisis intervention due to the fluidity of crisis counseling and the need for assessments to be done in a spontaneous, subjective, and interactive manner. From my perspective, such a view of assessment is needed for an overall perspective of the crisis. A crisis is complex in that it involves both dynamics within and outside of the individual. The assessment of the crisis situation is critical: It is a "launching pad" for the rest of the intervention in the crisis situation. As such, the crisis assessment needs to be tentative and flexible throughout crisis counseling, so that it allows a feedback loop of information that continually refines and recalibrates the assessment and interventions in the crisis situation.

An assessment of the BASIC (Behavioral, Affective, Somatic, Interpersonal, Cognitive) personality profile (Slaikeu, 1990) in a crisis counseling situation can guide the counselor in determining whether a specific aspect of one area needs to be examined more thoroughly and, if so, whether an instrument is needed to make such an assessment. For example, the client experiencing a crisis is incredibly emotional in his or her description of the crisis at hand. While the counselor knows that it is a crisis for the client and maintains a supportive, calm presence with the client, the counselor may "hear" components that indicate a possible PTSD. This clinical hunch may lead the counselor to ask more trauma-focused questions and may lead him/her to include an instrument to further clarify the presence of this disorder and its impact on the crisis.

The assessment area examined in this chapter is that of problem exploration according to Slaikeu's (1990) model: the factors leading up to the crisis, the client's strengths and weaknesses, and what occurred after the crisis. Specifically, the focus here is on the client's strengths and weaknesses, as shown by assessment instruments.

INSTRUMENT SELECTION GUIDELINES

In the selection of an instrument, some factors need to be considered. These factors include the instrument's use, the population for which it was developed, the groups used to determine the capacity of the instrument to evaluate the condition, the comparison norms, the administration options, the administration training needed, the computer scoring availability, and the cost (National Institute on Alcohol Abuse and Alcoholism, NIAAA; 1995). In a crisis counseling context, then, the counselor needs to consider these factors within the dynamics of the specific crisis counseling situation. For example, the selection and use of an instrument may be quite different for a counselor who is working with someone in crisis in a clinical office than for a counselor who is working at a disaster site. These differences may influence some or each of the factors listed above.

Also, the counselor wants to carefully choose a test based on its reliability and validity. As Miller (2010, p. 47) states:

> *Reliability* reflects the consistency of the instrument (the stability of the instrument) and *validity* reflects whether the test meets its intended purpose (it measures what it intends to measure). There are different types of reliability (test-retest, alternate form, internal consistency, Kuder-Richardson formula 20 coefficient, and Cronbach's coefficient alpha) and validity (content, construct, criterion-related, and predictive; Sattler, 1992). Typically, reliability coefficients of .80 or greater reflect adequate reliability (80% of the score is true and 20% is due to error). The validity of the instrument will address whether the instrument has been tested with the population to which the client belongs (e.g., is it a valid test to use with this client?). In addition, tests select targeted populations by establishing a cutoff score. A test with high sensitivity has few false negatives. A test with high specificity has few false positives.

Some other factors to take into account in test selection are as follows. First, remember that a test can be reliable without being valid. What this means is that a test can be consistent (reliable), but not be a valid measure of what is being measured. For example, if I hold up one finger and ask you repeatedly how many fingers I am holding up as a measure of your intelligence, you will continually answer "One." This test of holding up one finger is a reliable intelligence test, but it is not valid. It does not adequately measure the intelligence of the person responding on the test. Second, tests in a specific area may lack adequate reliability because an adequate instrument has not yet been developed. However, the counselor may choose to include such an instrument because it is the best that is available. The counselor using such an instrument needs to be aware of its limitations and must make sure its results are augmented by additional, reliable sources of information. Third, the counselor needs to select instruments from a consumer-wise stance. This means that even when using an instrument from a well-known and respected publisher of assessment instruments, the counselor needs to keep a critical examining eye on the instruments (according to the factors stated previously) rather than solely relying on the publisher.

MENTAL HEALTH/GENERAL TRAUMA

Overview

When doing a mental health assessment, particularly in a crisis situation, it is important to look at the baseline of the client's mental health functioning. One such baseline is the client's general mental status. The general mental status assessment reflects the client's "changes in orientation, intellectual functioning (language, memory, and calculation), thought content, judgment, mood, and behavior" (Patterson, Williams, Edwards, Chamow, & Grauf-Grounds, 2009, p. 60). The counselor should also assess factors such as the client's appearance, interactions, awareness of location and action, mood, language, attention, concentration, memory, delusions/hallucinations, judgment, and impulsiveness (Dilsaver, 1990).

The counselor is also encouraged to use the *DSM-IV-TR* to accurately assess mental health problems and use diagnostic criteria to determine whether another screening instrument needs to be used. Assessment publishers such as PAR™ (www.parinc.com), PsychCorp (Pearson) (www.psychcorp.com), and Western Psychological Services (WPS) (http://portal.wpspublish.com) can be consulted for screening instruments showing high reliability and validity—as discussed in the beginning of this chapter—that can be used in the assessment process. The reader is cautioned to select instruments that can be readily used in a crisis situation—for example, ones that are quick and efficient.

The main mental health concern addressed in this area is that of trauma, specifically PTSD. In the United States, 8 percent of adults show a lifetime prevalence of PTSD (*DSM-IV-TR*; American Psychiatric Association, 2000). PTSD can interfere with treatment (Mathias, 2003). PTSD has three types of symptoms: reliving the experience (nightmares, intrusive memories, etc.); attempting to avoid people, places, activities, and the like; and hypervigilance (Harvard Mental Health Letter, 2006). Trauma triggers can cause intense emotional reactions (Rothschild, 2000) that can lead to other problems, such as exacerbating the crisis situation or encouraging the development of another problem such as substance abuse. The very components of the crisis situation can even be a trigger for the trauma, thereby adding fuel to the fire of the crisis by enhancing the emotional reactivity of the client in response to the crisis. Because of the potential of PTSD to cause or increase the likelihood of the crisis situation, the counselor needs to be prepared to assess for the presence of PTSD in the client experiencing the crisis. Also, the counselor needs to make sure the client has a crisis plan if PTSD occurs outside of the crisis situation (Substance Abuse and Mental Health Services Administration [SAMHSA], 2000b).

Instruments

Short Portable Mental Status Questionnaire
This instrument has ten items and has an easy scoring process, with modifications for someone who has only a high school education.

Table 6.1   Short Portable Mental Status Questionnaire (SPMSQ)

1. What is the date today?
2. What day of the week is it?
3. What is the name of this place?
4. What is your telephone number (or address)?
5. How old are you?
6. When were you born?
7. Who is the [P]resident of the United States now?
8. Who was the president just before that?
9. What was your mother's maiden name?
10. Subtract 3 from 20 and keep subtracting 3 from each new number you get, all the way down.

For clients with high school education:
0-2 errors = intact mental function
3-4 errors = mild mental impairment
5-7 errors = moderate mental impairment
8-10 errors = severe mental impairment
Allow one more error if the client has only a grade school education. Allow one less error if the client has education beyond high school.

Adapted from Dilsaver (1990) and Pfeiffer (1975). Copyrights 1990 by the American Academy of Family Physicians and 1975 by the American Geriatrics Society/Wiley Periodicals, Inc. Adapted by permission.

Trauma Symptom Inventory (TSI)

This 100-item instrument assesses PTSD and other traumas. It has three validity scales (Response Level, Atypical Response, Inconsistent Response) that assist, respectively, in detecting those who deny common symptoms endorsed, an unusually high number of unlikely/bizarre responses, and inconsistent or random responses to similar content items. It has 10 clinical scales (Anxious Arousal, Depression, Anger/Irritability, Intrusive Experiences, Defensive Avoidance, Dissociation, Sexual Concerns, Dysfunctional Sexual Behavior, Impaired Self-Reference, Tension Reduction Behavior) that show internal consistency (Mean alpha coefficients of .86, .87, .84, .85 in sample populations—standardization, clinical, university, military, respectively) and reasonable validity in terms of convergent, predictive, and incremental. The test booklet can be reused because respondents complete an answer sheet separate from the booklet. It can be administered in an individual or group setting. It has a 4-point scoring scale ranging from 0 (never) to 3 (often). It is self-administered and can be read at the fifth-grade level. It takes approximately 20 minutes to complete and can be scored and profiled within 15 minutes. Information can be obtained at: http://www4.parinc.com.

Case Study 6.1 Mental Health/General Trauma

Your client, whom you have not seen before, has a disheveled appearance and answers your questions and comments in vague terms that seem only tangentially related to the topics you present in the first 10 minutes.

1. What indicators say it may be helpful to use a mental status exam before proceeding?
2. How would you integrate the exam into your session?
3. If appropriate, which aspects of the exam would you especially focus in on with your client?

EXERCISE 6.1 MENTAL HEALTH/GENERAL TRAUMA

Discuss with a colleague how your focus would shift in the session and why. Especially discuss how you would shift your priority in the assessment so that it does not negatively impact your client's trust in you.

ADDICTION

Overview

There are a high number of Americans who use alcohol and drugs: the 2008 National Survey on Drug Use and Health (Substance Abuse and Mental Health

Services Administration [SAMHSA]) reports that approximately 129 million Americans drink alcohol and 20.1 million used an illicit drug the month before their interview. Such high numbers indicate that counselors will frequently encounter clients who are using alcohol and drugs and, therefore, need to be prepared to assess whether use is a problem and, if it is, to what extent.

To elicit as much accurate information as possible in the interview assessment of the client's alcohol and drug use, the counselor needs to be especially nonjudgmental and empathic (Margolis & Zweben, 1998). This emphasis on openness is due to the tendency of alcoholics and drug addicts to use defense mechanisms such as denial when a counselor asks about usage (Griffin, 1991). The counselor assessing the alcohol and drug use is trying to obtain accurate information while also being aware that the client is not being honest about his/her use due to denial or self-protection.

Although it is beyond the scope of this book, the counselor is encouraged to examine his/her professional reactions to alcohol and drug use in individuals. The reader is encouraged to examine his/her own usage and, if necessary, obtain an assessment of his/her own usage by a licensed or certified alcohol/drug counselor. The reader is also encouraged to examine the impact of other individuals' alcohol and drug use on him/herself both personally and professionally. This examination may involve the counselor receiving therapy for personal "wounds" that have occurred as a result of personal and professional experiences dealing with alcoholics/drug addicts. Such careful, thorough examination, while difficult at times, can reduce the countertransference placed on the assessment of the client's alcohol and drug usage and can thereby enhance the welfare of the client.

Due to the frequency of the use of alcohol and drugs, as well as the tendency of those who have a substance abuse problem to deny the existence of a problem, the counselor may want to regularly incorporate a broad assessment instrument of alcohol and drug use into their crisis assessment process. Because of the frequency of the interaction between crisis situations and alcohol and drug use, a number of broad assessment instruments are included here.

Instruments

The following instruments can be used by a clinician to obtain a general overview of the client's alcohol/drug usage. Positive indicators of an alcohol/drug problem can be more extensively evaluated by applicable instruments. The following section is taken from Miller (2010) pp. 47–50.

Alcohol Use Disorders Identification Test

The Alcohol Use Disorders Identification Test (AUDIT; Saunders, Aasland, Babor, de la Fuente, & Grant, 1993) came out of a study in six nations. It came from the World Health Organization's interest in developing a tool that could be used in different cultural settings. It has ten questions: alcohol consumption (three questions), dependence symptoms (four questions), and alcohol-related problems (three questions). The questions can be answered as a part of an interview or responded to by paper and pencil. It takes about two minutes, and there is a Spanish version of the test. A score of 8 indicates at-risk drinking (see Table 6.2). It has test-retest reliability of . 86 and internal consistency of . 75 to . 94. It has shown construct, discriminant, and criteria-related validity.

Table 6.2 Alcohol Use Disorders Identification Test (AUDIT)

Please circle the answer that is correct for you.

1. How often do you have a drink containing alcohol?

| Never | Monthly or less | Two to four times a month | Two to three times a week | Four or more times a week |

2. How many drinks containing alcohol do you have on a typical day when you are drinking?

| 1 or 2 | 3 or 4 | 5 or 6 | 7 to 9 | 10 or more |

3. How often do you have six or more drinks on one occasion?

| Never | Less than monthly | Monthly | Weekly | Daily or almost daily |

4. How often during the last year have you found that you were not able to stop drinking once you had started?

| Never | Less than monthly | Monthly | Weekly | Daily or almost daily |

5. How often during the last year have you failed to do what was normally expected from you because of drinking?

| Never | Less than monthly | Monthly | Weekly | Daily or almost daily |

6. How often during the last year have you needed a first drink in the morning to get yourself going after a heavy drinking session?

| Never | Less than monthly | Monthly | Weekly | Daily or almost daily |

7. How often during the last year have you had a feeling of guilt or remorse after drinking?

| Never | Less than monthly | Monthly | Weekly | Daily or almost daily |

8. How often during the last year have you been unable to remember what happened the night before because you had been drinking?

| Never | Less than monthly | Monthly | Weekly | Daily or almost daily |

(continued)

Table 6.2 (Continued)

9. Have you or someone else been injured as a result of your drinking?

| No | Yes, but not in the last year | Yes, during the last year |

10. Has a relative or friend, or a doctor or other health worker been concerned about your drinking or suggested you cut down?

| No | Yes, but not in the last year | Yes, during the last year |

Note: Questions 1–8 are scored 0, 1, 2, 3, or 4 ("Never" to "Four or more times per week" respectively). Questions 9 and 10 are scored 0, 2, or 4 respectively.

Source: *Audit: Guidelines for Use in Primary Care*, second edition, by Babor and Higgins, 2002. Reprinted with permission. Copyright permission has been granted by Dr. Vladmir Poznyak (e-mail: poznyakv@who.ch), Department of Mental Health and Substance Dependence, World Health Organization, CH-1211 Geneva 27, Switzerland. Reprinted with permission of John Wiley & Sons, Inc.

CAGE

The CAGE (Ewing, 1984) has been used to determine whether a client has a problem with alcohol. It can be given verbally or in a paper-and-pencil format. It takes about one minute to administer. The first letter of each of the capitalized phrases spells out the acronym. The instrument can be used with individuals aged 16 or older, and appears to have internal consistency reliability and criterion validity (NIAAA, 1995). Fleming (2003) recommends that it be used with questions that explore the client's quantity and frequency of use, as well as binge drinking. A cutoff score of 2 is typically used. Internal consistency reliability is .89 (for a score of 2) with a sensitivity of 74 percent and specificity of 91 percent.

Michigan Alcohol Screening Test

The purpose of the Michigan Alcohol Screening Test (MAST; Selzer, 1971) is to detect the presence and extent of drinking in adults. This paper-and-pencil test is a convenient, efficient screening (not diagnostic) measure of drinking problems. It uses a yes/no format and has 25 items. It can be completed in approximately 10 minutes. The most popular scoring procedure assigns scores of 2 or 1 for each of the questions (0 if the response is nondrinking), except item number 7, which does not receive a score. Because item 7 ("Do you ever try to limit your drinking to certain times of the day or to certain places?") does not receive a score of 1 or 2, this item is sometimes eliminated in the test taking (Selzer, 1985).

To control for clients who appear to have alcohol problems when they actually do not, the counselor may need to gather more clinical information or modify the scoring system to make it more stringent. (The more conservative scoring system makes a score of 5 indicative of alcoholism.) The instrument appears valid; a number of studies show high agreement between MAST scores and previous alcohol-related problems. Studies report high internal consistency reliabilities of .83 to .95 and test-retest reliability over one to three days is .86 (Connors & Tarbox, 1985).

A shortened version of the MAST is called the SMAST (Short MAST; Selzer, Vinokur, & van Rooijen, 1975), shown in Table 6.3. Using stepwise multiple regression, 13 MAST items (1, 3, 5, 6, 8, 9, 11, 14, 16, 20, 21, 24, 25) were retained because they distinguished especially well between alcoholics and nonalcoholics, and one MAST item (24) was expanded to alcohol-related arrests. All items are scored one point if the answer indicates alcoholism. A total of three or more points

Table 6.3   The Short Michigan Alcoholism Screening Test (SMAST)

1. Do you feel you are a normal drinker? (By normal we mean you drink less than or as much as most other people.) (No)

2. Does your wife, husband, a parent, or other near relative ever worry or complain about your drinking? (Yes)

3. Do you ever feel guilty about your drinking? (Yes)

4. Do friends or relatives think you are a normal drinker? (No)

5. Are you able to stop drinking when you want to? (No)

6. Have you ever attended a meeting of Alcoholics Anonymous? (Yes)

7. Has drinking ever created problems between you and your wife, husband, a parent, or other near relative? (Yes)

8. Have you ever gotten into trouble at work because of drinking? (Yes)

9. Have you ever neglected your obligations, your family, or your work for two or more days in a row because you were drinking? (Yes)

10. Have you ever gone to anyone for help about your drinking? (Yes)

11. Have you ever been in a hospital because of drinking? (Yes)

12. Have you ever been arrested for drunken driving, driving while intoxicated, or driving under the influence of alcoholic beverages? (Yes)

13. Have you ever been arrested, even for a few hours, because of other drunken behavior? (Yes)

Note: Answers related to alcoholism are given in parentheses after each question. Three or more of these answers indicate probable alcoholism; two answers indicate the possibility of alcoholism; less than two answers indicate that alcoholism is not likely.

Reprinted with permission from *Journal of Studies on Alcohol*, vol. 36, pp. 117–126, 1975 (presently *Journal of Studies on Alcohol and Drugs*). Copyright by Alcohol Research Documentation, Inc., Rutgers Center of Alcohol Studies, Piscataway, NJ 08854.

means that alcoholism is probable, two or more points means it is possible, and less than two points means it is unlikely. With pregnant women, it has a risk drinking sensitivity of 11.4 percent and a specificity of 95.9 percent.

In addition, the Brief Michigan Alcoholism Screening Test (Brief MAST; Pokorny, Miller, & Kaplan, 1972) has 10 items. The Brief MAST has an overall sensitivity of 30 percent to 78 percent and a specificity of 80 percent to 99 percent.

Case Study 6.2 Addiction

Your client is talking with you about her crisis situation. You become aware of a strong smell of alcohol on her breath as she discusses her situation in a very intense, tearful manner.

1. How would you approach asking her about the smell of alcohol?
2. Would you use an assessment instrument to determine if she has an alcohol problem that needs to be further assessed? If so, which one?
3. What concerns would you have about bringing up a possible alcohol problem during the crisis counseling? What concerns would you have about not bringing up a possible alcohol problem during the crisis counseling? How might you walk the balance between the extremes of addressing it and not addressing it?

EXERCISE 6.2 ADDICTION

Jot down the concerns you have about bringing up a possible alcohol problem with your client. Now jot down the concerns you have in general about bringing up alcohol concerns with your clients. As you note these concerns, write in the margin personal and professional experiences you have had regarding confronting others on their alcohol/drug usage that may impact the concerns you have. Finally, process these concerns with someone whom you trust professionally (professor, colleague, supervisor, mentor, etc.) to address barriers you may have when bringing up such concerns with clients.

CO-OCCURRING DISORDERS

Overview

This section follows the general mental health and the addiction sections because it is common for another disorder to be present when alcohol and drugs are involved. SAMHSA (2007) estimates that 5 million Americans have a *co-occurring disorder* (COD). COD is common, complex (SAMHSA, 2002b), complicated, and reciprocal (DiClemente, 2003). A counselor who has a client in a crisis situation who displays general mental health problems or alcohol/drug use problems beyond the crisis situation would be well-advised to include a broad assessment instrument for mental health concerns.

The counselor also needs to keep in mind the possible interaction between the client's mental health and alcohol/drug use problems. The client in crisis might be using the alcohol/drugs to self-medicate the mental health problem; or the client might be receiving addictive drugs to treat the mental health problem. Because both mental health problems and substance abuse problems are caused by overlapping factors, such as brain deficits, genetic vulnerabilities, or stress/trauma exposure early in life (NIDA, 2008a), both conditions may be present in the client. Their co-existence means that the crisis counselor needs to be prepared to assess for both.

Instruments

At least minimally, the broad assessment instrument being encouraged for use here is the mental status exam discussed in the section on general mental health. As stated previously in the general mental health section, the counselor is encouraged to use the *DSM-IV-TR* to assess mental health problems, to use the diagnostic criteria to determine if another screening instrument is required, and to contact reputable assessment instrument publishers to locate additional screening instruments that show high reliability and validity and are both quick/efficient and applicable to a crisis counseling situation.

Case Study 6.3 Co-Occurring Disorders

Your client has a developmental crisis that is connected with his aging process. During your few sessions with him, he has told you that he is in addiction recovery and works a 12-step program that has helped him remain sober for 10 years. However, you begin to suspect that he has another diagnosis (PTSD) that has been untreated from his Vietnam experiences 40 years ago.

1. How would you integrate the assessment of his possible co-occurring disorder without overwhelming him as he deals with his current crisis?
2. Would you make the assessment shift obvious or subtle?
3. Would you use a specific instrument as a part of the assessment process?

EXERCISE 6.3 CO-OCCURRING DISORDERS

Write down the pros and cons for making the assessment shift obvious and then the pros and cons for making it subtle. Describe how this may impact your use of a specific assessment instrument and the impact on the therapeutic relationship.

INTIMATE PARTNER VIOLENCE

Overview

Intimate partner violence (IPV) is defined as verbal, psychological, or physical force used by a family member toward another family member (SAMHSA, 1997). The form of IPV discussed in this chapter is called patriarchal terrorism by some authors (Greene & Bogo, 2002). This is where violence is often more severe and is used to control the partner; the perpetrator is feared, and males are typically the perpetrators. Often, offenders are more likely to be using alcohol or drugs (Bureau of Justice, 2005); they may use the alcohol/drug use to excuse or justify their planned violence, or the alcohol/drug use may reduce their impulse control (Jacobson & Gottman, 1998). Battered women may have alcohol/drug use problems (Erbele, 1982) or may self-medicate through them (Gomberg & Nirenberg, 1991). Assessment of IPV needs to involve assessment of substance abuse problems in both perpetrators and survivors. It is necessary for the counselor to remember that while both problems may be present, the substance abuse does not cause the IPV. The overall safety of the survivor needs to be assessed in coordination with high accountability of behavior in the perpetrator.

Instruments

In the assessment of batterers, the counselor needs to: ask questions that are specific, concrete, and determine whether the person views the violence as justified; be direct/candid; learn typical excuses given for the violence; refuse to allow substance use to be blamed for the violence; and examine the relationship between substance use and violence (SAMHSA, 1997). The survivor needs to have a private interview in order to ensure safety, be asked about the violence concretely, and be told there is no excuse for the violence. The counselor needs to be aware of the possibility of child abuse also being present (SAMHSA, 1997). Generally, in the assessment process with perpetrators or survivors, the counselor needs to ask who has control over different aspects of the relationship and needs to remember that physical abuse is not the only expression of violence (survivors may not *look* battered).

The Duluth Intervention Project (Pence & Paymar, 1993) developed the commonly known Domestic Violence Wheel, which shows eight areas of IPV that can be used in an assessment of both perpetrators and survivors: isolation; minimizing, denial, and blame; using children; using male privilege; economic abuse; coercion and threats; intimidation; and emotional abuse. At the hub of the wheel is power and control. A helpful guide to assessing domestic violence, *A Guide for Conducting Domestic Violence Assessments* (Domestic Abuse Intervention Project, 2002), provides a domestic violence matrix and a risk assessment for women that focuses on the woman's safety.

Women's Experience with Battering (WEB) Scale

This instrument examines the experiences of battered women instead of specific abusive behaviors they experience in an attempt to unmask the nature of the battering in terms of its continuity and the relationship between the woman's experience and the events (the meaning she attaches to the violence). Focus groups were used to generate qualitative data that was then used to develop scale items and a survey to determine final scale items. Factor analysis of the original 40 items showed a strong single-factor solution, resulting in 10 items. It show high internal consistency reliability and good construct validity (DeVellis, Earp, & Smith, 1995). (See Table 6.4.)

Ontario Domestic Assault Risk Assessment (ODARA) [and] Domestic Violence Risk Appraisal Guide (DVRAG)

The 13-item Ontario Domestic Assault Risk Assessment (ODARA) scale was developed from 589 offenders (male-to-female violence) that were identified in

Table 6.4 Women's Experiences with Battering (WEB) Scale

1	2	3	4	5	6
Agree Strongly	Agree Somewhat	Agree A Little	Disagree A Little	Disagree Somewhat	Disagree Strongly

Following are a number of statements that women have used to describe their lives with their male partners. Please read each statement, and then circle the answer that best describes how much you agree or disagree in general with each one as a description of your relationship. If you are not now in a relationship think about the last man you were involved with. There are no right or wrong answers; just circle the number that seems to best describe how much you agree or disagree with each statement.

1. He makes me feel unsafe even in my own home.
2. I feel ashamed of the things he does to me.
3. I try to not rock the boat because I am afraid of what he might do.
4. I feel like I am programmed to react a certain way to him.
5. I feel like he keeps me prisoner.
6. He makes me feel like I have no control over my life, no power, no protection.
7. I hide the truth from others because I am afraid not to.
8. I feel owned and controlled by him.
9. He can scare me without laying a hand on me.
10. He has a look that goes straight through me and terrifies me.

Scoring: (1) reverse score the items (e.g., $1 = 6$; $2 = 5$; $3 = 4$; $4 = 3$; $5 = 2$; $6 = 1$); (2) add together the numbers representing the women's level of agreement or disagreement with each scale item. Higher scores indicate higher levels of psychological vulnerability. The range is 10 to 60.

police records and followed for almost 5 years on the average. It showed high inter-rater reliability (standard error of measurement of . 48) and predictive validity in terms of recidivism offenses, time up to the first recidivism, total injury caused, and severity of assaults. Each item is scored 0 or 1 with the total score being the sum of the item score (0 to 13). Some of the items are scored regarding events that occur at the index assault. The Domestic Violence Risk Appraisal Guide (DVRAG) consists of the 13 ODARA items (most of them are scored continuously rather than dichotomously) plus the score on the Hare Psychopathy Checklist. The ODARA is meant to be used when more time and information resources are available. When used together as a two-part system, the DVRAG is used when the ODARA score is 2 or more. These actuarial risk assessments provide helpful recidivism predictions. Hilton, Harris, and Rice (2010) provide overall information about the instrument, including the specific 13 items and scoring criterion. Hilton et al. (2010) serves as the manual, and there are no separate assessment sheets.

Case Study 6.4 Intimate Partner Violence

You are an on-call counselor who has been contacted to respond to a woman in the emergency room who has been raped. You meet with her and talk with her about her situation. As you talk with her, you find that she is in a relationship (that was not involved in the rape) that has the markings of intimate partner violence. While your main focus is on the rape, you are also concerned with the dynamics of this intimate relationship and believe you need to address these dynamics since she is living with her partner and she plans to return to that living situation when she leaves the emergency room.

1. How would you bring up the possibility of intimate partner violence with her?
2. How would you assess the violence without "scaring" her away from therapy?
3. What would be your philosophical approach in assessing the level of violence?

EXERCISE 6.4 INTIMATE PARTNER VIOLENCE

Allow yourself time to recall your personal and professional experiences with intimate partner violence. What are common themes (feelings, thoughts, behaviors) that emerge for you when you reflect on your experiences of being exposed to violence? What biases may come from these experiences as you work in the assessment of intimate partner violence in conjunction with a crisis situation?

SEXUAL ABUSE

Overview

Regarding the assessment of sexual abuse, it is important to remember that some diagnostic labels are overlapping. For example, in the area of sexual abuse, childhood sexual abuse is the best prediction of female alcohol dependence, and drug use can medicate the depression and low self-esteem of childhood sexual abuse survivors (Van Wormer & Davis, 2008). Childhood sexual abuse is considered to be a risk factor for adolescents and adults with regard to alcohol and drug problems (Downs & Harrison, 1998). Regarding rape, women experience it more frequently (90 percent of victims of reported rapes are women) and most of the time the victim knows the rapist (Bureau of Justice Statistics, 2004). Survivors of rape may increase their use of alcohol (McMullin & White, 2006) or prescription drugs (Sturza & Campbell, 2005). Rape survivors may also experience PTSD (Sturza & Campbell, 2005).

This same overlapping of abuse with substance use may occur with offenders. Sexual abuse offenders may use alcohol/drugs to overcome internal inhibitions about abusing (Finkelhor, 1986). They may also say they offended because they were using alcohol and drugs. However, while alcohol and drugs may assist them in offending, they do not cause them to offend.

Because of such overlapping areas, organizations such as SAMHSA (2000b) recommend that counselors screen for trauma when PTSD, major depression, or mood disorders emerge. This means, then, that the crisis counselor assessing for sexual abuse may want to select an instrument that screens for trauma in general, as discussed in the general mental health section of this chapter. Also, those working with clients who have alcohol and drug problems may want to broaden their assessment interview to include sexual violence in order to determine whether another problem besides the alcohol and drug problem is present.

Instruments

The following instrument can be used to obtain a general overview of the client's childhood trauma.

Childhood Trauma Questionnaire (CTQ) (CTQ Manual, 1998)

The *Childhood Trauma Questionnaire* has 28 items. It has internal consistency reliability ranging from .66–.92; and test-retest reliability ranging from .79–.86 for scales. It has shown construct, content, convergent, concurrent, and predictive validity.

The counselor can also use basic interviewing skills to elicit the story of possible sexual abuse. Asking a client, "Has anyone ever touched you in a way that felt sexual and was uncomfortable for you?" (Miller, 2010, p. 149) can facilitate gathering the sexual abuse survivor story from the client while not suggesting that the client has been sexually abused. Regarding the assessment of children for sexual abuse, the reader is encouraged to follow state laws on the process of reporting suspected child abuse. Briere (1989) reminds counselors that we do not have to be the litmus test of truth when we report suspected child abuse. As stated previously, counselors may want to assess for sexual abuse perpetrators by expanding their interview process to include this area.

Case Study 6.5 Sexual Abuse

Your client is pregnant and is concerned about some recent results she has heard from her doctor about possible complications in the delivery process. These complications sound as if they may cause a difficult delivery for her. She has come into counseling because her husband has a concern about how her anxiety about the delivery process in general may be impacting her as well as the baby. This recent news has solidified his insistence (and her willingness) to come in for counseling. As you talk with her about her concerns, she tells you that she was molested as a child by a family member, has struggled with anxiety around that for many years, and has never talked about it in therapy because she has not come to therapy before. Your clinical hunch is that her unresolved sexual abuse issues may be fueling her current anxiety.

1. Because she already has anxiety that feels at a crisis level for her, how would you bring up the possible sexual abuse issues?
2. What would be your philosophical approach in addressing the anxiety or the sexual abuse?
3. How would you help her manage her anxiety as you explore the area of sexual abuse with her?

EXERCISE 6.5 SEXUAL ABUSE

As you work with this client, what would draw you to using an assessment instrument as a part of the crisis counseling? What would invite you to avoid including such an instrument? Note your ambivalence in this situation and how the context of the crisis may shift you in one direction more than another.

EATING DISORDERS

Overview

Women in the United States make up 90 to 95 percent of clients who are diagnosed as having an eating disorder (APA, 1996b). Assessment of eating disorders requires obtaining information in general about interacting factors, such as sociocultural, personal, and demographic factors, to accurately assess that individual's eating disorder. While eating disorders are similar to other addictive behaviors (compulsiveness, powerlessness, preoccupation, avoidance of feeling, relief by substance abuse), food cannot be totally avoided. Because of overlapping tendencies with other addictive behaviors, counselors need to assess for substance use as well as eating disorders. Additionally, there appears to be a crossover between eating disorders and sexual abuse (MacDonald, Lambie, & Simmonds, 1995).

The *DSM-IV-TR* classifies eating disorders in three ways: anorexia nervosa, bulimia nervosa, and eating disorder not otherwise specified (NOS). The last category is used when criteria for either of the other two categories have not been met. Anorexia nervosa is where the client does not maintain a normal body weight, has fears of gaining weight, and has a distorted body perception. As stated previously, counselors need to assess for the contributing factors that are sociocultural, genetic, personality-based, and family interaction–based in relation to anorexia nervosa. Bulimia nervosa means that the client binge eats and often follows this behavior with purging (vomiting or using laxatives, diuretics, enemas) or fasting/exercising excessively. There are two types of this diagnosis: purging and nonpurging. Again, this eating disorder occurs more commonly in females. Once again, sociocultural, family, and stress factors need to be considered in the overall assessment process, and this area requires asking for information in a supportive, accepting manner.

Instruments

Eating Attitudes Test (EAT-26)©
This test has 26 items that assess the possibility of an eating disorder. It has three subscales (Dieting, Bulimia and Food Preoccupation, Oral Control). It takes about 10 minutes to complete; a score of 20 is of concern and involves physician consultation. The administrator does not need any training. It has shown high internal consistency of .97. Information can be obtained at http://river-centre.org.

Table 6.5   Eating Attitudes Test (EAT-26)©

Instructions: This is a screening measure to help you determine whether you might have an eating disorder that needs professional attention. This screening measure is not designed to make a diagnosis of an eating disorder or take the place of a professional consultation. Please fill out the below form as accurately, honestly, and completely as possible. There are no right or wrong answers. All of your responses are confidential.							
Part A: Complete the following questions:							
1) Birth Date	Month:		Day:	Year:	2) Gender:	Male	Female
3) Height Feet :		Inches:				☐	☐

(continued)

Table 6.5 (Continued)

4) Current Weight (lbs.):	5) Highest Weight (excluding pregnancy):					
6) Lowest Adult Weight:	7) Ideal Weight:					
Part B: Check a response for each of the following statements:	Always	Usually	Often	Some-times	Rarely	Never
1. Am terrified about being overweight.	☐	☐	☐	☐	☐	☐
2. Avoid eating when I am hungry.	☐	☐	☐	☐	☐	☐
3. Find myself preoccupied with food.	☐	☐	☐	☐	☐	☐
4. Have gone on eating binges where I feel that I may not be able to stop.	☐	☐	☐	☐	☐	☐
5. Cut my food into small pieces.	☐	☐	☐	☐	☐	☐
6. Aware of the calorie content of foods that I eat.	☐	☐	☐	☐	☐	☐
7. Particularly avoid food with a high carbohydrate content (i.e., bread, rice, potatoes, etc.)	☐	☐	☐	☐	☐	☐
8. Feel that others would prefer if I ate more.	☐	☐	☐	☐	☐	☐
9. Vomit after I have eaten.	☐	☐	☐	☐	☐	☐

Part B: Check a response for each of the following statements:		Always	Usually	Often	Some-times	Rarely	Never
10.	Feel extremely guilty after eating.	☐	☐	☐	☐	☐	☐
11.	Am preoccupied with a desire to be thinner.	☐	☐	☐	☐	☐	☐
12.	Think about burning up calories when I exercise.	☐	☐	☐	☐	☐	☐
13.	Other people think that I am too thin.	☐	☐	☐	☐	☐	☐
14.	Am preoccupied with the thought of having fat on my body.	☐	☐	☐	☐	☐	☐
15.	Take longer than others to eat my meals.	☐	☐	☐	☐	☐	☐
16.	Avoid foods with sugar in them.	☐	☐	☐	☐	☐	☐
17.	Eat diet foods.	☐	☐	☐	☐	☐	☐
18.	Feel that food controls my life.	☐	☐	☐	☐	☐	☐
19.	Display self-control around food.	☐	☐	☐	☐	☐	☐
20.	Feel that others pressure me to eat.	☐	☐	☐	☐	☐	☐
21.	Give too much time and thought to food.	☐	☐	☐	☐	☐	☐

(continued)

Table 6.5 (Continued)

Part B: Check a response for each of the following statements:		Always	Usually	Often	Some-times	Rarely	Never
22.	Feel uncomfortable after eating sweets.	☐	☐	☐	☐	☐	☐
23.	Engage in dieting behavior.	☐	☐	☐	☐	☐	☐
24.	Like my stomach to be empty.	☐	☐	☐	☐	☐	☐
25.	Have the impulse to vomit after meals.	☐	☐	☐	☐	☐	☐
26.	Enjoy trying new rich foods.	☐	☐	☐	☐	☐	☐
Part C: Behavioral Questions: In the past 6 months have you:		Never	Once a month or less	2–3 times a month	Once a week	2–6 times a week	Once a day or more
A	Gone on eating binges where you feel that you may not be able to stop? *	☐	☐	☐	☐	☐	☐
B	Ever made yourself sick (vomited) to control your weight or shape?	☐	☐	☐	☐	☐	☐
C	Ever used laxatives, diet pills, or diuretics (water pills) to control your weight or shape?	☐	☐	☐	☐	☐	☐
D	Exercised more than 60 minutes a day to lose or to control your weight?	☐	☐	☐	☐	☐	☐

E	Lost 20 pounds or more in the past 6 months?	Yes ☐	No ☐		

*Defined as eating much more than most people would under the same circumstances and feeling that eating is out of control.

©EAT-26: (Garner et al. 1982, *Psychological Medicine, 12*, 871–878); adapted by D. Garner with permission.

The EAT-26 has been reproduced with permission. Garner et al. (1982). The Eating Attitudes Test: Psychometric features and clinical correlates. *Psychological Medicine, 12*, 871–878.

Interpreting Eating Attitudes Test (Eat-26)® Scores
David M. Garner, PhD

(Suitable for Online Feedback)

The Eating Attitudes Test (EAT-26)® is probably the most widely used test used to assess "eating disorder risk" based on attitudes, feelings, and behaviors related to eating and eating disorder symptoms. It was used as a screening instrument in the 1998 National Eating Disorders Screening program and has been used in many other studies to identify individuals with possible eating disorders. However, the EAT-26 does not provide a diagnosis of an eating disorder. A diagnosis can only be provided by a qualified health care professional.

The version of the Eating Attitudes Test (EAT-26) you have just completed has three criteria for determining whether you should seek further evaluation of your risk of having an eating disorder. These are:

1. Your score on the actual EAT test items
2. Low body weight compared to age-matched norms
3. Behavioral questions indicating possible eating disorder symptoms or recent significant weight loss

If you meet one or more of these criteria, you should seek an evaluation by a professional who specializes in the treatment of eating disorders.

1. Your Eating Attitudes Test (EAT-26®) score is: ___
A score at or above 20 on the EAT-26® indicates a high level of concern about dieting, body weight or problematic eating behaviors. Because your score is

(continued)

above 20, you should seek an evaluation by a qualified health professional to determine whether your score reflects a problem that warrants clinical attention. However, please keep in mind that high scores do not always reflect over-concern about body weight, body shape, and eating. Screening studies have shown that some people with high scores do not have eating disorders. Regardless of your score, if you are suffering from feelings which are causing you concern or interfering with your daily functioning, you should seek an evaluation from a trained mental health professional.

EAT-26® SCORE

	Scoring System for the EAT-26					
	Always	Usually	Often	Sometimes	Rarely	Never
Score for questions 1–25	3	2	1	0	0	0
Score for question # 26	0	0	0	1	2	3

Add the scores for each item together for a total score.

2. Your body mass index (BMI) is: ___
If your BMI meets the criterion for "underweight," it is an important risk factor for a serious eating disorder. If your EAT-26® score is 20 or more, this increases your likelihood of having a serious eating disorder. If your BMI indicates that you are neither "underweight" nor "extremely underweight" compared to age/gender-matched norms, you could still have a serious eating disorder. It just means that it is unlikely that you have anorexia nervosa. If you believe that your body weight is a problem, then it would be good for you to consult with a qualified health professional for further clarification. See the note below for further explanation of BMI. (See Table 6.6.)

3. Behavioral Questions: If you scored in any of the checked boxed (√), you should seek an evaluation from a trained mental health professional. (See Table 6.7.)

Table 6.6 BMI Considered "Underweight" for Different Ages and Sexes According to Norms

Age	9	10	11	12	13	14	15	16	17	18	19	20	21+
Female (BMI)	14.0	14.5	14.5	15.0	15.5	16.0	16.5	17.0	17.5	18.0	18.0	18.5	19.0
Male (BMI)	14.0	14.5	15.0	15.0	16.0	16.5	17.0	17.5	18.0	18.5	19.0	19.5	20.0

Table 6.7 Behavioral Questions Form

In the past 6 months have you:	Never	Once a month or less	2–3 times a month	Once a week	2–6 times a week	Once a day or more
Gone on eating binges where you feel that you may not be able to stop?	☐	☐	√	√	√	√
Ever made yourself sick (vomited) to control your weight or shape?	☐	√	√	√	√	√
Ever used laxatives, diet pills, or diuretics (water pills) to control your weight or shape?	☐	√	√	√	√	√
Exercised more than 60 minutes a day to lose or to control your weight?	☐	☐	☐	☐	☐	√
Lost 20 pounds or more in the past 6 months?	Yes √		No ☐			

Please remember that the EAT-26© does not provide a diagnosis of an eating disorder. A diagnosis can only be provided by a qualified health care professional.

*Note on BMI: The EAT-26 includes specific questions on height, weight, and gender that can be used to compute Body Mass Index (BMI) for the purpose of determining if you are "at risk" for an eating disorder because your body weight is extremely underweight according to age-matched population norms. BMI is a formula for estimating body mass that takes both height and weight into account. It is calculated by dividing weight (in kilograms) by height in meters, and then divided again by height in meters (kg/m2). Alternatively, BMI can be calculated as weight (in pounds) divided by height in inches, then divided again by height in inches and multiplied by 703. We recommend that you seek a professional evaluation for a possible eating disorder if your body weight is "extremely underweight" according to age-matched population norms.

More Information on BMI

The National Health and Nutrition Examination Survey III (NHANES III, Kuczmarski, Ogden, Guo, Grummer-Strawn, Flegal, Mei, et al., 2002) has collected reference data to establish weight and height norms at different ages for girls/women and boys/men from birth to 20 years old. These norms indicate that BMI varies considerably with age and gender, with children between 5 and 8 years old having the lowest BMI values followed by a steady increase with age. The expected changes in BMI associated females and males as "underweight" (BMI between the 5th and 10th percentile for girls/women and boys/men from 9 to 20 years old) and "very underweight" (BMI less than the 5th percentile). A BMI cutoff of between the 5th and 10th percentile for different ages and sexes should be used to determine if you meet the "underweight" BMI referral criterion. For men and women 21 years old and older, the "underweight" category according to the NHLBI (1998) survey data were used to determine the "underweight" criterion for referral.

You can easily determine whether you meet the BMI thresholds in Table 6.8 by finding your height on the column on the left in Table 6.9 and the BMI on the bottom and follow the height and the BMI columns to where they intersect. This is the weight that you need to be at or below for the BMI you have selected.

Although BMI is a convenient and useful weight classification tool, it does have limitations. For example, BMI can overestimate fatness for people who are athletic. Also, some races, ethnic groups, and nationalities have different body fat distributions and body compositions; therefore, the NHANES data are not appropriate for all groups (Kuczmarski, Ogden, Guo, Grummer-Strawn, Flegal, Mei, et al., 2002).

Table 6.8 BMI Considered "Underweight" and "Very Underweight" Using Norms for Sex and Age

Age	9	10	11	12	13	14	15	16	17	18	19	20	20+
Female													
Very Underweight													
(less than or equal to)	13.5	14.0	14.0	14.5	15.0	15.5	16.0	16.5	17.0	17.5	17.5	17.5	18.5
Underweight													
(between)	13.6–14.0	14.1–14.5	14.1–14.5	14.6–15.0	15.1–15.5	15.6–16.0	16.1–16.5	16.6–17.0	17.1–17.5	17.6–18.0	17.6–18.0	17.6–18.5	18.6–19.0
Male													
Very Underweight													
(less than or equal to)	13.5	14.0	14.5	14.5	15.0	16.0	16.5	17.0	17.5	18.0	18.5	19.0	19.5
Underweight													
(between)	13.6–14.0	14.1–14.5	14.6–15.0	14.6–15.0	15.1–16.0	16.1–16.5	16.6–17.0	17.1–17.5	17.6–18.0	18.1–18.5	18.6–19.0	19.1–19.5	19.6–20.0

Data from the NHANES III survey, Kuczmarski, Ogden, Guo, Grummer-Strawn, Flegal, Mei,...Johnson, 2002.

Table 6.9 Body Weight and Height to Calculate Body Mass Index (BMI)

Height (in.)	Weight (lb.)													
50	50	52	54	55	57	59	60	62	64	66	68	70	78	89
51	52	54	56	58	59	61	63	65	67	68	70	73	81	91
52	54	56	58	60	62	64	65	67	69	71	73	76	85	96
53	56	58	60	62	64	66	68	70	72	74	76	79	88	100
54	58	60	62	64	66	69	71	73	75	77	79	82	91	104
55	60	63	65	67	69	71	73	76	78	80	82	85	95	108
56	63	65	67	69	72	74	76	78	81	83	85	88	98	111
57	65	67	70	72	74	76	79	81	83	86	88	91	101	115
58	67	70	72	74	77	79	82	84	86	89	91	94	105	119
59	70	72	75	77	79	82	84	87	89	92	94	97	108	124
60	72	74	77	80	82	85	87	90	92	95	97	100	112	128
61	74	77	80	82	85	88	90	93	96	98	100	104	116	132
62	77	80	82	85	88	90	93	96	99	101	104	107	120	136
63	79	82	85	88	91	93	96	99	102	105	107	110	124	141
64	82	85	88	91	93	96	99	102	105	108	110	114	128	145
65	84	87	90	93	96	99	102	105	108	112	114	118	132	150
66	87	90	93	96	99	102	106	109	112	115	118	121	136	155

(continued)

	14.0	14.5	15.0	15.5	16.0	16.5	17.0	17.5	18.0	18.5	19.0	19.5	22.0	25.0
67	90	93	96	99	102	106	109	112	115	118	121	125	140	160
68	92	96	99	102	105	109	112	115	119	122	125	128	145	165
69	95	98	102	105	109	112	115	119	122	126	128	132	148	170
70	98	101	105	108	112	115	119	122	126	129	132	136	153	175
71	101	104	108	111	115	118	122	126	129	133	136	140	157	180
72	103	107	111	114	118	122	125	129	133	137	140	144	162	185
73	106	110	114	118	122	125	129	133	137	140	144	148	166	190
74	109	113	117	121	125	129	133	136	140	144	148	152	171	195
75	112	116	120	124	128	132	136	140	144	148	152	156	175	200
76	115	120	124	128	132	136	140	144	148	152	156	160	180	205
BMI (kg/m)	14.0	14.5	15.0	15.5	16.0	16.5	17.0	17.5	18.0	18.5	19.0	19.5	22.0	25.0

Table 6.10 3rd, 5th, and 10th Percentiles for Females and Males by age from the NHANES III

Age	Female Percentile			Male Percentile		
	3rd	5th	10th	3rd	5th	10th
9	13.5	13.7	14.2	13.7	14.0	14.3
10	13.7	14.0	14.5	14.0	14.2	14.6
11	14.1	14.4	14.9	14.3	14.6	15.0
12	14.5	14.8	15.4	14.6	14.9	15.4
13	15.0	15.3	15.9	15.1	15.5	16.0
14	15.4	15.8	16.4	15.7	16.0	16.5
15	15.9	16.3	16.9	16.2	16.6	17.1
16	16.4	16.8	17.4	16.8	17.1	17.7
17	16.8	17.2	17.8	17.3	17.7	18.3
18	17.2	17.6	18.2	17.9	18.2	18.9
19	17.4	17.8	18.4	18.3	18.7	19.4
20	17.4	17.8	18.5	18.7	19.1	19.8

http://www.cdc.gov/nchs/about/major/nhanes/growthcharts/datafiles.htm

---

Case Study 6.6 Eating Disorders

You are meeting with your client in her home in response to a crisis call to the organization for which you work. As you meet with her about her crisis, you notice that many high-calorie snack foods are strewn throughout the house (living room, bathroom, kitchen, etc.) and many of the packages are opened, as though they have recently been eaten from. Your client lives alone and is extremely slender. While you are meeting with her, she goes to the bathroom for an extended period of time and comes back smelling of vomit. You suspect that she has thrown up and is bulimic.

1. How would you approach your concerns within the context of the crisis?
2. How would you address the concerns without losing focus on the crisis?
3. Could you use an assessment instrument in this setting? If not, what would the setting need to be in order to use an assessment instrument, and what assessment instrument might you use in that setting?

EXERCISE 6.6 EATING DISORDERS

Does the type or degree of an eating disorder impact your comfort in working with it in a crisis situation? Does the type of crisis or the setting in which the crisis counseling is occurring impact your comfort in addressing this issue? What would be the criteria that would guide your use of an instrument as a part of crisis counseling (type/degree of eating disorder, type/setting of crisis)?

SUICIDE

Overview

Being suicidal is described as a complex, stressful process; the client is weighing the pros and cons of killing him/herself because he/she lacks better solutions (Shea, 2002). Counselors need to connect with the part of the individual that wants to be alive, but in order to do so, the counselor must first be able to assess that the client is suicidal. In this area, there is again an overlap between substance abuse/mental health problems and suicide: (a) chemically dependent individuals commit suicide at four times the national average (Buelow & Buelow, 1998); (b) 65 percent of suicide attempts are related to alcohol (Kinney, 2003); and (c) 90 percent of suicides are connected with mental illness/substance abuse disorders (Goldsmith, Pellmar, Kleinman, & Bunney, 2002). Counselors need to be sensitive to this overlapping when assessing for suicide.

Assessing suicide is challenging and anxiety producing for counselors (Schechter & Barnett, 2010). In the suicide assessment, the counselor needs to be flexible and collaborative while gathering information about the level of risk and both risk and protective factors of the client (McKeon, 2009). Most suicidal (as well as homicidal) clients send out clues to others (James, 2008). The risk factors for suicide include (McKeon, 2009):

- Mental disorders (mood disorders, schizophrenia, anxiety disorders, borderline personality disorder)
- Alcohol/substance use disorders
- Sense of hopelessness
- Impulsive/aggressive tendencies
- Trauma/abuse
- Previous attempts
- Loss of relationship/job
- Lethal means access
- Isolation socially
- Sense of being a burden
- Having problems asking for help
- Experiencing barriers to health care

Generally, the counselor can assess for suicidal tendencies by asking clients three questions (Miller, 2010, p. 101):

1. Are you thinking of hurting yourself? (reflects openness to topic discussion).
2. How would you hurt yourself? (addresses means of the attempt).
3. What stops you from hurting yourself? (taps client's values, sense of hope and meaning).

With regard to a suicide plan, the counselor needs to be direct in asking about suicidal ideas, lethality of method, availability of means, and specificity of the plan (Hoff, Hallisey, & Hoff, 2009). When assessing lethality, the counselor can ask him/herself: "Can I go home tonight and get a good night's sleep trusting this person won't harm themselves?" This self-reflective question may assist the counselor in determining if everything that needs to be done by the counselor is being done. It is imperative for counselors to document the safety plan carefully and to use consultation and supervision wisely.

Instruments

The overall caution in discussing assessment instruments is to remember that there is no formula that the counselor can use psychometrically to be precisely accurate in assessing the level of suicide risk (Kanel, 2007; McKeon, 2009). Given this general limitation, the counselor may find it helpful to use the following instruments as one source of information in assessing suicide risk.

Adult Suicidal Ideation Questionnaire (ASIQ)

This self-report questionnaire can be used during intake or treatment to clarify whether there is serious suicidal ideation. It has 25 items and can be used with college students and adults in a general assessment of suicidal ideation. It takes about 10 minutes to complete. Items are rated on a 7-point scale, and it has a built-in scoring key. It provides a total score with a corresponding *T* score and percentile score; the total score can be compared to a cutoff score that allows for identification of individuals in need of further evaluation of suicide risk. It was normed on a sample of 2,000 adults (18 and older) that included psychiatric outpatients, normal adults, and college students. It has an internal consistency and test-retest reliability coefficients that range from .96–.97 and .85–.95, respectively, depending on the sample. For additional information, contact www .sigmaassessmentsystems.com.

Beck Depression Inventory (BDI)

The test has 21 items and can be self-administered. It assesses depressive symptoms. It takes about 10 minutes and clients can read at the sixth-grade level. It is computerized and comes in a shorter version as well as a BDI-II. It has reliability consistency that ranges from .73 to .95. For further information, contact: www .beckinstitute.org.

Case Study 6.7 Suicide

Your client is elderly, has recently lost his spouse, and sees no reason to go on living. You have visited him in his new assisted living facility once before, but it is during this visit that he has told you that in addition to the tremendous grief he has experienced with regard to the loss of his wife, he also does not want to live. In your assessment of this client, you are concerned that he has the motivation to kill himself, has decided on the means with which to kill himself, and has nothing that is stopping him from taking such action.

1. Would you need to assess his suicidal state further?
2. Do you have enough information to take action?
3. What action options would you consider taking?

EXERCISE 6.7 SUICIDE

What are your personal views about suicide? How are these views reflected in your professional practice?

HOMICIDE

Overview

In terms of homicidal tendencies, there is encouragement in the assessment process to look into the following factors (Hoff, Hallisey, & Hoff, 2009): statistics (more men than women), personality (higher aggressiveness), and situations (weapon availability), and their interaction with one another. The same overall questions can be adapted from the suicide assessment (Miller, 2010, p. 102):

1. Are you thinking of hurting someone?
2. How would you hurt this person?
3. What stops you from hurting this person?

As in the suicide assessment, these questions will reflect an openness toward discussing the topic and assessing the lethality of the situation. Kanel (2007) adds asking whether: the client is engaged (actively or passively) in violent/dangerous behavior, has a background in such behavior, or has acted on violent plans in the past. Again, the counselor can use the self-reflective question under the suicide section to determine if everything that needs to be done by the counselor is being done ("Can I go home tonight and get a good night's sleep trusting this person won't harm another?"). Also, as in the section on suicide, it is imperative for counselors to document the plan carefully and to use consultation and supervision wisely.

Instruments

As with IPV and suicide assessment, there is no psychometric instrument that can be used to definitively assess for violence. Again, the assessment process is general in nature and relies on the clinical judgment of the counselor. Probably the best predictor of violent behavior is whether the client has been violent in the past.

In the assessment process, the counselor needs to look at the need for hospitalization and medication, but also needs to notify the person the client has threatened to harm. This type of crisis situation overrides confidentiality, as reflected in *Tarasoff v. Regents of the University of California* (Bersoff, 1976).

Case Study 6.8 Homicide

You are counseling a client who has lost everything he had in a recent hurricane. He has lost his office as well as his home, and he has a family to support. While he is openly discussing his grief with you, he tells you he is extremely angry at the local insurance agent who sold him a policy that did not include hurricane coverage for either his home or workplace. He tells you he wants to kill the agent. You have known

---

your client for a short time (a few sessions) and have not assessed a history of violence. You are aware that other people in the community have complained about this agent (you have heard these stories outside of sessions from trustworthy people in the community, especially during the recovery of the community following the hurricane).

1. What aspects of your client's reaction would concern you around lethality?
2. How would you assess the level of his lethality further?
3. What information would you need to have to believe you have sufficient concern to warn the insurance agent of the client's intent to kill him?

EXERCISE 6.8 HOMICIDE

What are your general concerns about applying the duty to warn practice during a crisis situation? How would you handle the concerns you have? Are there any preventatives or rehearsals you can do to prepare for such situations in advance?

SUMMARY

This chapter addressed eight diagnoses that are common to crisis counseling work: general mental health, addiction, co-occurring disorders, intimate partner violence, sexual abuse, eating disorders, suicide, and homicide. Each area included a brief overview, an instrument summary or theoretical/philosophical approach, a case study, and an exercise. Also, a general overview of assessment and instrument guidelines was provided to assist the reader in instrument selection.

QUESTIONS

1. What are some common diagnoses that may appear in crisis counseling?
2. What are some of the assessment instruments related to these diagnoses that may be used in a crisis counseling situation?
3. Questions to ask oneself: "While working with the case studies and exercises, which diagnoses and assessment instruments did I realize that I am comfortable working with? Why? Which diagnoses and assessment instruments are less comfortable for me and why?"

SUGGESTED READINGS

General Mental Health/General Trauma

Briere, J., & Scott, C. (2006). *Principles of trauma therapy*. Thousand Oaks, CA: Sage.

This book is divided into two sections: trauma effects and assessment and clinical interventions.

Foa, E. B., Keane, T. M., Friedman, M. J., & Cohen, J. A. (2009). *Effective treatments for PTSD: Practice guidelines from the International Society for Traumatic Stress Studies* (2nd ed.). New York, NY: Guilford.

This book is divided into five sections: assessment and diagnosis (two chapters); early interventions (three chapters); treatment for chronic PTSD (15 chapters; children/adolescents/adults, various treatment approaches); treatment guidelines (18 sections); and conclusions.

Hien, D., Litt, L. C., Cohen, L. R., Miele, G. M., & Campbell, A. (2009). *Trauma services for women in substance abuse treatment.* Washington, DC: American Psychological Association.

This book has three sections: the relationship between trauma and substance abuse; the impact of trauma on functioning; and strategies for implementation.

Ogden, P., Minton, K., & Pain, C. (2006). *Trauma and the body: A sensimotor approach to psychotherapy.* New York, NY: Norton.

This book is divided into two sections: theory and treatment. The theoretical section has seven chapters that look at thoughts, feelings, and sensimotor reactions to trauma. The treatment section has five chapters that provide the counselor with information on how to apply the theory to clinical practice with trauma survivors.

Rothschild, B. (2000). *The body remembers.* New York, NY: Norton.

This book is divided into two sections: theory and practice. The theoretical portion describes the main impacts of trauma on the mind and body. The practice section provides the counselor with practical suggestions on working with trauma survivors.

Addiction

Dimeff, L. A., Comtois, K. A., & Linehan, M. M. (2009). Co-occurring addiction and borderline personality disorder. In R. K. Ries, D. A. Fiellin, S. C. Miller, & R. Saitz (Eds.) *Principles of addiction medicine* (4th ed., pp. 1227–1237). Philadelphia, PA: Wolters Kluwer/Lippincott Williams & Wilkins.

This chapter provides a concise overview of DBT as applied to a substance-abusing borderline population.

Dimeff, L. A., & Linehan, M. M. (2008). Dialectical behavior therapy for substance abusers. *Addiction Science & Clinical Practice, 4,* 39–47.

This article provides a concise overview of DBT as applied to a substance abusing borderline population.

Goldstein, E. G. (2004). Substance abusers with borderline disorders. In S. L. A. Straussner (Ed.) *Clinical work with substance-abusing clients* (2nd ed.) (pp. 370–391). New York, NY: Guilford.

This chapter discusses characteristics and causes of borderline personality disorders as well as assessment and treatment strategies.

Margolis, R. D., & Zweben, J. E. (1998). *Treating patients with alcohol and other drug problems: An integrated approach.* Washington, DC: American Psychological Association.

This 358-page book has an excellent section on techniques a counselor can use to encourage abstinence.

Miller, G. A. (2010). *Learning the language of addiction counseling* (3rd ed.). Hoboken, NJ: Wiley.

This book provides a summary of addiction counseling. It has 14 chapters (introduction, theories, assessment of addiction, assessment of co-occurring disorders, treatment, treatment-related issues, relapse prevention, self-help groups, current and evolving therapies, culturally sensitive counseling, spirituality, chronic pain, personal and professional development, preparation of certification and licensure). The text has numerous case studies and exercises to facilitate application of the material.

Schenker, M. D. (2009). *A clinician's guide to 12 step recovery: Integrating 12-step programs into psychotherapy.* New York, NY: Norton.

This book has 12 chapters that are designed to educate the clinician about the core components of 12-step recovery programs and how to integrate them with one's clinical practice. Chapters address topics such as the history of AA, what happens in meetings, common treatment issues as they relate to AA, and critiques and challenges.

Shaw, B. F., Ritvo, P., & Irvine, J. (2005). *Addiction & recovery for dummies.* Hoboken, NJ: Wiley.

This book has 20 chapters divided into five sections: the detection of addiction, taking initial steps, treatment approaches, a recovery life, and 10 ways to help a loved one and self-help resources. It is written for a non-professional.

Co-Occurring Disorders

Center for Substance Abuse Treatment (CSAT) (2005). *Substance abuse treatment for persons with co-occurring disorders.* Treatment Improvement Protocol (TIP) Series, No. 42. DHHS Publication No. (SMA) 05-3922. Rockville, MD: Substance Abuse and Mental Health Services Administration.

The manual provides a general overview of treatment for these disorders.

Center for Substance Abuse Treatment (CSAT) (2008). *Managing depressive symptoms in substance abuse clients during early recovery.* Treatment Improvement Protocol (TIP) Series, No. 48. DHHS Publication No. (SMA) 05-3922. Rockville, MD: Substance Abuse and Mental Health Services Administration.

This manual is the first TIP manual using a new format that describes working with this population in three parts for: substance abuse counselors (Part 1—counseling methods and frameworks), program administrators (Part 2—provision of administrative support for Part 1 to be integrated), and clinical supervisors (Part 3—online literature review that is updated every six months for five years and can be accessed at www.kap.samhsa.gov).

Daley, D. C., & Moss, H. B. (2002). *Dual disorders: Counseling clients with chemical dependency and mental illness* (3rd ed.). Center City, MN: Hazelden.

This book has 15 chapters that provide an overview of dual disorders and the treatment (including group treatment) and recovery process (including relapse prevention) as well as chapters that focus on the family, specific disorders (personality, antisocial, borderline, depression, bipolar, anxiety, schizophrenia, cognitive) and specific program development issues.

Evans, K., & Sullivan, J. M. (2001). *Dual diagnosis: Counseling the mentally ill substance abuser* (2nd ed.). New York, NY: Guilford Press.

This book provides suggestions on the practice of working with this population.

Hamilton, T., & Samples, P. (1994). *The twelve steps and dual disorders*. Center City, MN: Hazelden.

This book describes how the 12 steps can be effectively used with this population.

Hazelden (1993). *The dual disorders recovery book*. Center City, MN: Hazelden.

This book focuses on the 12-step program of dual disorders (Dual Recovery Anonymous) through the stories of individuals.

L'Abate, L. L., Farrar, J. E., & Serritella, D. A. (1992). *Handbook of differential treatments for addictions*. Boston, MA: Allyn & Bacon.

This book provides information on a variety of addictions that the authors describe as: socially destructive (alcohol, substance abuse, tobacco use, domestic violence, sexual abuses and offenses), socially unacceptable (interpersonal/love, eating disorders), and socially acceptable (gambling, workaholism, exercise, spending, religion, codependency).

McGovern, M. (2009). *Living with co-occurring addiction and mental health disorders*. Center City, MN: Hazelden.

This book is written to the person struggling with these disorders. It has 14 chapters that explain basic concepts of dual diagnosis and its treatment.

Mueser, K. T., Noordsy, D. L., Drake, R. E., & Fox, L. (2003). *Integrated treatment for dual disorders*. New York, NY: Guilford Press.

This is an excellent workbook that generally describes co-occurring diagnosis and then provides information on working with this population in the assessment and treatment process, including individual, group, and family therapy. Its appendix contains 16 educational handouts and 20 assessment and treatment forms.

National Institute on Drug Abuse (NIDA) (2008a). Comorbidity: Addiction and other mental illnesses. *Research Report Series*. Rockville, MD: NIDA.

This 11-page publication provides an excellent summary of co-morbidity.

Smith, T. (2008). *A balanced life: 9 strategies for coping with the mental health problems of a loved one*. Center City, MN: Hazelden.

This book is written for the family and friends of a loved one who struggles with mental illness. It provides nine strategies to help the individual cope with the daily realities of this situation within a balanced lifestyle. It incorporates a Higher Power concept.

Solomon, J., Zimberg, S., & Shollar, E. (Eds.) (1993). *Dual diagnosis: Evaluation, treatment, training, and program development* (pp. 39–53). New York: Plenum Press.

This book covers theory, research, and practice with co-occurring diagnosis. Specific suggestions are made regarding assessment and treatment of the dually diagnosed.

Substance Abuse and Mental Health Services Administration (1994). *Assessment and treatment of patients with coexisting mental illness and alcohol and other drug abuse* (DHHS Publication No. 94-2078). Rockville, MD: Author.

This publication has nine chapters that provide basic information on co-occurring diagnosis and treatment (issues, collaboration, medication) and a separate chapter on specific diagnoses (mood disorders, anxiety disorders, personality disorders, psychotic disorders).

Substance Abuse and Mental Health Services Administration (2002). *Report to Congress on the prevention and treatment of co-occurring substance abuse disorders and mental disorders* (www.samhsa.gov). Rockville, MD: Author.

This report is divided into five chapters: characteristics/needs, impact of federal block grants, prevention, evidence-based practices, and five-year action blueprint.

Watkins, T. R., Lewellen, A., & Barrett, M. C. (2001). *Dual diagnosis: An integrated approach to treatment*. Thousand Oaks, CA: Sage.

This book covers general issues related to co-occurring diagnosis and then provides separate chapters on assessment and treatment on specific disorders in relation to substance abuse (schizophrenia, depression, bipolar, personality disorders, anxiety disorders).

Intimate Partner Violence

Suggested Readings (Professional)

Domestic Abuse Intervention Project (2002). *A guide for conducting domestic violence assessments*. Duluth, MN: Author.

This manual has four sections (using the assessment guide, assessing social risks of battered women, preparing for the assessment, assessment interview format) and ten appendices. It provides a domestic violence matrix and a risk assessment for women that focuses on the woman's safety.

Edelson, J. L., & Tolman, R. M. (1992). *Intervention for men who batter: An ecological approach*. Newbury Park, CA: Sage.

This manual is designed to provide practical suggestions to the counselor who wants to counsel batterers.

Goodman, M. S., & Fallon, B. C. (1995). *Pattern changing for abused women*. Thousand Oaks, CA: Sage.

This text provides an overview of domestic violence counseling theory and approaches. The accompanying workbook has helpful exercises that a counselor can use in working with this population; one especially helpful handout is "Your Bill of Rights."

Graham-Bermann, S. A., & Edleson, J. L. (Eds.) (2001). *Domestic violence in the lives of children*. Washington, DC: American Psychological Association.

This book is divided into three sections: understanding children's exposure to intimate partner violence, the role of families and social support, and preventive intervention initiatives and evaluations.

Hilton, N. Z., Harris, G. T., & Rice, M. E. (2010). *Risk assessment for domestically violent men*. Washington, DC: American Psychological Association.

This book provides information on the Ontario Domestic Assault Risk Assessment (ODARA) and the Domestic Violence Risk Appraisal Guide (DVRAG), which can be used to predict recidivism in male domestic violence offenders. It has seven chapters that provide an overview and six appendices on the instruments, including one specifically on scoring criteria for the ODARA and one for the DVRAG.

Hines, D. A., & Malley-Morrison, K. M. (2005). *Family violence in the United States*. Thousand Oaks, CA: Sage.

This book has 12 chapters that address: definition issues, cultural contexts, religious contexts, child physical abuse, child sexual abuse, child neglect, wife abuse, husband abuse, GLBT abuse, elder abuse, hidden types of abuse, and effective responses.

Holden, G. W., Geffner, R., & Jouriles, E. N. (Eds.) (1998). *Children exposed to marital violence*. Washington, DC: American Psychological Association.

This book covers theoretical and conceptual issues, research, and applied issues.

Knapp, S. J., & VandeCreek, L. (1997). *Treating patients with memories of abuse: Legal risk management*. Washington, DC: American Psychological Association.

This book presents suggestions on how to treat clients who have been abused from a risk management perspective. It provides helpful guidelines for practice in working with this population.

Leventhal, B., & Lundy, S. E. (1999). *Same-sex domestic violence*. Thousand Oaks, CA: Sage.

This book is divided into four sections: personal stories, legal perspectives, organizing coalitions/building communities, and providing services.

Miller, G., Clark, C., & Herman, J. (2007). Domestic violence in a rural setting. *Journal of Rural Mental Health, 31*, 28–42.

This journal article provides a summary of barriers that face intimate partner violence survivors in a rural setting, along with specific counseling examples. Recommendations are made to rural healthcare professionals.

Minnesota Coalition for Battered Women (1992). *Safety first: A guide for battered women*. St. Paul, MN: Author.

This is a useful book for survivors of intimate partner violence because it provides both theoretical and practical information and suggestions.

Schechter, S. (1987). *Guidelines for mental health practitioners in domestic violence cases*. Washington, DC: National Coalition Against Domestic Violence.

This booklet has basic information on intimate partner violence (definition, misconceptions, indicators) as well as clinical suggestions on working with this population.

Substance Abuse and Mental Health Services Administration (1997). *Substance abuse treatment and domestic violence*. Rockville, MD: Author.

This manual summarizes the knowledge base of intimate partner violence (male batterers to female survivors), the relationship between substance abuse and intimate partner violence, and how to screen for it in treatment. It also provides instruments that can be used for assessment.

Substance Abuse and Mental Health Services Administration (2002). *Domestic violence and the new Americans: Directory of programs and resources for battered refugee women* (CMHS-SVP-0061). Rockville, MD: Author.

This book provides information about services and programs available by state.

Trickett, P. K., & Schellenbach, C. J. (1998). *Violence against children in the family and the community*. Washington, DC: American Psychological Association.

This book has five sections: developmental consequences, causes of different forms of violence, effective interventions, prevention, and effectiveness of interventions.

Suggested Readings (Personal)

NiCarthy, G. (1987). *The ones who got away: Women who left abusive partners*. Seattle, WA: Seal Press.

This book has 33 stories of women from all different walks of life who left their abusers. There is also a chapter on the lessons the women who leave provide and a chapter on why they left and how they were able to stay away.

NiCarthy, G. (1997). *Getting free: You can end abuse and take back your life*. Seattle, WA: Seal Press.

This book provides general information on intimate partner violence with exercises to facilitate the survivor's awareness. There are chapters on teen abuse, lesbian abuse, and emotional abuse.

White, E. C. (1994). *Chain, chain, change: For black women in abusive relationships*. Seattle, WA: Seal Press.

This book has nine chapters that attempt to provide information enabling the reader to assess whether she is in a violent relationship and explore actions she may choose to take. There is a chapter on lesbians and abuse also.

Sexual Abuse

Suggested Readings (Professional)

Cunningham, C., & MacFarlane, K. (1991). *When children molest children: Group treatment strategies for young sexual abusers.* Orwell, VT: The Safer Society Press.

This book contains simple activities for children ages 4 to 12 that counselors can use in addressing sexual offender behaviors in young children. It has three sections (interventions, skills/competencies, progress measures) with accompanying exercises the counselor can use in group counseling.

Finkelhor, D. (1986). *A sourcebook on child sexual abuse.* Beverly Hills, CA: Sage.

This book provides an excellent general overview on sexual abuse.

Gonsiorek, J. C., Bera, W. H., & LeTourneau, D. (1994). *Male sexual abuse.* Thousand Oaks, CA: Sage.

This book covers basic information on male sexual abuse with specific counseling suggestions.

Schwartz, M. F., & Cohn, L. (Eds.) (1996). *Sexual abuse and eating disorders.* New York, NY: Brunner/Mazel.

This book provides an excellent overview of the overlap of the issues between sexual abuse and eating disorders.

Substance Abuse and Mental Health Services Administration (2000b). *Substance abuse treatment for persons with child abuse and neglect issues.* Rockville, MD: Author.

The seven chapters in this manual cover areas that include working with these issues: screening, assessment, treatment, therapeutic issues, breaking the cycle, and legal concerns.

Suggested Readings (Personal)

Bass, E. (Ed.) (1983). *I never told anyone: Writings by women survivors of child sexual abuse.* New York, NY: Harper Perennial.

This book has 33 stories of survivors of sexual abuse that are organized by the type of perpetrator (fathers, relatives, friends/acquaintances, strangers).

Bass, E., & Davis, L. (1988). *The courage to heal.* New York, NY: Harper & Row.

This book was written for female survivors. It has five sections (taking stock, the healing process, changing patterns, survivor supporters, and courageous women) that provide information as well as questions and exercises to assist the survivor in the healing process.

Lew, M. (1988). *Victims no longer: Men recovering from incest and other sexual child abuse.* New York, NY: Harper & Row.

This book has five sections (general information, information about men, survival, recovery, and other people/resources). Each section provides information and the story of a survivor.

Lew, M. (2004). *Victims no longer: The classic guide for men recovering from sexual child abuse*. New York, NY: Harper Paperbacks.

This book describes how culture inhibits men's ability to see abuse and obtain treatment for it.

Mendel, M. P. (1995). *The male survivor*. Thousand Oaks, CA: Sage.

This book has eight chapters that each provide information on male sexual abuse and are accompanied by a survivor's story. The final chapter discusses the male survivor in general.

Eating Disorders

Schwartz, M. F., & Cohn, L. (Eds.) (1996). *Sexual abuse and eating disorders*. New York, NY: Brunner/Mazel.

This book provides an excellent overview of the overlap of the issues between sexual abuse and eating disorders.

Stromberg, G., & Merrill, J. (2006). *Feeding the fame*. Center City, MN: Hazelden.

This book tells the stories of 17 celebrities who struggled with eating disorders and are in the process of recovery. It does an excellent job of personalizing and demystifying the struggle with eating disorders. The celebrities come from all types of careers (political, journalistic, acting, writing, modeling, religious, entertaining, sports, paranomalistic).

Thompson, J. K., Heinberg, L. J., Altable, M., & Tantleff-Dunn, S. (1999). *Exacting beauty: Theory, assessment, and treatment of body image disturbance*. Washington, DC: American Psychological Association.

This book provides an excellent overview of theoretical approaches (societal/ social, interpersonal, feminist, behavioral, cognitive, and integrative) that explain eating disorder prevalence. It has 36 scales, surveys, and questionnaires that can be used with this population.

Suicide

Hoff, L. A., Hallisey, B. J., & Hoff, M. L. A. (2009). *People in crisis: Clinical and diversity perspectives* (6th ed.). New York, NY: Routledge.

This book is an overview of crisis work. It is divided into three sections: under-standing crisis intervention, specific crises, and suicide/homicide/catastrophic events.

James, R. K. (2008). *Crisis intervention strategies*. Belmont, CA: Thomson Brooks/Cole.

This book provides an overview of crisis intervention. It has four sections: theory and application, handling specific crises, workplace, and disaster. There is a specific chapter related to addiction.

McKeon, R. (2009). *Suicidal behavior*. Cambridge, MA: Hogrefe & Huber.

This short text of 96 pages is divided into four sections: description, theories and models, risk assessment and treatment planning, and treatment. It also has a case vignette, a case example, recommendations for further reading, and two appendices of tools and resources.

Shea, S. C. (2002). *The practical art of suicide assessment: A guide for mental health professionals and substance abuse counselors*. Hoboken, NJ: Wiley.

This book has three sections: an overview, suicidal ideation, and assessment. It has helpful appendices on assessment documentation, safety contracts, and suicide prevention websites.

Homicide

Hoff, L. A., Hallisey, B. J., & Hoff, M. L. A. (2009). *People in crisis: Clinical and diversity perspectives* (6th ed.). New York, NY: Routledge.

This book is an overview of crisis work. It is divided into three sections: understanding crisis intervention; specific crises; and suicide, homicide, or catastrophic events.

James, R. K. (2008). *Crisis intervention strategies*. Belmont, CA: Thomson Brooks/Cole.

This book provides an overview of crisis intervention. It has four sections: theory and application, handling specific crises, workplace, and disaster. There is a specific chapter related to addiction.

MANUALS/WORKBOOKS

General Mental Health/General Trauma

Linehan, M. M. (1993a). *Cognitive-behavioral treatment of borderline personality disorder*. New York, NY: Guilford.

This book comprehensively describes this treatment approach.

Linehan, M. M. (1993b). *Skills training manual for treating borderline personality disorder*. New York: Guilford.

This book comprehensively describes this treatment approach in terms of skills, teaching strategies, and discussion topics in groups.

Linehan, M. M. (in press). *Skills training manual for disordered emotional regulation*. New York, NY: Guilford.

Marra, T. (2004). *Depressed & anxious: The dialectical behavior therapy workbook for overcoming depression & anxiety*. Oakland, CA: New Harbinger.

This book has nine chapters. The first is an overview of DBT. The remaining eight are meant for the client to use as exercises (dialectics of anxiety and depression, feelings, "there must be something wrong with me," meaning making, mindfulness skills, emotional regulation, distress tolerance skills, and strategic behavioral skills).

Najavits, L. M. (2002). *Seeking safety: A treatment manual for PTSD and substance abuse*. New York, NY: Guilford.

The manual has a chapter that provides an overview of PTSD and substance abuse and a chapter that discusses how to conduct the treatment. The remainder of the manual focuses on treatment topics.

Rosenbloom, D., & Williams, M. B. (1999). *Life after trauma: A workbook for healing*. New York, NY: Guilford.

This workbook is meant for trauma survivors in general. It has eight sections that have accompanying exercises to facilitate awareness in trauma survivors. It also has a prologue with suggestions on how to use the book and an epilogue on long-term healing. Finally, it has appendices on recommended readings, the psychotherapy process, and suggestions to counselors on how to use the book.

Williams, M. B., & Poijula, S. (2002). *The PTSD workbook*. Oakland, CA: New Harbinger.

This book has 15 chapters. Each chapter has exercises that facilitate awareness about the impact of the trauma on the survivor and ways to heal from the trauma.

Addiction

Documentation Resources

Berghuis, D. J., & Jongsma, A. E. (2002). *The addiction progress notes planner*. Hoboken, NJ: Wiley.

This book is a guide to documenting the therapeutic process and can assist in eligibility determination of reimbursable treatment. It complements *The Addiction Treatment Planner, Second Edition* (2001) also published by Wiley.

Finley, J. R., & Lenz, B. S. (1999a). *The chemical dependence treatment documentation sourcebook*. New York, NY: Wiley.

This book has more than 80 forms that cover the continuum of addiction treatment and can be readily copied. It also has a disk of the forms.

Finley, J. R., & Lenz, B. S. (1999b). *Chemical dependence treatment homework planner*. New York, NY: Wiley.

This 302-page book has 53 homework assignments that can be readily copied. It also has a disk of the assignments.

Finley, J. R., & Lenz, B. S. (2003). *Addiction treatment homework planner* (2nd ed.). Hoboken, NJ: Wiley.

This book has 78 homework assignments for chemical and nonchemical addiction treatment issues. It has all the forms on a CD.

Jongsma, A. E., & Peterson, L. M. (2003). *The complete adult psychotherapy treatment planner*. Hoboken, NJ: Wiley.

This book covers numerous diagnoses and has two sections specifically on chemical dependency: chemical dependence and chemical dependence-relapse. For each one it provides: behavioral definitions, long-term goals, short-term objectives/therapeutic interventions, and diagnostic suggestions. It provides a section on how to write a treatment plan as well as two sample treatment plans.

Perkinson, R. R., & Jongsma, A. E. (1998). *The chemical dependence treatment planner*. New York, NY: Wiley.

This 248-page book provides guidelines for writing treatment plans as well as specific goals and objectives that can be used in treatment plan writing.

Resources (Workbooks)

Hazelden (2005a). *Client recovery workbook*. Center City, MN: Author.

This 143-page workbook has five sections: getting started, you and your team, 12-step and other group meetings, AA/NA/CA recovery basics, and getting ready to go off probation/parole or leaving the safety of the drug court. It has 52 exercises, each of which has an introduction and a set of questions.

Hazelden (2005b). *Client cognitive skills workbook*. Center City, MN: Author.

This 148-page workbook has eight parts: mapmaking, criminal and addiction history, becoming aware of your inner maps, learning to think about your thinking, learning to think about your behaviors, socialization, what works/what doesn't, and how to change. It has 45 exercises designed to facilitate self-exploration.

Hazelden (2005c). *Client life skills workbook*. Center City, MN: Author.

This 100-page workbook has four parts: have a plan, plan the work, the many parts of the plan, and work the plan. There is a good, simple explanation of the Stages of Change model on page 11. It looks at recovery in a holistic way. There are 52 exercises designed to facilitate the client's self-exploration.

Substance Abuse and Mental Health Services Administration (SAMHSA) (1996). *Counselor's manual for relapse prevention with chemically dependent criminal offenders* (Technical Assistance Publication Series 19; DHHS Publication No. SMA 96-3115). Rockville, MD: Author.

This 181-page booklet provides general information on addiction, relapse prevention treatment, a guide to professionals on how to use the workbook, and an appendix workbook on relapse prevention that has 27 exercises.

Co-Occurring Disorders

Center for Substance Abuse Treatment (CSAT) (2003). *Co-occurring disorders: Integrated dual disorders treatment: Implementation resource kit*. Rockville, MD.

Intimate Partner Violence

Fall, K. A., & Howard, S. (2004). *Alternatives to domestic violence* (2nd ed.). New York, NY: Brunner/Routledge.

This is a homework manual for participants in a battering intervention group. It has 12 chapters meant to facilitate self-awareness through exercises for each chapter.

Goodman, M. S., & Fallon, B. C. (1995). *Pattern changing for abused women*. Thousand Oaks, CA: Sage.

This text provides an overview of intimate partner violence counseling theory and approaches. The accompanying workbook has helpful exercises that a counselor can use in working with this population; one especially helpful handout is "Your Bill of Rights."

Minnesota Coalition for Battered Women (1992). *Safety first: A guide for counselors and advocates.* St. Paul, MN: Author.

This workbook provides very helpful guidelines on working with survivors of domestic violence.

Rosenbloom, D., & Williams, M. B. (1999). *Life after trauma: A workbook for healing.* New York: Guilford.

This workbook is meant for trauma survivors in general. It has eight sections that have accompanying exercises to facilitate awareness in trauma survivors. It also has a prologue with suggestions on how to use the book and an epilogue on long-term healing. Finally, it has appendices on recommended readings, the psychotherapy process, and suggestions to counselors on how to use the book.

Sexual Abuse

Carter, W. L. (2002). *It happened to me: A teen's guide to overcoming sexual abuse.* Oakland, CA: New Harbinger.

This book has five sections with exercises in each section meant to help teenagers become aware of their reactions to sexual abuse they have experienced.

Davis, L. (1990). *The courage to heal workbook.* New York: Harper & Row.

This workbook is designed for women and men who have survived sexual abuse. It has three sections (healing survival skills, taking stock, and healing aspects). Each section has subsections with specific exercises meant to help the survivor learn about self and heal from the sexual abuse.

Rosenbloom, D., & Williams, M. B. (1999). *Life after trauma: A workbook for healing.* New York, NY: Guilford.

This workbook is meant for trauma survivors in general. It has eight sections that have accompanying exercises to facilitate awareness in trauma survivors. It also has a prologue with suggestions on how to use the book and an epilogue on long-term healing. Finally, it has appendices on recommended readings, the psychotherapy process, and suggestions to counselors on how to use the book.

Videotapes/DVDs

General Mental Health/General Trauma

Cavalcade Productions (Producer) (1998a). *Trauma and substance abuse I: Therapeutic approaches* [video]. Available from www.calvacadeproductions.com

This 46-minute video discusses ways to work with substance abuse trauma survivors.

Cavalcade Productions (Producer) (1998b). *Trauma and substance abuse II: Special treatment issues* [video]. Available from www.calvacadeproductions.com

This 40-minute video discusses the issues of countertransference, codependency, crisis, and relapse.

Cavalcade Productions (Producer) (2005). *Numbing the pain: Substance abuse and psychological trauma* [video]. Available from www.calvacadeproductions.com

This 30-minute video examines how substance abuse has assisted survivors in their lives and the ways therapy can provide challenges and benefits to the survivor.

CNS Productions (Producer) (2008). *In & out of control* [video]. Available from www.cnsproductions.com

This 38-minute video provides general information about emotional, physical, and sexual violence.

Addiction

A&E (Producer). *Investigative reports: Inside Alcoholics Anonymous* [DVD]. Available from www.aetn.com

This 50-minute DVD provides an overview of Alcoholics Anonymous.

Films for the Humanities & Sciences (Producer) (2004). *Understanding addiction* [DVD]. Available from www.films.com

This 24-minute DVD provides overall information about addiction with one individual's story of recovery highlighted.

Hazelden (Producer) (2004). *The Hazelden Step Series for Adults* [DVD]. Available from www.hazelden.org

These three DVDs are each 12 minutes in length, and each covers one of the first three steps of Alcoholics Anonymous.

HBO Documentary Films (Producer) (2007). *Addiction* [4 DVDs]. Available from www.hbo.com/documentaries

This four-DVD set is divided into: (a) disks 1 & 2 (90 minutes), which focus on "What is Addiction?"; "Understanding Relapse"; "The Search for Treatment: A Challenging Journey"; and "The Adolescent Addict"; and (b) disks 3 & 4 (270 minutes), which have four interviews with addiction professionals, three sections on treatment, one section on drug court, and one about a mother.

Co-Occurring Disorders

See General Mental Health section above.

Intimate Partner Violence

Domestic Abuse Intervention Project (Producer) (2011a). *Power & control: A woman's perspective* [video]. Available from www.theduluthmodel.org

This one-hour video discusses power and control issues from a woman's perspective through interviews with survivors.

Domestic Abuse Intervention Project (Producer) (2011b). *Power & control: The tactics of men who batter* [video]. Available from www.theduluthmodel.org
This 40-minute video discusses power and control issues from a man's perspective through interviews with perpetrators.

New Day Films (Producer). *To have and to hold* [video]. Available from www.newday.com
This 20-minute film interviews men who have assaulted their wives.

Sexual Abuse

Fanlight Productions (Producer) (2006). *Talk to me* [DVD]. Available from www.fanlight.com
This 33-minute DVD is a summary of powerful stories of teenagers who have been sexually abused.

KB Films (Producer). *The healing years* [DVD]. Available by e-mailing: kbfilms@compuserv.com
This 52-minute DVD has a summary of different women's stories of sexual abuse and incest. A former Miss America tells her story.

WEB SITES

General Mental Health/General Trauma

Behavioral Tech. www.behavioraltech.org
This Web site provides information on workshops, training (intensive, on-line), and educational products related to DBT.

Seeking Safety. www.seekingsafety.org
This Web site provides general information about the Seeking Safety approach. It includes article and training information on the topic.

Addiction

National Association of Drug Court Professionals (NADCP). www.nadcp.org
The National Association of Drug Court Professionals (NADCP) provides general information about their organization at this Web site.

National Drug Court Institute. www.ndci.org
The National Drug Court Institute provides education, research, and scholarship for drug court intervention programs. This Web site provides information on how to access these resources.

Restorative Justice. www.restorativejustice.org
The Restorative Justice Web site provides resources such as crime victim support. The focus of this group is to repair the harm done by crime.

The National Institute on Alcohol Abuse and Alcoholism (NIAAA). www.niaaa
.nih.gov

The NIAAA Web site provides general information on alcohol use as well as
resources helpful to the counselor.

National Institute on Drug Abuse (NIDA). www.nida.nih.gov

The NIDA Web site provides general information about drug abuse as well as
numerous resources.

Substance Abuse and Mental Health Services Administration (SAMHSA). www
.samhsa.gov

The SAMHSA Web site assists in treatment location and services as well as providing resources (publications, etc.) on substance abuse.

Co-Occurring Disorders

National Institute on Drug Abuse. www.drugabuse.gov

This Web site provides general information on drug abuse and addiction.

National Institutes of Mental Health. www.nimh.nih.gov

This Web site provides information on understanding and treating mental illness.

Substance Abuse and Mental Health Services Administration (SAMHSA). www
.samhsa.gov

This Web site provides a variety of information and resources on substance
abuse and mental health.

Treatment Improvement Exchange (TIE) (SAMHSA funded). www.treatment.org

This Web site provides information on the treatment of addiction with a special
topics section that addresses concerns such as co-occurring disorders, gambling,
and homelessness.

Intimate Partner Violence

The Domestic Violence Initiative for Women with Disabilities. www.dviforwomen.org

This Web site provides information regarding domestic violence within the
disabled population of women.

The Domestic Abuse Intervention Project. www.theduluthmodel.org

This Web site provides overall information on intimate partner violence from the
Duluth Model-Domestic Abuse Intervention Project.

National Latino Alliance for the Elimination of Domestic Violence. www
.dvalianza.org

This Web site provides information on intimate partner violence in the Latino
population.

The Institute on Domestic Violence in the African-American Community. E-mail:
nidvaac@umn.edu, www.dvinstitute.org

This Web site provides information on family violence in the African-American community and provides an avenue where individuals can state their perspectives.

Jewish Women International. www.jwi.org

This Web site provides information on programs, education, and advocacy within the Jewish population.

Minnesota Coalition for Battered Women. www.mcbw.org

This organization provides general information, books, stickers, pins, posters, referrals, trainings, research, networking, and legislative lobbying.

Mending the Sacred Hoop: Technical Assistance Project. www.msh-ta.org

This Web site provides training and technical assistance to American Indians and Alaskan Natives in the effort of eliminating intimate partner violence in this population.

National Coalition Against Domestic Violence. www.ncadv.org

This Web site provides information helpful at the regional, state, and national levels. Information includes safe homes/shelters, policy development and legislation, public education, and technical assistance.

Sacred Circle National Resource Center to End Violence against Native Women. www.sacred-circle.com

This Web site provides information on intimate partner violence in American Indian and Alaskan Native tribal communities.

Sexual Abuse

Rape

Rape, Abuse, & Incest National Network (RAINN). E-mail: info@rainn.org, Web site: www.rainn.org

This Web site provides information on rape, abuse, and incest, regarding services, education, and advocacy.

Sacred Circle-National Resource Center to End Violence against Native Women. www.sacred-circle.com

This Web site provides information on sexual assault in American Indian and Alaskan Native tribal communities.

Sexual Abuse

Posttraumatic Stress Disorder Alliance. www.ptsdalliance.org

This Web site is for the Posttraumatic Stress Disorder Alliance. It has general information on PTSD as well as articles and support group information.

Rape, Abuse, & Incest National Network (RAINN). E-mail: info@rainn.org; Web site www.rainn.org

This Web site provides information on rape, abuse, and incest regarding services, education, and advocacy.

Sacred Circle-National Resource Center to End Violence against Native Women. www.sacred-circle.com

This Web site provides information on sexual assault in American Indian and Alaskan Native tribal communities.

SAMHSA (Substance Abuse and Mental Health Services Administration). www. samhsa.gov

This website provides the TIP series and their related products. Two helpful, free brochures are *Helping Yourself Heal*. One is written for recovering men (DHHS Publication No. SMA04-3969) who have been abused as children and one for recovering women (DHHS Publication No. SMA06-4132).

S. E. S. A. M. E. (Stop Educator Sexual Abuse, Misconduct, and Exploitation). E-mail: Babe4justice@aol.com; Web site: www.sesamenet.org

This Web site is for the group S. E. S. A. M. E. (Stop Educator Sexual Abuse, Misconduct, and Exploitation), whose goal is to be a national voice for preventing sexual exploitation, abuse, and harassment of students by teachers and school staff.

Survivorship. E-mail: info@survivorship.org; Web site: www.survivorship.org

This Web site provides resources for survivors of ritualistic abuse, mind control, and torture.

Suicide

American Association of Suicidology (AAS). www.suicidology.org

One can join this organization. The Web site has facts, warning signs, support groups, crisis centers, a bulletin board (members only), and a bookstore.

American Foundation for Suicide Prevention (AFSP). www.afsp.org

This Web site has statistics and suicide survivor information.

SA/VE-Suicide Awareness/Voices of Education. www.save.org

This Web site has suicide prevention education, advocates for suicide survivors, and information on developing a group for suicide survivors.

Suicide Prevention Action Network (SPAN) USA. www.spanusa.org

If You Are Thinking About Suicide . . . Read This First. www.metanoia.org/suicide

This Web site attempts to reduce the stigma around having suicidal thoughts so that the reader is open to receiving help.

CHAPTER SEVEN

Current Additional Therapies and Concepts

LEARNING OBJECTIVES

1. To learn four types of therapy (brief therapy, motivational interviewing, positive psychology, and grief therapy) and how they may apply to crisis counseling.
2. To use therapeutic techniques from these models within the context of crisis counseling.
3. To apply a spiritual focus to crisis counseling.

> Just as despair can come to one only from other human beings, hope too can be given to one only by other human beings.
>
> —*Elie Wiesel*

This chapter examines four types of therapy and their related techniques: brief therapy, motivational interviewing, positive psychology, and grief therapy. These approaches complement and overlap one another. This is why the case studies and exercises are grouped together at the end of the chapter—to provide the reader with the opportunity to compare and contrast the therapies. Also included in the discussion of these therapies are the stages of change model and the concept of client resilience. The therapies, techniques, and related concepts will be housed in the approach to crisis counseling. Three types of therapy (brief, motivational interviewing, positive psychology), the stages of change model, and the concept of client resilience are brief summaries of these areas as described in Miller (2010). The section on spirituality draws heavily from Miller's (2003) work also.

The reader is cautioned that there are numerous lists provided in this chapter. The danger in organizing a chapter in this manner is that after a few lists are provided, we may have a tendency to stop reading them carefully. Because lists are so helpful in outlining specific aspects of therapy concepts and techniques, I have chosen to include a number of lists. My hope is that the reader can work with the number by pausing before each list and recognizing the import of this framework in elucidating significant points.

Brief therapy has a philosophy highly compatible with crisis counseling, because assessments need to be done quickly, efficiently, and yet humanely. *Motivational interviewing* emphasizes the "drawing out" of the client's story through a welcoming and hopeful approach critical to crisis work. *Positive psychology* focuses on the strengths of the client, rather than the client's pathology, in an attempt to encourage change. *Grief therapy* within crisis counseling addresses the losses the client is experiencing both during and following the crisis.

The concepts of client resilience and the stages of change model are presented because of their usefulness in crisis counseling. *Client resilience* is important to examine, because the counselor in a crisis counseling situation needs to have clarity about the client's history and current status of resilience in order to draw on strengths within and outside the client. The *stages of change model* can help the counselor match the appropriate intervention level with the client's readiness for change in the situation.

Finally, the spiritual aspect of counseling is included to facilitate the effectiveness of the application of the crisis intervention theories and techniques: Keeping the client's spirit "alive" is integral to the client experiencing a resurgence of hope in the crisis situation.

BRIEF THERAPY

Brief therapy has been called *solution-focused therapy* and *planned short-term psychotherapy* with the different terms resulting from managed care and theoretical orientation influences (Bloom, 1997). Overall, it: (a) focuses on increasing coping abilities to manage future situations better and does so within a specific number of sessions that focus on specific goals (Nugent, 1994), and (b) uses a concrete definition of the problem to guide counseling that focuses on specific change with plans for the change (Littrell, 1998). Counselors using this theory also view clients' complaints as legitimate in and of themselves, believe that therapy can be too long, and think that it (therapy) is just one important part of a client's life.

Through the various terminology and theoretical orientations, the following are common aspects of brief therapy (Koss & Shiang, 1994 as described in Miller, 2010, pp. 255–256):

1. Intervention is prompt and early.
2. Therapists are active and directive.

3. Goals are specific and time limited.
4. Therapy focus is on the here and now.
5. Limited goals are to reduce symptoms and enhance coping.
6. Therapists remain focused on goals, quickly assess problems and resources, obtain necessary information to work with the situation, and have a flexible intervention approach.

Preston (1998) suggests the following six components as a framework of brief therapy: (as summarized in Miller, 2010, p. 258)

1. Rapid assessment
2. Deciding upon a focus
3. Setting time limits
4. Targeted treatment strategies
5. Homework
6. Developing additional sources of support

It is critical to note that brief therapy does not mean that the counselor has simply seen the client briefly; rather, brief therapy has intentional counseling session limits where the counselor and client agree that the problem will be addressed within a specific brief time framework. This approach has been (and still is) viewed as the antithesis of counseling work by some counselors who believe the client is seen for as long as it takes to address the problem, which cannot be determined at the onset of therapy; they may believe that counseling in the brief format lacks quality and effectiveness. These beliefs may have been reinforced by traditional training in the counseling field where effective counseling was equated with therapeutic alliance strength, resolution of resistance and transference/countertransference, counseling termination issues, and improved life functioning (Talmon, 1990).

However, changes in the counseling field from the 1960s into the 1990s have resulted in an openness to the use of brief therapy. Because of the community mental health movement in the 1960s, as many clients as possible needed to be counseled efficiently, effectively, and promptly (Bloom, 1997). In the 1980s, reduced financial resources and increased cost of and demand for counseling services facilitated an interest in the application of brief therapy, and in the 1990s, it was seen as efficient, effective, and less expensive (Nugent, 1994).

The brief therapy approach requires a shift in perspective where behaviors are viewed as changing through small, successive changes that are supported over time by others and eventually lead to larger changes. We need to look at how we view change and what we believe is required for change to occur (Littrell, 1998). We essentially serve as consultants where we teach clients to be their own counselors; the core of therapy may occur outside of sessions in their daily lives.

In this changed perspective, assessment and counseling overlap (Talmon, 1990), and a here-and-now approach is adopted that recognizes that we do not know how long we will see a client, so we need to view each session as the only known chance to have an impact on the client's life. One aspect of a here-and-now approach is _therapist immediacy_: the counselor discloses to the client (in the session) feelings about the client, the therapeutic relationship, or the counselor's self in relation to the client (Kasper, Hill, & Kivlighan, 2008). The belief underlying this approach is that clients reenact their interpersonal conflicts in therapy and such disclosure can draw out interpersonal conflicts, thereby providing the client a chance to change behavior within the counseling context.

There are three reasons counselors may be more open to using brief therapy theories and techniques. First, the financial constraints imposed on counseling by mental health agencies and managed health care systems typically limit the number of sessions allowed for counseling. Second, increased caseloads due to budget constraints or a counselor's desire to see a large number of clients can be professionally and ethically handled by provision of a balanced, realistic perspective of what can be accomplished in counseling. Third, counselors believe that they can achieve counseling goals in a shorter time period that can meet the welfare of the client.

Main Concepts

Assessment

Brief therapy may not work for every client in a crisis situation; by its nature, crisis counseling is inherently time-limited, making it an excellent match with brief therapy. However, the counselor also needs to assess the client's match with brief therapy by assessing his or her motivation, working alliance ability, relationship history, capacity for experiencing and reflecting on thoughts and feelings, and focusing ability (Bloom, 1997).

Nonetheless, counselors can approach the crisis counseling situation by following the specific components of brief therapy: minimizing historical questions, being active and direct, intervening promptly, focusing on the here and now with specific time-limited goals, and enhancing the coping abilities of the client by assessing their strengths and resources.

Treatment

The acronym FRAMES represents six aspects in brief therapy treatment: feedback, responsibility, advice, menu, empathy, and self-efficacy (W. R. Miller & Sanchez, 1994). Give _feedback_ in a nonjudgmental approach. Encourage _responsibility_ by assisting the client in viewing him/herself as being responsible for his/her choices. If giving _advice_ to the client, ask the client for permission to give it and then, again, give the advice in a nonjudgmental manner. The _menu_ component means that the counselor provides the client with options for changing behavior. _Empathy_ is where the counselor communicates that he/she is listening to the client's story in an attempt to help establish a therapeutic alliance. _Self-efficacy_ is encouraged by the counselor: The client sees that his/her self can persist after the behavior

152

change. This model can be used to guide the approach taken in the crisis work within a brief therapy framework.

There are various theoretical perspectives on brief therapy. Bloom (1997) divides these various approaches into three categories: psychodynamic, cognitive and behavioral, and strategic and systemic. A few techniques from each of these approaches are discussed in this section for crisis counseling application.

Techniques

Psychodynamic

In psychodynamic brief therapy, human behavior is seen as motivated (but the person is not aware of the motivation), personality is shaped by biology and experiences, thought/feeling/behavioral disturbance is a result of contradictory feedback, and early experiences play a part in reactions (Marmor, 1968).

In Bloom's focused single-session therapy (1997), the counselor is attempting to help the client uncover something of significance and begin a therapeutic process.

The author suggests counselors:

1. Focus on a problem.
2. Present simple ideas.
3. Be active in the latter part of the session (avoid self-disclosure, ask open-ended questions, learn the language the client speaks, provide simple information, and have the responsibility of the communication lie with the client).
4. Explore and present tentative interpretations.
5. Use empathy.
6. Be aware of the time.
7. Minimize factual questions.
8. Do not focus too much on the event that brought the client to counseling.
9. Avoid side issues.
10. Do not overestimate what the client knows about himself or herself (as stated in Miller, 2010, p. 260).

These suggestions can help the crisis client become more clear about the problem and help the counselor in the assessment, treatment, and referral process. Some of these suggestions require clarification in the crisis counseling context.

In a crisis counseling situation, the problem may be evident in the crisis. However, the crisis may house a variety of problems requiring the counselor to assist the client in prioritizing the problems and choosing one or a few on which to focus. Also, the counselor may need to adjust the focus by taking into account why the person has been referred for counseling (self-referred vs. other-referred) so both the client and referral source wishes are being met through the problem focus. Second, simple, brief, and straightforward information and ideas are necessary in crisis counseling. Personally, I encourage students and counselors to think of the few minutes following a car accident or a near car accident, and how much new information they could handle being told in that time frame. That analogy may guide the counselor in providing the right amount and type of information to the client who may be overwhelmed by the crisis situation.

To start the therapeutic process, Bloom (1997) suggests the counselor learn the myths operating about self and others, credit the client with work done leading up to the session, be aware of the client's strengths, assist in the development of social supports, educate the client with necessary information, refer for additional counseling as required, and have a follow-up plan. It is easy to see how these suggestions apply to crisis counseling. The focus is to help the client diminish the barriers to effective coping and enhance the bridges to effective coping that exist both within and outside of the client.

The techniques used from Davanloo's theory (Bloom, 1997; Davanloo, 1980) are the triangle of conflict or the triangle of person. The three endpoints on the *triangle of conflict* are labeled impulse, anxiety, and defense. An unacceptable impulse increases anxiety, resulting in a defensive reaction. The counselor needs to look for the defensive reaction in the client and trace the anxiety that stirred the defensive reaction to its impulse. For example, in a crisis situation where a person has lost all of their belongings to a house fire, the client may have relapsed into an addictive chemical behavior, such as abusing alcohol/drugs. This use was meant to reduce the anxiety that came from the unacceptable impulse of the client to strike out in anger at the world for the injustice experienced through the house fire (e.g., the fire was caused by the heating source of the apartment complex). Such a tracking may guide the counselor in realizing that the client needs assistance in developing ways to effectively express anger that are not damaging to him/herself.

In the *triangle of person*, the three endpoints on the triangle are the past, present, and future. Significant people in the client's life are present at each endpoint. From this perspective, the client may react to the counselor in a manner that is similar to how they might react to those significant individuals from the past or present. This can help the counselor understand the client's transference issues, thereby allowing the counselor to work with them more effectively. For example, if the counselor is male, and the client is in a crisis situation where she was raped by a male, if the client has a history of untrustworthy males in her life, the counselor can anticipate possible negative transference from the client, thereby inhibiting a therapeutic alliance. Such awareness may help the counselor approach the client in a gentle, slow, supportive manner respectful of the issues that stem from the countertransference. The counselor may also use this information to encourage the client to be aware of a tendency, at least in the near future, of (in this case) a difficulty in trusting males.

Additionally, I have used this concept in therapy to assist in helping the client find supportive individuals, natural healers, in his/her life. By clarifying individuals who have been influential and supportive to the client, both in terms of the past and present, the counselor can encourage the client to reach out to natural healers who are currently in his/her life and/or to add natural healers, based on past positive experiences, into his/her life. For example, a client in a crisis situation may have connected with a religious leader and community that were very helpful to them. While this leader and community may still be available, the client lost contact with them over time. The counselor may encourage the client to explore resuming contact with the leader and community and add them to their current support network in handling the crisis situation.

Cognitive and Behavioral

In this theoretical orientation, the focus is on the present, where the counselor assesses current problems, designs goals, reduces problem pressure, and increases self-efficacy (Bloom, 1997). Two approaches, Ellis's rational emotive psychotherapy (1962) and Beck's (1976) cognitive restructuring therapy, are explored.

Ellis's theory of rational emotive psychotherapy (RET) (Bloom, 1997; Ellis, 1962) presents that client actions are the results of their beliefs. Counseling is direct and active, and may involve homework, bibliotherapy, and confrontation of problems in cognition, emotion, and/or behavior by exploring the beliefs occurring between the client's experience and emotion. In crisis counseling, the crisis may have stirred irrational beliefs that are negatively impacting the coping abilities of the client. RET techniques of homework assignments, bibliotherapy, and in-session confrontation can be used to assist in intervening on the client's irrational beliefs.

For example, a client who has discovered that his wife has had an affair may be struggling with the irrational belief that he is not a competent lover. The counselor may suggest that the client view his history of his sexual experiences as a homework assignment. The client may return to the session and report that he became aware that prior to his second marriage he did not have difficulty being sexual in relationships, but in this marriage, the tendency to overwork because of increased financial burdens caused changes in the relationship dynamic, which resulted in his being away from home more and having more communication difficulties with his wife. The focus in counseling, then, could shift to the more accurate problems of overworking and decreased contact with his wife.

Beck's work (Beck, 1976; Bloom, 1997) is similar to Ellis's in that it explores the relationship between the client's thoughts and feelings. In this work, depression is seen as a product of client distortions of the self, the world, and the future that together result in a sense of hopelessness. The client's schema—his or her way of viewing the world—has an emphasis on failure and a minimization of success. In this therapy, the client's automatic thoughts (the first thoughts in reaction to a situation), life event explanations, and assumptions made about the world are examined in counseling in order to guide interventions that run counter to negative thought patterns; this can result in a sense of hope. Here it is not presence of the problems alone that determine the client's behavior, but the client's view and level of hopelessness about the problem that make the difference. The counselor can use questions in session to increase client awareness of thoughts and assumptions, as well as homework assignments such as a record-keeping log where automatic thoughts that occur between the event and the client's reaction to it are tracked.

Such a log can be quite elaborate or simple (depending on the client's motivation, comfort with journal keeping, and one's life situation), but needs to include categories such as date, situation description, feeling, automatic thought, and possibly intensity of feeling (on a scale of 1 to 10, or 1 to 100). A category of responding thought needs to be added after the automatic thought category; this can be added after the client keeps the log so the counselor and client together can develop responding thoughts to the negative, automatic ones. Some clients may have an easier time recording their feelings or their thoughts. I encourage them to make their best guess in the category that is difficult for them and we can fine-tune these distinctions in their counseling. In crisis counseling, such a log can provide the client with a sense of hope, self-control, and increased self-observation skills, thereby increasing their life choices. An example of this may be when a client has had a difficult work situation in which she felt continually attacked by her supervisor, which resulted in a crisis at work where she was almost fired, causing her to seek counseling through an employee assistance program. Her homework assignment was to track the work situations that raised her anxiety in a cognitive-behavioral log format. In doing so, she discovered negative automatic thoughts ("No matter what I do it will not be good enough to keep them from firing me") and negative underlying assumptions ("I have always failed at every job I have ever had"). These negative automatic thoughts led her to behave in a self-defeating manner in the workplace. By learning to counter her automatic thoughts through responding thoughts developed in therapy ("I am only responsible for putting forth the best effort I can"), she was able to stave off being fired, because her behavior reflected a more positive, hopeful, collaborative attitude.

Strategic and Systemic

The specific theory addressed in this section is De Shazer's solution-based brief therapy (Bloom, 1997; De Shazer, 1985). This orientation, which began in the mid-1970s, emphasizes the solutions rather than the problems in marriages and families. It attempts to change the perceptions and behaviors of clients and help them gain better access to their strengths. The counselor looks at the symptoms of the problem, but also looks for the exceptions to the problem, when it does not exist, and based on this information helps the client intervene on the problem by developing specific goals. One common technique is to ask the miracle question in a session: "If a miracle occurs tonight while you are asleep and the problem is eliminated, how will you know the next morning? How will others know? What will you be doing differently or saying differently?" Such a question underscores for the client what constitutes healthy functioning, and the solutions to the problem are determined by the client (Kingsbury, 1997). As with the cognitive-behavioral therapies, sessions often involve homework to help the client find successful problem resolution (Huber & Backlund, 1992) and support for the change (Preston, 1998).

Also, scaling questions (scales of 1 to 10 or 1 to 100) can be used to describe issue intensity experienced by the client, determine client progress, and track behavior that has helped with problem resolution (Berg, 1995). For example, after asking the miracle question, the counselor can use scaling questions to clarify the information: "On a scale of 1 to 10, 10 being the highest point, in what settings do you have the greatest urge to abuse your child, and what point on the scale would you assign to each of those settings?" And: "In the past week, using a scale of 1 to 10 again, scale the most stressful interaction you had with your child and describe that experience." Finally, asking clients questions about their significant others can be helpful to the counseling process (e.g., how they rate their significant others, how they rate the client's progress in counseling, and where they see the client in terms of change) (Berg, 2000).

Overall, the counselor is helping the client develop a goal focus, explore the problem the client desires to change, explore when the problem does not happen (exceptions), and what the client will be doing differently once the problem is resolved (Littrell, 1998). In exploring exceptions to problems, the counselor wants to help the client "demystify" how the exception occurs, so the client realizes the behavior does not happen in a vacuum and can choose to take the action more often in a conscious, deliberate manner that builds on small changes.

MOTIVATIONAL INTERVIEWING

Motivational interviewing (MI) (W.R. Miller & Rollnick, 2002) originated in addiction treatment in the 1970s and 1980s, when the common treatment for addicts was highly confrontational and the client was seen as fully responsible for treatment and recovery motivation and needing to "hit bottom" in order to be motivated for change (DiClemente, Garay, & Gemmell, 2008). Since that time, MI has become quite popular in the counseling field in general and now has an international organization of trainers and a Web site (www.motivationalinterview .org). In its popularity, different myths about MI have arisen, leading to Miller and Rollnick's (2009) article stating what MI is not:

1. Anchored in the transtheoretical model (TTM)
2. "A way of tricking people into doing what they don't want to do" (p. 131)
3. A technique
4. A decisional balance (an examination of the pros and cons of change, but more of trying to find the client's motivation to change)
5. Requiring assessment feedback (MI was paired with structured personal feedback based on intake assessment treatment in Project Match that was called Motivational Enhancement Therapy)
6. A form of cognitive-behavior therapy
7. Simply client-centered counseling

8. Easy (but it is simple)
9. What counselors are already doing
10. A panacea designed to address all the client problems a counselor faces (Miller, 2010, p. 251)

Main Concepts

What is MI then? As number 3 above states, it is more than technique. Its techniques are very helpful to clients, but it is larger than techniques. Maybe we could think of it like the human body: it would be wrong to think of the human body only in terms of its arm; the body is a system, and one of its helpful parts is an arm. MI is a spirit, a style of counseling that is based on a relational component of empathy, and its "helpful parts" are its techniques. The technical aspect of it, the techniques, comes from the evocation and reinforcement of change talk (Miller & Rose, 2009).

Clients typically approach counseling with ambivalence about receiving help (DiClemente, Garay, & Gemmell, 2008). MI works with this ambivalence, which is viewed as normal and natural in response to change, by exploring it and resolving it, thereby inviting behavior change. It is an interaction (Sorbell, 2009)—a welcoming approach to clients that intends to plant seeds of hope for change in them and invite change from them. It is an "agenda-driven, directive style [used] while maintaining a non-confrontational approach" (Tober and Raistrick, 2007, p. 6). It has been described as: optimistic, hopeful, strengths-based (Van Wormer & Davis, 2008), practical, accessible, and grounded in theory and research (Arkowitz, Westra, Miller, & Rollnick, 2008). The words *collaboration*, *evocation*, and *autonomy* are key words in this theory (W. R. Miller & Rollnick, 2002; Adams & Madson, 2006).

MI has been found to be useful throughout the counseling process—engagement, assessment, and treatment—especially when change ambivalence arises (Harvard Mental Health Letter, 2011). There are four general principles of MI (Miller & Rollnick, 2002): empathy, discrepancy, self-efficacy, and resistance. *Empathy* needs to be accurate and involve nonpossessive warmth and genuineness (Rogers, 1951). The counselor needs to practice reflective listening and an ability to let go of assumptions and a tendency to give advice (the "righting reflex," Miller & Rollnick, 2002), as well as encourage the client to do most of the talking about the change process (Sorbell, 2009). Such a nonargumentative, respectful approach, paired with a genuine desire to understand the client's point of view, invites an open discussion of the problem. This allows the counselor to make a more accurate assessment and thereby develop a more accurate treatment approach with the client, thus motivating them to change. Empathy facilitates motivation, a readiness to change (Sorbell, 2009), has been described as elusive (Shaw, Ritvo, & Irvine, 2005) and complex (DiClemente, Garay, & Gemmell, 2008). With MI, clients are invited to change, drawn to change by what they love because this is how we are as humans: We change for what we love. Therefore, counselors need to find out what clients love in order to help them act in their best interest. Note that some clients need to be taught what to love, because their values are so deeply distorted as a result of their life experiences; with such clients, often, finding them placements in inpatient treatment settings can be beneficial because behaviors that are self- and other-enhancing can be reinforced.

Discrepancy is important, because it can also encourage a motivation to change. When there is conflict between a client's behavior and his/her values, it is often the behavior that will change (W. R. Miller & Rollnick, 2002). Counselors can encourage change motivation by focusing on the discrepancy between who the client is and who the client wants to be.

Self-efficacy is a related concept. Self-efficacy means that the client has confidence that a change can be made (W. R. Miller & Rollnick, 2002). The client views him/herself as being able to persist at change and use internal and external supports to make that happen; the counselor helps the client have and maintain the belief that change is possible (Miller & Rollnick, 2002), that there is hope for change. Finally, the counselor needs to assess how important the change is to the client, as well as how confident the client is that the change can be made. This aspect of the assessment can help the counselor determine the client's values that may motivate change. For example, if a client is engaged in high-risk sexual behavior and is in a crisis situation due to finding out he/she may have HIV/AIDS, the counselor may respond by assessing importance and confidence regarding a decrease in high-risk sexual behavior. In so doing, the counselor may discover that while the client does not view it as important to make the change, he/she does have confidence that he/she can make such a change. The client may rate the importance as a 2 on a scale of 1 to 10, but confidence in his/her ability to make the change as a 10. This information tells the counselor that the client, if motivated by values (e.g., caring about others' lives or his/her own), has the confidence that a change can be made. Therefore, the counselor needs to determine which of the client's values might encourage such a behavior change. A large discrepancy with change viewed as important and high self-efficacy regarding the change will result in a lowered tendency in the client to use defense mechanisms (denial, rationalization, or projection) (W. R. Miller & Rollnick, 2002).

In MI, *resistance* is seen as natural and is "marked" in the session by the counselor: The counselor uses it as a "traffic signal" to do something different. Rather than confronting the client directly on the resistance, the counselor uses the appearance of resistance as a signal to join the client in an attempt to understand the resistance and then approach the discussion of the problem in a manner that involves rolling with the resistance (W.R. Miller & Rollnick, 2002).

In addition to these general principles of MI, there are six specific traps counselors need to avoid in session:

1. Engaging in a question-and-answer format
2. Taking sides on the change issue

3. Playing the expert
4. Labeling the problem
5. Developing a premature focus
6. Blaming the client for the behavior (W. R. Miller & Rollnick, 2002, as cited in Miller, 2010, p. 253)

These concepts are easily applicable to crisis counseling. In crisis counseling, the counselor is approaching the session with a desire to welcome the client and provide him/her with a sense of hope. An acceptance of the client and provision of hope for living through the crisis can be an umbilical cord of nurturance to the client who feels adrift. The client can "catch" the contagious "germs" of acceptance and hope from the counselor at a time that he/she feels an ebb of those within him/herself.

Techniques

There are a number of MI techniques that can be used in crisis situations. W.R. Miller and Rollnick (2002) encourage the use of the **OARS+** strategies:

1. Asking *Open* questions
2. *Affirming* the client (in terms of change attempts, strengths, etc.)
3. Listening *Reflectively*
4. *Summarizing*
5. + Eliciting *change talk* (Miller, 2010, p. 253)

Open questions, questions or statements that elicit the client's story, are those that avoid resulting in dichotomous answers. *Affirmations* are genuine comments made by the counselor that emphasize the strengths of the client—what is "good" or "right" about the client. *Reflections* are comments made by the counselor that reflect and restate what the client says in the session, letting the client know that he or she has been heard correctly. *Summary* statements are essentially a longer reflection. These can be thought of as a "paragraph" of reflection statements that are again trying to convey to the client that his/her story has been heard accurately. The use of the OARS will facilitate the expression of the crisis story, helping the counselor make the most accurate assessment possible, thereby allowing for a more personalized and effective treatment for the crisis. Also, the OARS acronym can be used by the counselor to keep a session balanced in terms of inclusion of each of the OARS components. This may be critical in crisis counseling, where the counselor may be facing his/her own anxiety about handling the crisis situation effectively in the face of intense emotions.

Change talk means that in the session, the client is talking about the problem in terms of changing it. Here the client recognizes there is a problem, shows concern for it, is planning to change it, and has an optimism about the change (Miller & Rollnick, 2002).

The client shows *Desire* to make the change ("I want to do this . . ."), an *Ability/* self-efficacy to make the change ("I can see myself doing this . . ."), *Reason* for the change ("I need to change because . . ."), *Need* for the change("I need to do something . . ."), and *Commitment* to make the change ("I will make this change.") (DARN-C), which encourage change talk (Miller, 2004).

Seven techniques for eliciting change talk in a client are (Miller, 2010, pp. 253–254):

1. *Asking evocative questions*: These questions encourage expressions of the client's views and concerns.
2. *Using the importance ruler*: Ask the client to rate on a scale—from 0 (not at all) to 10 (extremely)—the importance of change in the behavior, and to follow it with questions: "Why are you at a___ and not zero?" and "What would it take for you to go from ___ to a [a higher number]?" This scale can also be used to ask the client how confident he or she is about making the change.
3. *Exploring the decisional balance*: The client weighs the pros and cons of change, and you help the client explore this balance.
4. *Elaborating*: When the client gives a reason to change, ask for clarification, an example, or a description of when the change last occurred. Or ask, "What else?"
5. *Querying extremes*: Ask the client for extremes in terms of concerns about his/ her behavior (and others'), or the best consequences that could result from making a change.
6. *Looking back*: The client looks back to a time when the problem behavior didn't exist and compares it to the present.
7. *Looking forward*: The client looks to the future to describe how a change would impact the future or what it will be like in the future if no change is made.

Each of these seven techniques can be used as needed in the crisis counseling situation. In using these techniques, it is important to not overwhelm the client with too much information gathering or too many problems to address in the crisis situation. Again, focusing on the aspects of the crisis that seem of most import is helpful to both the client and the counselor in handling the crisis situation.

STAGES OF CHANGE MODEL

Because clients come to counseling with different levels of motivation, the stages of change model underscores the importance of counselors matching interventions with client motivation level. This model is the best known aspect of the transtheoretical model (TTM) that was developed in the early 1980s (Miller & Rollnick, 2009). People change when the right process happens at the right time (Prochaska, DiClemente, & Norcross, 1992). The model is presented here because when it emerged in the early 1980s, it came alongside motivational interviewing (MI). While this model and MI are different models, the fit between them is a natural one (Miller & Rollnick, 2009).

Main Concepts

● The stages of the model are: *precontemplation, contemplation, preparation, action, maintenance,* and *termination.* In the *precontemplation* stage, the client does not intend to change the behavior, has little awareness that it is a problem, and is resistant to change (Prochaska & Norcross, 2002). In the *contemplation* stage, the client is aware of a problem and, while thinking seriously about changing the problem, has not made a commitment to do so. In the *preparation* stage, the client has plans to take action within a month and has tried unsuccessfully to take action in the past year. In the *action* stage, the client is addressing the problem by changing behavior, experiences, and/or the environment. In the *maintenance* stage, there is prevention of relapse and change has been consistent for at least six months. In the *termination* stage, relapse does not need to be prevented, because the change is complete.

Techniques

Four general recommendations to counselors working with the stages of change are as follows (Prochaska & Norcross, 2001):

1. Assess the client's stage level.
2. Avoid treatment of every client as being in the action stage.
3. Set realistic goals with clients.
4. Match the change process with the stage.

Two related concepts that counselors need to consider as general factors in counseling: *decisional balance* and *self-efficacy* (DiClemente, 2003). Decisional balance means that the client is weighing the benefits and costs of change, which can impact the stages of change. The client's self-efficacy—how much they view themselves as able to persist at change—impacts the action and long-term change stages. Specific processes, interventions, can be used to assist clients in moving from one stage to another (Prochaska & Norcross, 2002).

1. *Precontemplation to Contemplation*: Here *consciousness raising* techniques such as bibliotherapy and confrontation may help the client realize that maybe both change and therapy could be helpful to him/her. The techniques of *self-reevaluation* (examining what they value and how they view themselves) and *dramatic relief* (experiencing feelings about both problems and solutions through grief exercises or role-plays) can also encourage client movement from one stage to another.

2. *Contemplation to Preparation*: Techniques that facilitate *self-liberation* (the client starts to believe that change can happen through commitment/willpower) by encouraging decisions and commitment.

3. *Preparation to Action*: Here techniques of *reinforcement* and *counterconditioning* (replacing behaviors with healthier ones) are useful.

4. *Action to Maintenance*: *Stimulus control* techniques help the client be aware of relapse.

Counselors in crisis situations can use knowledge of these stages of change to help choose interventions that match the client's stage level. Appropriate matching can result in a reduction of resistance and treatment dropout, as well as increase treatment effectiveness through appropriate treatment plan development (Washton & Zweben, 2006).

POSITIVE PSYCHOLOGY

Positive psychology has existed for more than 100 years (Taylor, 2001), but has become more strong since the 1990s when it began to focus on positive subjective experiences (such as hope and "flow"), personality traits (strengths in a person's character and life virtues such as perseverance and wisdom), and social institutional qualities that can strengthen both experiences and traits (Robbins, 2008; Seligman, Steen, Park, & Peterson, 2005). It encourages psychology to look more completely at the individual rather than to focus on the client's suffering. In the past, psychology may have had a leaning toward a negative focus on the individual because of a need to assist people in survival, a tendency to assume people had conditions they needed to live, and the evolution of American culture (now, comparatively, a more stable, prosperous, and peaceful country) that has more room to examine the positive aspects both within and outside of the individual (Seligman and Csikszentmihalyi, 2000).

Main Concepts

Human beings need a positive reason to live, and this psychology theory attempts to encourage people to live and flourish instead of simply existing (Keyes & Haidt, 2003). It promotes what is good in life (being happy, finding meaningful work, volunteering for good causes). Happiness means the person has positive emotions and experiences engagement with and meaning in life (Seligman, 2002). The goal of positive psychology is to promote the good in life (stay happy, find meaningful work, volunteer for good causes) (Kogan, 2001).

It aims to assist clients in developing positive emotions, experiences, and traits (Harvard Mental Health Letter, 2008). In individuals who are already healthy, it tries to enhance their well-being and optimal functioning through a "build what's strong approach" (Seligman, as quoted in the Harvard Mental Health Letter, 2008). Instead of asking "What is wrong about people?" positive psychology asks "What is right about people?" It draws on the work of humanistic psychologists such as Maslow (character strengths and virtues of self-actualized people) and Rogers (fully functioning individuals) (Robbins, 2008). It believes that certain characteristics both within and outside the person (courage, future-mindedness, optimism, interpersonal skill, faith, work ethic, hope, honesty, perseverance, and capacity for flow and insight) help buffer against mental illness (Seligman and Csikszentmihalyi, 2000).

Some of the terms of positive psychology—*valued experiences*, *positive individual traits*, and *civic virtues*—require explanation. *Valued experiences* are related to the past (well-being, contentment, satisfaction), the future (hope and optimism), and the present (flow and happiness). Flow, one of the valued experiences, means the person focuses on a task involving concentration, skill, and perseverance, where the individual enjoys the activity for its own sake and experiences a sense of harmony and self-integration during the activity (Csikszentmihalyi, 1990). There are a number of *positive individual traits* (capacity for love and vocation, courage, interpersonal skill, aesthetic sensibility, perseverance, forgiveness, originality, future-mindedness, spirituality, talent, and wisdom). *Civic virtues* are related to a group of individuals and include responsibility, nurturance, altruism, civility, moderation, tolerance, and work ethic.

Through the application of this theory to counseling, clients can become more self-assured in the world by being alert, open, and finding problem solutions by allowing the problem to emerge. Counselors can assist clients in goal setting, increasing awareness of themselves and their world, taking enjoyment in the here and now, and experiencing immersion in their activities—all of which can provide a client with hope for living.

One of the limits of positive psychology is that it requires more research. As a result, the current encouragement to counselors is to include the techniques of it in traditional therapy (Harvard Mental Health Letter, 2008). For example, at the University of Pennsylvania it is being used to increase positive emotions and client strengths and sense of meaning.

Crisis counseling lends itself well to the concepts of positive psychology. In a crisis, the individual has a tendency to focus on the negative, and the counselor can assist the client in finding some positive aspects of the situation. It is important for the counselor to stay realistic and respectful in this process, however, because otherwise the client may feel as though they are not being heard, are being judged, or are simply being disrespected by the counselor, resulting in a reduced chance for a therapeutic alliance. If the counselor can respectfully, gently, and firmly point out factors such as client strengths and resources, this approach can serve as an encouragement to the client in the face of a situation(s) that can feel overwhelming.

Techniques

Four guiding principles for integrating positive psychology into therapy are (Kauffman, 2006):

1. Changing the focus in counseling to a positive one
2. Encouraging the language of strength

3. Balancing the positive and negative
4. Developing strategies that are hope-building

Additional suggestions are:

1. Look at the strengths and resources of the client by expanding the assessment process to gather such information (Harris, Thoresen, & Lopez, 2007).
2. Reframe weaknesses as strengths (Gelso & Woodhouse, 2003).
3. Examine language and problem conceptualization (Harris et al., 2007).
4. View symptoms as logical responses, given the client's historical life context (Gelso & Woodhouse, 2003).

Finally, Seligman et al. (2005) provide five specific examples of positive psychology techniques: gratitude visit, three good things in life, you at your best, using signature strengths in a new way, and identifying signature strengths:

> In the *gratitude visit* exercise, the client has one week to write and send a letter of gratitude to someone they have never thanked for their kindness. *Three good things in life* requires the client to write down three things that went well in a day and why—for one week. *You are at your best* has the client write a story about a time they were at their best and look for the strengths in the story and review the story once each day. *Using signature strengths in a new way* means taking the inventory of character strengths online (http://www.authentichappiness.org), receiving feedback on one's top five strengths and then for one week using one of these in a new and different way each day. *Identifying signature strengths* is a shorter version of the previous technique where the client simply uses their strengths more often in a week. (Miller, 2010, pp. 245–246)

As stated in the previous section of main concepts, the counselor needs to use these techniques of positive psychology thoughtfully with regard to crisis situations. For example, asking a client experiencing a crisis to participate in the homework assignment of *three good things in life* may not fit appropriately with the person's life context, and may come across as inappropriate and disrespectful. As with all counseling techniques, the concept of timing of the intervention is a large part of determining its appropriateness and effectiveness.

GRIEF THERAPY

Grief therapy is discussed in this chapter because often, people in crisis situations are faced with loss that needs to be addressed as a part of the crisis. Grief is an interesting phenomenon; it seems to have a force of its own that needs to be respected as it ebbs and flows within an individual's life. In this work, it is very critical to listen to the client's story so the counselor makes sure that the losses heard in the story are actually the client's and not the projections of the counselor on the client's story. The clarifying strategies of listening skills that are basic to counseling need to be used here. Also, approaches such as MI can be used to assure the counselor that the client is being heard.

When practicing grief therapy, the counselor can experience a sense of being overwhelmed, such as in practicing sex therapy if one is not an expert in this area. However, the counselor needs to approach this area as they would any area of counseling. First, the commitment in counseling is to the welfare of the client and practicing within one's area of competence. If the counselor is committed to both of these guidelines, then the counselor can more comfortably put on the lens of grief therapy in counseling. One can integrate this lens into any theory of counseling used typically by the counselor; it is important that we do not underestimate doing that with which we are comfortable. A statement from the martial arts that can guide this view is: It is better to practice one technique a thousand times than to practice a thousand techniques once. The framework is meant to focus the lens of grief therapy on the issues presented in the session within the counseling framework with which we are comfortable.

Second, because issues such as grief and trauma processing overlap in counseling, it can be confusing to sort out what issue belongs to what area (Neimeyer & Wogrin, 2008). For example, a client who is experiencing depersonalization may be experiencing it as a result of PTSD related to the crisis or a significant loss. Another client may experience symptoms of depression that are more connected to grief than to a depression that stands alone. While an accurate diagnosis is important, it is critical that the difficulties being presented are addressed from the framework that is most appropriate for the client and that best fits the counselor. For example, the counselor may be working with a client who has PTSD symptoms of depersonalization related to the crisis, and shift to talking with the client about the losses that are being and have been experienced through the crisis.

The reader, then, is encouraged to read this section with a view of "Take what you like and leave the rest." Derive from the narrative those concepts and techniques of the large body of grief work that seem most useful within your practice and your population. For example, play therapy may be especially effective with traumatized children (Webb, 2001).

Especially important is to not overwhelm the client with grief work in addition to issues presented. Depending on the type of crisis, the client's level of internal and external resources, and the reality of the client's current life, grief work in itself can overwhelm the client, who may already be experiencing feelings of being overwhelmed. It is more beneficial for the counselor to have the lens of grief work focused and then determine whether it is clinically appropriate, including the timing of the interventions, to process the grief directly with the client and at that time. Once again, the importance of the welfare of the client is paramount.

Main Concepts

What is grief? The simple definition being used here is that it is a reaction to a change or loss that is significant to the individual; in that way, it is part of the person's healing process. It is strong emotion that incorporates the feelings of helplessness and passivity and an emotion that the client cannot control (Leming & Dickinson, 1998). It manifests itself in:

- *Feelings* (sadness, anger, guilt/self-reproach, anxiety, loneliness, fatigue, helplessness, shock, yearning, emancipation, relief, numbness)
- *Physical sensations* (hollowness, tightness, oversensitivity to noise, depersonalization, breathlessness, weakness, decreased energy, dry mouth)
- *Cognitions* (disbelief, confusion, preoccupation, sense of deceased's presence, hallucinations)
- *Behaviors* (sleep and appetite disturbances, absent-minded behavior, social withdrawal, dreams of the deceased, avoidance of reminders of the deceased, searching and calling out, sighing, restless overactivity, crying, visiting places/carrying objects that are reminders of the deceased, treasuring objects belonging to the deceased) (Worden, 2009)

Also, there may be:

- Susceptibility to illness
- Problems with memory and concentration
- Despair
- Depression
- Loss of pleasure (Stroebe, Hansson, Stroebe, & Schut, 2001)

In terms of relationships, grief involves attachment that come from a need of security and safety that we develop early in our lives, and the greater our loss potential, the greater the power of our reactions and the type (Bowlby, 1977). Engel (1961) proposed that when we lose someone, it is similar to physical trauma that draws us from a healthy state, and mourning the loss can bring us back to a balanced state through the process of mourning. Mourning, then, is an adaptation to loss, involving four tasks (Worden, 2009). First, the individual needs to accept the reality of the loss. Clients may show denial here in various ways: leaving items of the deceased around, denying the meaning of the loss to them, forgetting the person selectively, and denying that the death is irreversible. Second, the client needs to work through the pain of the grief. Barriers to working through the grief include receiving messages that block the expression of the grief ("Don't feel sorry for yourself"), refusing to feel the emotions, and finding a geographical cure. Third, the person needs to adjust to the environment in which the deceased person is missing. The client needs to adjust to the deceased person no longer acting a role in his/her life; he/she also needs to adjust to a new sense of him/herself, and a new sense of the world without the deceased person in it. Fourth, the client needs to "emotionally relocate" the deceased and proceed with his/her life. Here the barrier is when the client *does not love* again.

These tasks of mourning are not necessarily limited to relationships that end in physical death. They can also apply to relationships that have simply ended or that are broken to a point of nonrepair for the client. The lack of physical death does not necessarily impact the loss experienced by the client in the crisis situation; it only makes it different. An example of this may be a personal crisis (e.g., partner's affair in a committed relationship) or a professional crisis (e.g., betrayal of a significant co-worker/boss in a workplace), where the individual is still living in the world, but the loss experienced is the loss of the relationship as it was known. The tasks still need to be addressed and respected in the client's journey through the counseling process. In fact, the client may have even more difficulty allowing him/herself to grieve, because while there is a "death," the death is not necessarily seen or respected by others.

Both the counselor and the client may experience a need to predict what is going to happen in the grief process, as well as how long it is going to last (Friedman & James, 2009). Such a need may result in simplistic, formulated approaches to grief, such as Kubler-Ross's five stages of dying (1968)—approaches that may actually end up warping the client's process of grief. Rather, it is critical to see the grief process as a messy and unique one.

Grief needs to be viewed from a larger perspective—one that holds that it is a natural result of loss experienced by the client in relation to numerous life events (moving, job loss, homelessness, acquired disability, incarceration) (Shallcross, 2009). Grief is normal and natural when we experience loss. Factors such as the loss of meaning to the client or the time and intensity of the relationship loss may directly impact the level of feelings experienced in the loss.

Grief therapy assists the client in meaning reconstruction through the concepts of narrative truth, discourse and rhetoric, the tacit dimension, the relational self, and evolutionary epistemology (Neimeyer, 2002). In *narrative truth*, the loss interrupts our creation of our life story, causing us to reorganize and rewrite the narrative of our life in an intelligent, continuous manner that ties our past to our future. Counseling can provide a safe place to reorganize one's life story. In *discourse and rhetoric*, the client uses language to express the construction of the meaning of the loss in terms of family, community, and culture. Here the counselor needs to watch for gaps in the client's story or inconsistencies between word use and emotional expressions, and work with those in a manner that "unfreezes" the client (e.g., role-playing). The *tacit dimension* means that we use words that are suggestive, that have a texture that requires additional exploration. We need to look at how we make meaning out of the transitions in our lives that inherently redefine how we identify ourselves and others and how we interact with the world. The counselor needs to listen carefully and help the client create a new dialogue. In the *relational self aspect*, the loss of relationships may change our self-narrative and strain our sense of identity in relation to our connection with others. Here the counselor can assist the client by providing a therapeutic relationship in which the client examines his or her identity with the counselor, validating this narrative change. Finally, in *evolutionary epistemology*, human beings experiment with new ways of being that are selectively chosen to fit into the social world. Loss challenges the client to find parts of the self-narrative that can be retained or to experiment with new identities that work better in the current context of one's life. Reflection and questioning counseling techniques can assist clients with this process.

Related to narrative therapy is a sensitivity to the use of the client's metaphors that may be used to describe the grief experience. Metaphors assist in the negotiation of the client's reality of the loss (Nadeau, 2006). A counselor, then, attuned to the metaphors used by the client, can understand more deeply the grief as it is experienced by the client.

The counselor can use the specific techniques presented below to facilitate the client through the grief process. At the same time, the counselor needs to recognize the individual's unique way of processing, consider the messages and influences of the client's culture on the grief process, and help the client process the shattered assumptions/meanings and assist them in finding new meanings (Shallcross, 2009). The interventions also need to be developmentally appropriate (Sandovai, Scott, & Padilla, 2009).

Techniques

Shallcross (2009) summarizes the work of various counselors and experts in the field of grief work as the following:

- Identifying client strengths
- Honoring the relationship, but moving on in life
- Recognizing that the grief may resurface
- Using three-generation genograms to trace loss/grief experiences
- Writing a dialogue letter
- Using a keepsake in session to stimulate discussion
- Making booklines that document the grief journey
- Creating resilient images in the client's mind
- Journaling
- Using the empty chair technique
- Providing opportunities for emotional expression through art
- Practicing rituals

Worden (1991) adds the following techniques to this list:

- Using language that evokes emotional responses from clients and a reality check for them
- Role-playing
- Cognitive restructuring
- Developing a memory book

If a counselor is thoughtful in applying the lens of grief therapy to crisis work, the client can benefit from such application with a greater clarity of the issues being faced and addressed in terms of loss. Neimeyer and Wogrin (2008) advocate a counseling approach that combines knowledge of bereavement, counseling training, and a counselor having an informed, humble recognition of his/her role in the grief change process.

CLIENT RESILIENCE

Resilience is one of the concepts that is closely related to the five therapies discussed in this chapter. It is necessary to discuss because in crisis counseling, an individual's resilience can make a significant difference in their surviving the crisis and in how they survive it. Resilience has been defined as getting up once more than we are knocked down and being ordinary rather than magical (Masten, 2001). It has also been defined as "the process of adapting well in the face of adversity, trauma, tragedy, threats, or even significant sources of stress—such as family and relationship problems, serious health problems, or workplace and financial stressors" (Discovery Health Channel & American Psychological Association [APA], 2002, p. 2).

The definition of resilience includes both outcome and dynamic process definitions (Ryff & Singer, 2003). *Outcome* looks at how the individual improves mentally or physically after a challenge, while the *dynamic process* definition describes the individual as having a successful engagement with the events and experiences of difficulties that face the individual. Related to these definitions are the ideas of "reserve capacity" and "thriving." *Reserve capacity* means that the person has the potential to change, to grow (Staudinger, Marsiske, & Baltes, 1995). *Thriving* states that the person is improved after a trauma (Ryff & Singer, 2003). People who thrive appear to have psychological and social factors that protect them: "coping strategies, flexible self-concepts, quality relationships with others, positive comparison processes" (Ryff & Singer, 2003, p. 23).

The person's growth following a trauma may cause a shift in self-perception and view/philosophy of life, a respect of self-vulnerability, more intimate relationships, as well as deepened appreciation of significant others and self-disclosure (Tedeschi & Calhoun, 1995).

Main Concepts

The Discovery Health Channel and APA (2002) report five main concepts of resilience:

1. People can learn to be resilient, to "bounce back."
2. The development of resilience is personal and unique.
3. Being resilient does not preclude difficult times.
4. Resilience is not something that is extraordinary.
5. Resilience is ongoing, requiring time and effort (Miller, 2010, p. 246).

Techniques

Resilience requires the examination of both internal and external factors with regard to the client. Clients can learn through counseling to assess and name these factors so that they can intentionally "play to their strengths" when they face adverse situations, which can result in an increase of hope. Clients can learn to be resilient no matter what life hands them. Counselors can assist in this process by helping clients name and assess their deficits and helping them find self-protective and adaptive responses (Leadbeater, Dodgen, & Solarz, 2005), such as coping/problem-solving skills and social supports (National Institute of Drug Abuse [NIDA], 2006). Also, counselors can help clients increase their resilience by:

1. Learning/using new coping strategies
2. Developing a flexible self-concept
3. Having quality relationships
4. Developing positive comparison processes (Ryff & Singer, 2003)

Positive comparison processes involve both intra- and inter-feedback loops. The intra-feedback loop is the client's self-talk. The client needs to become aware of the self-talk that is occurring. This self-talk is connected to the inter-feedback loop, from which the client receives feedback on the effectiveness of coping strategies and the kinds of relationships needed in such demanding circumstances. Counseling can provide the client with such feedback.

A counselor can use the following two frameworks to enhance client resilience. In the first framework, a counselor can assist the client in developing:

- Caring and supportive relationships
- The capacity to create realistic plans and to take necessary steps to create those plans
- A positive self-view and confidence
- Communication and problem-solving skills
- The ability to manage intense feelings and impulses (Discovery Health Channel & APA, 2002)

A second framework the counselor can use to build resilience in the client is the following 10-item list (adapted from the Discovery Health Channel and American Psychological Association, 2002):

Ten Ways to Build Resilience

1. Make connections.
2. Avoid seeing crises as insurmountable problems.
3. Accept that change is a part of living.

4. Move toward your goals.
5. Take decisive actions.
6. Look for opportunities for self-discovery.
7. Nurture a positive view of yourself.
8. Keep things in perspective.
9. Maintain a hopeful outlook.
10. Take care of yourself.

The Discovery Channel and APA's packet titled *Aftermath: The Road to Resilience*, in conjunction with their *The Road to Resilience* project, provides community-based tools and information to facilitate resilience in individuals and communities. Professionals can access this information by calling (800) 964-2000 or visiting www.apa.org/helpcenter/index.aspx.

There are three general ways counselors can assist clients in increasing their resilience (Miller, 2010, p. 248):

1. *Develop a more positive view of themselves.* Individual tendencies (e.g., being positive) are important in having resilience (Eisenberg & Wang, 2003).
2. *Develop supportive relationships.* Interpersonal relationships that nurture the person's qualities that are resilient are a critical component of resilience (Caprara & Cervone, 2003).
3. *Learn to make plans, learn problem-solving skills, and learn to manage intense feelings.* Human strength, resilience, is framed as persevering, "hanging on" and "letting go," and experiencing growth changes in oneself (Carver & Scheier, 2003).

As stated earlier, crisis counseling needs to be anchored in client resilience. Helping clients find and enhance their resilience can make all the difference in the outcome of crisis counseling, because it operates as a reserve tank for the client who is living in the crisis situation.

SPIRITUALITY

The reader may ask why there is a focus on spirituality in crisis counseling and at this point in the chapter. A crisis in our lives "shakes us up." It causes us to be catapulted into existential issues that we have not experienced or that we thought we had previously explored and to some degree resolved. As we experience these existential issues, we may reach for answers to our questions, solutions for our problems that can lead to other problems. Our reaching out for assistance may be frantic and chaotic, depending on the level of desperation we feel for the need for some type of umbilical cord to anchor us in the existential void we are experiencing. For example, substance abuse may be a form of self-medicating in response to the presence of PTSD symptoms (Saladin, Back, and Payne, 2009). This is an example of trauma resulting in clients reaching out for something to assist them and developing another problem in addition to the crisis problem.

This is why exploring the spiritual life of the client is important in a crisis situation. Spirituality has historically offered support to marginalized people (Van Wormer & Davis, 2008) and life transitions and experiences can impact one's spirituality (Tisdell, 2003). Therefore, the exploration of a client's spirituality might expand the client's "reserve capacity" through intentional inclusion of spiritually related resources in response to the crisis, as well as prevent the development of additional problems in response to the crisis.

The counselor needs to look at how to facilitate this integration of spirituality — how to invite the client into healing and wholeness through the encouragement of a spiritual life, practice, and perspective to assist in day-to-day living. This integration means the counselor, with each client in crisis, needs to explore this sensitive area *with* the client. Particularly, the counselor needs to determine *if* the area needs to be explored in the context of the crisis, *when* it needs to be explored in the crisis, and *how* it needs to be explored.

The reader of this text who is skeptical of its inclusion is simply encouraged to keep an open mind to the possibility that the inclusion of this focus in counseling is an attempt to serve the best interest of our clients. For the reader who has a specific practice (e.g., religious orientation), the encouragement is also to keep an open mind as to how to include this dimension appropriately within the counseling context. All counselors need to practice within their area of competence and with respect to our own personal and professional values of spirituality.

Main Concepts

Spirituality is defined here as that which "keeps our spirit alive." It comes from the Latin word *spiritus* (breath of life). This discussion is anchored in the definition given for spirituality from the 1996 Summit on Spirituality, sponsored by the American Counseling Association's (ACA) division of the Association of Spiritual, Ethical, and Religious Values in Counseling (ASERVIC):

> Spirit may be defined as the animating life force, represented by such images as breath, wind, vigor, and courage. Spirituality is the drawing out and infusion of spirit in one's life. It is experienced as an active and passive process. Spirituality is also defined as a capacity and tendency that is innate and unique to all persons. This spiritual tendency moves the individual toward knowledge, love, meaning, peace, hope, transcendence, connectedness, compassion, wellness, and wholeness. Spirituality includes one's capacity for creativity, growth, and the development of a value system. Spirituality encompasses a variety of phenomena, including experiences, beliefs, and practices. Spirituality is approached from a variety of perspectives, including psychospiritual, religious, and transpersonal. While spirituality is usually expressed through culture, it both precedes and transcends culture (Position Paper, n.d., para. 3).

Barriers

Three barriers will be discussed in this section. The first is the *amount of exposure* the counselor has had to the area of spirituality. Many times counseling theory, research, and training have not been adequate in addressing these issues (Richards & Bergin, 1997). This means that counselors might miss, avoid, or be inadequate in addressing these concerns in sessions. The counselor may not meet the needs of the client due to biases and/or inadequate knowledge.

The second barrier stems from the first. The counselor may have *countertransference issues* regarding spirituality, in which the counselor's biases and views impact the counseling process of assessment and treatment of spirituality. These may be positive or negative in their influences, or a "mixed bag" of positive and negative personal/professional views and experiences whose contents impact the counseling in different ways depending on the client or the type of crisis issue. For example, the counselor may have been raised in a specific religion that has been positive, negative, or mixed in its positive and negative impact on the counselor. This experience can unknowingly or knowingly affect the counselor's degree of comfort and approach in addressing the spiritual aspect of the client's life. A specific "type" of client view of spirituality or crisis may pull from the counselor either positive, negative, or a combination of positive/negative countertransference stemming from the religious upbringing of the counselor.

The counselor can work with these barriers by seeking out information on how to integrate spirituality in counseling in terms of theory, research, and practice. The counselor can also examine biases/views by reading, training, and engaging in dialogue with colleagues, mentors, or supervisors in the area of spirituality. An increase of self-awareness will reduce the countertransference operating in the crisis situation. Finally, the counselor needs to be careful to *practice within the area of his/her competence* by working within the limits of his/her knowledge base. It is helpful to obtain training in the area of spirituality and then use techniques from the training with clients who provide informed consent, as well as be willing to recognize one's own limits (regarding knowledge, skills, biases) and consult with and refer to spiritual/religious experts.

Bridges

One of the core bridges to the integration of spirituality in counseling is the concept of resilience. As stated previously, an aspect of thriving in response to a crisis is that the person improves (Ryff & Singer, 2003). A person may improve based on their "reserve capacity" (change and growth potential) (Staudinger, Marsiske, & Baltes, 1995). Because a spiritual resource may assist the client in changing and growing in response to the crisis, the counselor needs to explore this aspect of his/her life with the client.

Also, *post-trauma growth* may result in self-perception and life philosophy changes, an increased awareness of and working with a self-vulnerability, deepened relationships, deepened appreciation of loved ones, and deeper self-disclosure (Tedeschi & Calhoun, 1995). First, self-perception changes and life philosophy changes may

174

draw on the client's spiritual views that influence both these areas. Clients may see themselves and life differently because of the experience of the crisis and may look to the spiritual realm to understand these shifts. Second, the client may view him/herself as more vulnerable than before the crisis. This increased sense of vulnerability, human frailty, may result in a different way of treating oneself. Spiritually, the client may treat self with a greater compassion and kindness. Finally, the crisis may result in a qualitative depth shift in terms of relationships, loved ones, and self-disclosure. The client, through the crisis, may learn the importance of reaching out to others for support and may find individuals who become more significant within the crisis or may recognize more deeply how much those individuals love him/her because they stayed and loved the client during the crisis. They saw the client at their "worst"—their "meltdown" moments—and at their most vulnerable time treated them with love and compassion. The increase in self-disclosure may occur during the crisis when the reaching out to others occurred and remained with the client following the crisis, resulting in an increased genuineness with others. With the spiritual lens in place, the counselor may assist the client in naming these shifts and addressing the impact of them on the client's life from a spiritual perspective.

Techniques

Spiritual development is fluid and spiral (Tisdell, 2003) and is impacted by life transitions and experiences such as crises. The counselor needs to assess the client's spiritual identity by asking how the spiritual realm is a refuge for the client, what healing rituals the client practices or has practiced, identifying safe spiritual places, and identifying spiritual community. The reader is reminded that spirituality may or may not be connected with a specific religion. The assessment needs to look at the client's past, present, and future spiritual and religious experiences, how the crisis has impacted the client's spiritual/religious life, and how the client's spiritual/religious perspective may assist the client through the crisis.

Although there are numerous techniques that can be used to assess and treat this aspect of the client's story and the previous techniques discussed in the therapy sections in this chapter can be easily adapted to this area, the following is a review of the techniques a counselor can use to facilitate resilience from a spiritual perspective. Resilience is used as a focus in this discussion because it is critical to surviving and healing from a crisis situation.

In the first framework discussed under the resilience section, a counselor can assist the client in developing:

- Caring and supportive relationships *within a spiritual/religious community*
- The capacity to create realistic plans and to take necessary steps to create those plans *with the support of the spiritual/religious community*
- A positive self-view and confidence *from a spiritual perspective*

- Communication and problem-solving skills *that may involve the additional resource of the spiritual/religious community*
- The ability to manage intense feelings and impulses (Discovery Health Channel & APA, 2002) *using spiritual resources such as readings and the spiritual/religious community*

Within the second framework of Ten Ways to Build Resilience (adapted from the Discovery Health Channel and American Psychological Association, 2002) outlined earlier in this chapter, each of the items can be connected with one's spiritual/religious philosophy and spiritual/religious community. Note that the spiritual perspective will be indirectly discussed in the case example in Chapter 9, where a community of support, a wellness center, is used to foster self-care, that is, resilience.

The client's spiritual philosophy, readings that are connected to that philosophy, and the support of a community that espouses such views can be a powerful part of the client's reserve capacity in the face of the crisis situation. Asking the client what they are reading, watching on television/computer, and so on, as well as whose presence they find reassuring and encouraging can improve the client's intra- and inter-feedback loops in the crisis situation. This encourages the client to view self as a "vessel" and examine what he/she puts in the vessel. Such an empowering view of the impact of one's choices can provide the client with a sense of power during a crisis that elicits a strong sense of powerlessness.

As stated previously in the section on resilience, counselors, then, can help clients increase their resilience from a spiritual perspective by helping them develop a more positive view of themselves, develop supportive relationships, and learn to make plans, develop problem-solving skills, and manage intense feelings.

SUMMARY

Four therapies have been discussed in this chapter: brief therapy, motivational interviewing, positive psychology, and grief therapy. Also, the infusion of a spiritual focus into counseling was presented, as well as the stages of change model and the concept of resilience. Each of these areas was outlined in terms of how they can assist in the crisis counseling situation.

QUESTIONS

1. Define:
   Brief therapy
   Motivational interviewing
   Stages of change
   Positive psychology
   Grief therapy

Resilience

Spirituality

2. What are the four types of therapy (and their main concepts) that can be applied to crisis counseling?

3. What are some of the core techniques of these types of therapy that can be used in crisis counseling?

4. How can spirituality be integrated into crisis counseling?

Case Study 7.1 Brief Therapy

Your client is a veteran who experienced the trauma of rape while serving in a war.

Recently she experienced PTSD symptoms when she was at a bar and was aggressively approached by a man who wanted to take her to a motel room to have sex. She has contacted you for counseling because she has found herself suicidal, drinking more often and in greater amounts, as well as having difficulty eating and sleeping. She is overwhelmed by the reactions she is having and is angry at herself for not being "stronger."

1. In terms of brief therapy, how would you prioritize the problems she is presenting?

2. What message(s) would you want to convey to her as she talks about the crisis?

3. How would you use the *triangle of person* technique with her?

Case Study 7.2 Motivational Interviewing

Your client has been referred to you for counseling by his wife of 20 years, who is angry about the amount of alcohol and drugs he has been using for the last 5 years. He tells you that she has threatened to leave him for the first time when he recently received a DUI. He also tells you that he does not see himself as having a drinking problem, has not received any feedback from others that he has a problem, and does not want to change his drinking behavior. He said he does love his wife and does not want to lose her, and he believes that if he does not quit drinking entirely, she will leave him for good.

1. How would you show empathy for him in his situation?

2. How might you point out discrepancies in his story, or would you avoid doing this and if so, why?

3. If you sensed he was resistant to looking at his drinking, how would you use the OARS to help enhance the development of a therapeutic relationship?

Case Study 7.3 Positive Psychology

Your client has recently been laid off from a factory plant where he worked for 18 years. He was two years short of retirement benefits and will receive no benefits and has lost all healthcare coverage for his family. He is very depressed (but not suicidal) and has come to the local mental health center for services. He has lost interest in activities he used to enjoy (car racing, fishing), has stopped his community involvement, and describes himself as a worn-out, useless, middle-aged male.

1. How might you use the concept of flow with this client?
2. What are some positive individual traits he has that you would explore?
3. How might you encourage community involvement for him?

Case Study 7.4 Grief Therapy

Your client has recently experienced a deep betrayal from a co-worker and friend of 18 years, in which the co-worker broke her confidence (and distorted the truth) by telling her boss of some issues she has at the workplace that made her look "bad" to her boss and her co-worker look "good." She presents herself in counseling as being depressed (trouble eating, sleeping) in response to the betrayal at the workplace. She no longer views herself as a viable, effective employee, but sees herself as being incompetent and difficult to work with following the confrontation of her boss. She does not know if she can continue to work at the agency, but during the current economic times, she does not see how she can find another job. She views her situation as hopeless and she feels trapped for various reasons: not being able to leave her profession at her age, not being able to find a new job, and needing to face her co-worker and her boss each day. She tends to minimize the loss and blame herself for the situation even existing.

1. How would you explain her situation through narrative reconstruction?
2. How would you generally approach her loss through the lens of grief counseling?
3. What specific techniques might you use to help her in counseling?

Case Study 7.5 Spirituality

Your client believes that his life was saved in a trauma situation (recent car accident) because God wants him to be alive. All he wants to talk about in the counseling session is related to his spiritual/religious views. He wants to explore with you his purpose in living, but he does not have a specific spiritual/religious framework or community with which he is involved. You sense an almost "evangelical," overly intense, overly focused passion from your client as he discusses his crisis situation with you from his spiritual perspective.

1. What would be your general approach in working with this client?
2. What would make you hesitant about yourself (personal/professional counter-transference) as you work with the client?
3. Where would you begin in the session in processing the client's concerns, and how would you respect your professional limitations and act in the best interest of the client throughout the session?

EXERCISES

Exercise 7.1 Brief Therapy

Imagine that you are working with the client in Case Study 7.1 for only one session. What would you attempt to do in that one session? Note your priorities and the messages you would want to send and discuss these with a colleague.

Exercise 7.2 Motivational Interviewing

With the client in Case Study 7.2, which change talk technique might you employ in your session with him and why? Discuss the technique and your rationale with a colleague.

Exercise 7.3 Positive Psychology

Write down the pros and cons for using each of the five positive psychology techniques discussed in this chapter with the client in Case Study 7.3.

Exercise 7.4 Grief Therapy

Think of a life transition that was deeply meaningful to you—one that shattered your self-perspective. Write down the messages you received from others during that period of time. If you had been your counselor during that time of transition, what approaches might you have used to assist yourself through the grieving process?

Exercise 7.5 Spirituality

List three strengths you have in working in the area of spirituality. Then list three weaknesses you have in working in this area. How may you draw on your strengths in terms of your current or anticipated work role, environment, and population? How might you reduce the impact of your weaknesses in terms of your current or anticipated work role, environment, and population?

Suggested Readings

Brief Therapy

Bloom, B. L. (1997). *Planned short-term psychotherapy: A clinical handbook* (2nd ed.). Boston, MA: Allyn & Bacon.

This book provides a comprehensive summary of the three main branches of short-term therapy: psychodynamic, cognitive and behavioral, and strategic and systemic. For each of the three main branches, the author provides helpful examples that can be used by the counselor in sessions.

Pichot, T., & Smock, S. A. (2009). *Solution-focused substance abuse treatment*. New York, NY: Routledge.

This book has nine chapters that apply solution-focused therapy to substance abuse treatment. The topics include an overview of treatment and solution-focused therapy, assessment, case management, group therapy, practice issues, and forms and handouts.

Motivational Interviewing

Miller, W. R., & Rollnick, S. (2002). *Motivational interviewing* (2nd ed.). New York, NY: Guilford Press.

This second edition has 25 chapters divided into four sections: context, practice, learning motivational interviewing, and applying motivational interviewing. The book is helpful in understanding the "spirit" of motivational interviewing and provides techniques of motivational interviewing that can easily be applied by the clinician.

Rosengren, D. B. (2009). *Building motivational interviewing skills: A practitioner workbook*. New York: Guilford Press.

This workbook is designed for counselors to develop the skills of motivational interviewing.

Stages of Change

Connors, G. J., Donovan, D. M., & DiClemente, C. C. (2001). *Substance abuse treatment and the stages of change*. New York, NY: Guilford.

This book has chapters addressing: overview, the stages of change, assessment, treatment planning, individual treatment, group treatment, couple/family treatment, special needs populations, relapse, and future directions.

DiClemente, C. C. (2003). *Addiction and change*. New York, NY: Guilford.

The book has four sections related to the stages of change model: understanding addiction, the road to addiction, quitting an addiction, and designing interventions.

Prochaska, J. O., DiClemente, C. C., & Norcross, J. C. (1992). In search of how people change. *American Psychologist, 47*, 1102–1114.

This article provides a description of the stages of change model.

Positive Psychology

Aspinwall, L. G., & Staudinger, U. M. (2003). *A psychology of human strengths: Fundamental questions and future directions for a positive psychology*. Washington, DC: American Psychological Association.

This book has 23 chapters that provide an overview of human strengths from a positive psychology perspective.

Csikszentmihalyi, M. (1990). *Flow*. New York, NY: Harper Perennial.

This book provides an in-depth description of this concept.

Harvard Mental Health Letter (May 2008). Positive psychology in practice. *Harvard Mental Health Letter, 24*, 1–3.

This short newsletter succinctly provides a current overview of positive psychology.

Keyes, C. L. M., & Haidt, J. (Eds.) (2003). *Flourishing: Positive psychology and the life well-lived*. Washington, DC: American Psychological Association.

This book has 13 chapters that provide an overview of positive psychology in five sections: rising to life's challenges, engaging and relating, finding fulfillment in creativity and productivity, looking beyond oneself, and looking ahead.

Lopez, S. J., & Snyder, C. R. (Eds.) (2003). *Positive psychological assessment: A handbook of models and measures*. Washington, DC: American Psychological Association.

This book provides an overview of research in positive psychology within five areas: cognitive, emotional, interpersonal, religious/philosophical, and positive processes/outcomes/environments.

Seligman, M. E. P., & Csikszentmihalyi, M. (2000). Positive psychology: An introduction. *American Psychologist, 55*, 5–14.

This article provides a helpful overview of the general concepts of positive psychology.

Grief Therapy

Harvard Health Publications (2010). *Coping with grief and loss*. Boston, MA: Harvard University.

This booklet provides an overview of grief and ways to cope with it; it includes a section on the terminally ill and a section on making arrangements related to the loss of someone.

Lewis, C. S. (1961). *A grief observed*. San Francisco, CA: Harper.

This book focuses on issues related to life, death, and faith one faces in loss.

Neimeyer, R. A. (2002). The language of loss: Grief therapy as a process of meaning reconstruction. In R. A. Neimeyer (Ed.), *Meaning reconstruction & the experience of loss*. Washington, DC: American Psychological Association.

This book chapter provides a helpful outline and techniques of using narrative therapy within the context of grief work.

Worden, W. (1991). *Grief counseling & grief therapy*. New York, NY: Springer.
This book provides an excellent overview of grief counseling.

Resilience

Csikszentmihalyi, M. (1990). *Flow*. New York, NY: Harper Perennial.
This book provides an in-depth description of this concept.

Miller, B. (2005). *The woman's book of resilience: 12 qualities to cultivate*. York Beach, ME: Conari Press.
This book has 12 chapters that are meant, through text and exercises, to assist the reader in developing resilient qualities.

Spirituality

Cashwell, C. S., & Young, J. S. (2005). *Integrating spirituality and religion into counseling: A guide to competent practice*. Alexandria, VA: American Counseling Association.
This book has 10 chapters that generally look at integration, assessment, counselor awareness, life span development, cultural, therapy goals, and working within one's limits as a counselor.

Fallot, R. D. (1998). *Spirituality and religion in recovery from mental illness*. New York, NY: Jossey-Bass.
This book has nine chapters that examine integration of spirituality in counseling, assessment, individual and group issues, and use of the spiritual community as a resource for clients.

Favier, C., Ingersoll, R. E., O'Brien, E., & McNally, C. (2001). *Explorations in counseling and spirituality*. Belmont, CA: Wadsworth/Thomson Learning.
This book has 10 chapters that focus on common themes between these areas, including evil, suffering, guilt, assessment, interventions, and self-assessment of the counselor. It has a specific chapter on the spirituality of the 12 steps. Its seven appendices include meditations, a client assessment form, a counselor self-assessment exercise, and a spiritual wellness inventory.

Fukuyama, M. A., & Sevig, T. D. (1999). *Integrating spirituality into multicultural counseling*. Thousand Oaks, CA: Sage.
This book has nine chapters that examine worldviews, developmental models, expressions of spirituality, issues (content, process), and an integrative model.

Griffith, J. L., & Griffith, M. E. (2002). *Encountering the sacred in psychotherapy: How to talk with people about their spiritual lives*. New York, NY: Guilford.
This book has 10 chapters that cover ways of hearing, approaches, metaphor, stories, beliefs and practices, community, destructiveness, and living beyond medical and psychiatric illnesses.

Miller, G. A. (2003). *Incorporating spirituality in counseling and psychotherapy: Theory and techniques*. Hoboken, NJ: Wiley.

This textbook has eight chapters (introduction, historical development, Western religions, Eastern religions, theoretical integration with cultural implications, counseling focus integration, ethical issues, specific treatment techniques), all of which involve case studies and exercises that can be used by counselors for self-awareness or within the context of counseling.

Miller, G., Clark, C., & Choae, L. H. (2008). Women and spirituality. In L. H. Choate (Ed.) *Girls' and women's wellness* (pp. 221–240). Alexandria, VA: American Counseling Association.

This book chapter provides an overview of spirituality and women that includes discussion of related factors such as age and ethnicity.

Miller, W. R. (Ed.) (1999). *Integrating spirituality into treatment*. Washington, DC: American Psychological Association.

This book has 13 chapters divided into four sections: an overview, addressing spirituality in treatment, specific spiritual issues, and training.

Sperry, L., & Shafranske, E. P. (Ed.). (2005). *Spirituality oriented psychotherapy*. Washington, DC: American Psychological Association.

This book has 15 chapters divided into three sections: theoretical foundations, contemporary approaches (related to specific theoretical frameworks), and commentary/critical analysis.

West, W. (2000). *Psychotherapy & spirituality*. Thousand Oaks, CA: Sage.

This book has nine chapters that discuss spirituality in terms of an overview, a part of therapy, issues related to the integration, and the general practice of spirituality in counseling.

Manuals

General

Berg, I. K., & Reuss, N. H. (1998). *Solutions: Step by step*. New York, NY: Norton.

This 185-page manual describes solution-focused therapy and discusses special treatment situations (codependents, relapsers, mandated clients, women, etc.) as they relate to substance abuse. It provides examples of interactions through transcripts. Its appendix contains 16 worksheets that can be used with clients (including a recovery checklist and worksheet that examines recovery from a holistic perspective).

Brief Therapy

Cohen-Posey, K. (2000). *Brief therapy client handouts*. New York, NY: Wiley.

This 185-page manual has exercise worksheets for working on relationship issues (emotions, family, marriage, parenting) and disorder-related issues (panic, OCD, moods, anger, ADD/ADHD, self-discovery). A computer disk is included.

Schultheis, G. M. (1998). *Brief therapy homework planner*. New York, NY: Wiley.

This 221-page manual has 62 homework assignments that match 30 behaviorally based problems from *The Complete Adult Psychotherapy Treatment Planner* (2nd ed.) that can be used to facilitate the solution-focused approach in counseling. It has a separate section on relapse prevention. A computer disk is included.

Grief Therapy (Client-Oriented Books)

Bozarth, A. R. (1990). *A journey through grief*. Center City, MN: Hazelden.

This 51-page book speaks to the person grieving. It provides practical "how to" suggestions.

Gilbert, K. (2001). *From grief to memories: A workbook on life's significant losses*. Silver Spring, MD: Soras Corporation.

This 208-page book has numerous exercises that clients can use in the grief process. It provides helpful resources at the end of the book.

Kemp, C. O. (2000). *A book of hope for the storms of life: Healing words for troubled times*. Franklin, TN: The Wisdom Company.

This short book is written from a Christian perspective and is meant to be uplifting to someone in grief.

Lewis, C. S. (1961). *A grief observed*. San Francisco, CA: Harper.

This 76-page book focuses on the issues related to life, death, and faith that one faces in loss.

Neeld, E. H. (1990). *Seven choices*. Austin, TX: Centerpoint Press.

In this 345-page book, the author describes seven phases that mark the grieving process. Based on her experience of having lost her husband to death, the author discusses these seven phases through her story and those of others and ends each section by discussing the choice of value in this phase.

Rich, P. (2001). *Grief counseling homework planner*. New York, NY: Wiley.

This 240-page book has 63 homework assignments that can be used with clients (disk included).

Wise, L. (2001). *Inside grief*. Incline Village, NV: Wise Press.

This 109-page book has 44 stories and poems in an anthology covering many different forms of loss. It is a very powerfully written book that could be used in bibliotherapy with clients.

York, S. (2000). *Remembering well: Rituals for celebrating life and mourning death*. San Francisco, CA: Jossey-Bass.

This 216-page book has nine chapters that offer family members and helping professionals ideas on planning services and rituals that both honor the person who is deceased and fit those attending the service. There are three resources at the end of the book: blessing and preparing a body, five services people created, and readings/prayers/blessings.

Zonnebelt-Smeege, S. J., & DeVries, R. C. (2001a). *The empty chair*. Grand Rapids, MI: Baker Books.

In this 222-page book, the authors write from a Christian perspective on the loss of a spouse based on both of their personal experiences. It is written to the grieving person. It contains "Helpful Suggestions" sections throughout the book.

Zonnebelt-Smeege, S. J., & DeVries, R. C. (2001b). *Getting to the other side of grief: Over coming to loss of a spouse*. Grand Rapids, MI: Baker Books.

This 91-page book is written from a Christian perspective for people in the pain of grief as it relates to death. It has five sections divided into three parts (reflections on personal experiences, suggestions on managing grief, a Christian meditation and prayer). There are two nice candle-lighting ceremonies at the end (one that is secular and one that is Christian).

WORKBOOKS

Brief Therapy

Araoz, D. L., & Carrese, M. A. (1996). *Solution-oriented brief therapy for adjustment disorders: A guide for providers under managed care*. Philadelphia, PA: Brunner/Mazel.

This 162-page book outlines working with adjustment disorders (according to the *DSM-IV*) in terms of diagnosis and therapy. It has an especially helpful chapter titled "Teaching Patients Self-Therapy," which includes nine cognitive-behavioral practices clients can use.

Cade, B., & O'Hanlon, W. H. (1993). *A brief guide to brief therapy*. New York, NY: Norton.

This 202-page book provides an overview of the theory of brief therapy and a description of common techniques such as framing, pattern, paradox, and metaphor interventions.

DeJong, P., & Berg, I. K. (2002). *Interviewing for solutions* (2nd ed.). Pacific Grove, CA: Brooks/Cole.

This 324-page book applies the solution-focused approach to interviewing and later sessions. It has an appendix of tools for protocols (feedback, first session, later session, involuntary clients, crisis interviews) as well as helpful questions with goal development, exceptions, involuntary clients, and coping.

Halford, W. K. (2001). *Brief therapy for couples*. New York, NY: Guilford Press.

This 288-page book describes self-regulatory couple therapy (SRCT) that enhances a couple's self-directed change. A framework for less than 25 sessions is provided with intervention guidelines.

Littrell, J. M. (1998). *Brief counseling in action*. New York, NY: Norton.

This 246-page book provides counselors with theoretical explanations of solution-focused therapy with exercises that can be used to facilitate its application with clients. There is also a modification of the stages of change model with client quotations, which is helpful in understanding the stages, as well as a four-item assessment of a client's stage level.

Metcalf, L. (1998). *Solution-focused group therapy*. New York, NY: Free Press.

This 242-page book applies the solution-focused approach to group therapy with ideas and worksheets for group work. It has a chapter on out-of-control behaviors, including eating disorders and alcohol and drug use. There is a helpful exercise on one's perception of how change happens as well as an admission interview and group process notes for both client and counselor.

VIDEOTAPES/DVDS

Motivational Interviewing

American Psychological Association (Producer) (2003) *Drugs and alcohol abuse: William Richard Miller, Ph.D.* (APA Psychotherapy Videotape Series III) [Videotape]. Available from www.apa.org/pubs/videos

The entire video is over 100 minutes and is broken into three segments: a discussion between the host and Dr. Miller, a therapy session with a real client, and a question-and-answer period with Dr. Miller regarding the session.

Moyers, T. B., Ph.D. (Producer) (1998). *Motivational interviewing: Professional training videotape series* (A-F) [Videotapes]. Available from www.motivationalinterview.org

This six-tape series (A–F) provides basic information on motivational interviewing through lecture/discussion by Miller and Rollnick and role-play situations with clients struggling with habitual patterns of behavior. The six tapes cover: (a) Introduction to Motivational Interviewing (41 minutes); (b) Phase 1: Opening Strategies (2 cassettes) — Part 1 (OARS) (39 minutes) and Part 2 (Change Talk) (51 minutes); (c) Handling Resistance (62 minutes); (d) Feedback and Information Exchange (55 minutes); (e) Motivational Interviewing in Medical Settings (48 minutes); and (f) Phase 2: Moving Toward Action (37 minutes). The tapes that cover the "core" MI techniques are the B tapes.

Stages of Change

Hazelden (Producer) (2004). *Stages of change* [DVD]. Available from www.hazelden
.org

This two-hour video is a thorough overview of the Stages of Change model in a lecture format.

Grief Therapy

Fanlight Productions (Producer). (1992). *Encounters with grief*. Available from www
.fanlight.com

This 13-minute film tells the stories of a mother, widow, and widower regarding death.

Fanlight Productions (Producer) (1997). *Grief in America*. Available from www.fan light.com

This 55-minute film tells seven stories from the lives of individuals who vary in terms of age, ethnicity, and religion. It has an educational focus and explores the impact of unresolved grief and the role of religion.

Fanlight Productions (Producer) (1998). *Surviving death: Stories of grief*. Available from www.fanlight.com

This 47-minute film has seven individuals from different ethnic groups (Caucasian, Chinese, Native American) discuss their experiences with loss and recovery that ended on a hopeful note.

Spirituality

HBO Home Video (Producer) (1996). *How do you spell God?* Available from Amazon .com or other vendors for VHS films.

This 32-minute film has children from different religions (Christianity, Judaism, Buddhism, Islam) talk about their views of God. It is interspersed with three animated stories that elaborate on different perspectives.

New Era Media (Producer) (1987). *It's in every one of us*. Available from Amazon .com or other vendors for VHS films.

This five-minute video blends pictures of different people throughout the world with the music and lyrics of David Pomeranz's song, "It's in Every One of Us."

PBS & HBO Home Video (Producers) (2002). *Frontline: Faith & doubt at Ground Zero*. Available from Amazon.com or other vendors for videos/DVDs.

This 120-minute video looks at the impact of 9/11 on individuals' spiritual lives struggling with questions such as good and evil.

Simple Truths (Producer) (2006). *The dash*. Available from www.simpletruths.com

This five-minute DVD uses visual images with the poem "The Dash," by Linda Ellis, to encourage the exploration of how we spend our lives.

WEB SITES

Brief Therapy

Solution-Focused Brief Therapy Association: www.sfbta.org

This Web site provides information on research, products, trainings, and conferences related to solution-focused brief therapy.

Motivational Interviewing

Addiction Technology Transfer Center: www.nattc.org

This Web site provides information on one's local Addiction Technology Transfer Center (ATTC), which has access to the *Motivational Interviewing Assessment:*

Supervisory Tools for Enhancing Proficiency (MIA:STEP) *products* (Briefing Materials, MI Assessment Protocol, Teaching Tools for Assessing and Enhancing MI Skills, Supervisor Tape Rating Guide, Demonstration Materials, and Supervisor Training Curriculum) and *Promoting Awareness of Motivational Incentives* (PAMI) *products* (video, PowerPoint presentations, and a tool kit).

Motivational Interviewing: www.motivationalinterview.org
This Web site provides information on clinical issues, has a library, and contains training-related information.

Positive Psychology

American Psychological Association: www.apa.org
This general Web site has links to different divisions' focus on positive psychology.

Positive Psychology at School of Behavioral & Organizational Sciences at Claremont Graduate University in California: www.cgu.edu/pages/4571.asp
This Web site provides information on the two concentrations in positive psychology, developmental and organizational, at the master's and doctoral levels, as well as information on the Quality of Life Research Center (QLRC), an institute for research in positive psychology.

Positive Psychology Center at University of Pennsylvania: www.positivepsychology .org, www.ppc.sas.upenn.edu
These Web sites are for the Positive Psychology Center at the University of Pennsylvania in Philadelphia. They provide general information on positive psychology, opportunities in this area of study, conferences, educational programs, teaching and research resources, and research information.

Grief Therapy

American Hospice Foundation: www.americanhospice.org
This Web site provides onsite training workshops, articles, resources, and publications.

Ashley Foundation: www.theashleyfoundation.org
This Web site helps teenagers face cancer with education and support.

Association for Death Education and Counseling: www.adec.org
This Web site provides education, care, research, and counseling information regarding death.

The Compassionate Friends: www.compassionatefriends.org
This is the Web site for the national nonprofit self-help support group for families grieving the death of a child.

Counseling for Loss and Life Changes: www.counselingforloss.com

This Web site provides counseling resources as well as articles and books.

The Grief Recovery Institute: www.grief-recovery.com

This Web site provides programs and workshops for individuals dealing with loss, as well as articles, books, and other resources. It also provides training for professionals.

National Hospice and Palliative Care Organization: www.nhpco.org

This Web site focuses on end of life care and facilitating access to hospice care.

Spirituality

American Psychological Association (APA) Division 36: Psychology of Religion: www.apa.org/about/division/div36.html

This division of APA's Web site provides information and resources for the integration of spirituality into one's practice of psychology.

Association for Spiritual, Ethical, and Religious Values in Counseling (ASERVIC): www.aservic.org

This division of the American Counseling Association has a Web site that provides a variety of information and resources for the counselor who is interested in integrating spirituality into their practice. There are also state affiliations of the national group.

CHAPTER EIGHT

Working With Different Cultures

LEARNING OBJECTIVES

1. To learn general multicultural counseling approaches and information that can be used in crisis counseling work.
2. To practice applying these approaches through case studies and exercises.
3. To personalize the application of these approaches and information, given one's own personal and professional orientation to working with others.

Thank you for being.

— *Traditional greeting of the Seneca*

This greeting captures the essence of the best of multicultural counseling: a welcoming, accepting approach where the client is allowed to "be" where he/she is—emotionally, physically, cognitively, and spiritually—without judgment. This chapter is meant to be an overview of multicultural counseling. For this reason, a general overview is provided on core aspects of multicultural counseling as it relates to counseling in general and to counseling specific populations. Some general multicultural models and counseling approaches are presented. In addition, significant influencing factors on the crisis situation, as related to specific populations (age, gender, sexual orientation, ethnicity) are presented. Specific approaches that can be used with the general population and with these specific populations are discussed.

By no means should this chapter be considered a summary of all of the information on multicultural counseling, but it is an attempt to highlight some of the aspects of and approaches to multicultural counseling as they relate to crisis counseling work, especially with specific populations. There is a lot of information regarding multicultural counseling, but little is written (except in some specific areas such as disaster mental health counseling) as it applies to crisis counseling. In light of this, case studies and exercises are provided to assist the reader in applying this information to counseling specific populations in crisis situations.

The reader is encouraged to keep an open mind as information is presented and to think critically about how this information can be useful in the crisis counseling contexts in which the reader currently works or intends to work. As stated in previous chapters, the reader is encouraged to examine him- or herself from this perspective. Because self-awareness diminishes the impact of countertransference, it cannot be emphasized enough. The counselor's heightened self-awareness is particularly important in the crisis counseling context, because the therapist needs to develop a therapeutic relationship as quickly as possible.

While the counselor needs to be self-aware about personal and professional factors that can impact the crisis counseling context, he/she must also have an "other-awareness" of how the client's multicultural traits can influence the client's openness to the use of different internal and external resources, as well as what resources are available. To offer assistance that is in the best interest of the client requires the counselor to have the highest possible awareness of both self and the client in terms of multicultural factors influencing the client's crisis situation.

This chapter begins with a general overview of multicultural counseling and then expands to explore significant factors such as age, gender, sexual orientation, and ethnicity. As stated previously, case studies and exercises are included in each specific population explored in order to assist the reader in self-exploration and in applying the concepts to working with specific populations within the crisis context.

DEFINITION OF MULTICULTURAL

Every counselor needs to learn how to work across differences, because whatever one *is*, that means one *is not* something else. For example, if one is male, then one is not female. Therefore, each counselor needs to develop an approach (or approaches) that will facilitate the development of bridges across the differences between the counselor and client. The capacity to build interrelationship bridges is critical to effective counseling in general, and is even more important in a crisis counseling context where the counselor needs to build these bridges as quickly as possible.

One of the difficulties with multicultural counseling is that even the definitions vary. Here, *multicultural* is defined as working with differences. Differences, for example, may be in ethnicity or sexual orientation; whatever the context of the differences between client and counselor, the emphasis is on the fact that there are differences between the two.

Reid and Kampfe (2000) provide an excellent summary of the history of multicultural counseling. The authors state that it began seriously in the early 20th century as counselors examined the needs of minority clients as they related to the counselors' vocation. In the 1950s, following legislation making segregation illegal, counselors focused on assimilating into mainstream America, using techniques that came from a mainstream perspective with little or no success because the client's cultural contexts were not considered. The 1964 Civil Rights Act opened discussions on how factors such as race impacted the therapeutic relationship, and more counselor diversity resulted in an openness to being more sensitive to diversity issues. Increased cultural tolerance of differences was reflected in counseling, and desegregation of schools showed the deficiency of what was known about crosscultural clients. The expansion of the definition of minority groups to women, gays/lesbians, and disabled individuals occurred in the 1970s. In the 1980s and 1990s, multicultural counseling theory showed a refinement of the theory, because counselors who came from different cultures helped develop it, resulting in an increased sensitivity to culture. For example, Amodeo and Jones (1997) include regional, religious, social class, age, and resettlement differences in their multicultural perspective.

[Section taken from Miller (2010) pp. 274–275.]

OVERVIEW OF MULTICULTURAL COUNSELING

"Culture is the sum total of a group's life ways" (el-Guebaly, 2008, p. 45). Cultural differences need to be valued, not feared (McFadden, 1999). Because our view of the world shapes how we assess and the action we take, counselors need to be aware, knowledgeable, and have multicultural counseling skills to help clients (Lee, 2003). Counselors need to look at how people are alike and different at the same time (Edwards, Johnson, & Feliu, 2003). Lopez et al. (1989) describe four stages of counselor development in terms of cultural sensitivity:

1. The counselor is unaware of cultural differences.
2. The counselor has increased awareness of the client's culture from his or her own perspective, but may not see it from the client's view.
3. The counselor is hypervigilant in cultural considerations, yet may not see how the client's behavior is connected to culture.
4. The counselor is more culturally sensitive by developing hypotheses about behavior based on the client's culture but is also open to testing these hypotheses.

Multicultural counseling involves counseling strategies to build bridges between the cultural differences of counselor and client. This type of counseling can be very difficult because of the struggle to understand the world from a completely different viewpoint. A person's culture is often fused with who that person is as an

193

individual. Even for those people who have had cultural experiences different from those with whom they were originally exposed, it is difficult at times to understand how individuals think and act the way they do.

Multicultural counseling, then, involves specific challenges to the counselor. It requires the counselor to have an awareness of self, others, and different cultures, as well as to be flexible, open, perceptive, and willing to learn in order to build a bridge between the differences. It does not require counselors to personally give up their value systems to work with clients, but it does require counselors to know their limitations and be willing to refer clients with whom they cannot work.

Because each person is a product of the culture in which he or she was raised, all counselors need to learn to work with individuals who are different from themselves. No one can be all things to all people. Three items are important to keep in mind with multicultural counseling. First, it may be more comfortable to work with people of some cultures than with others. No counselor can work with all individuals from all cultures equally well. Second, there is a danger that when a counselor learns things about different cultures, the counselor will end up stereotyping individuals based on what was learned about that culture. It is most important that the therapist hear the individual's story of what it was like for him or her to grow up in the United States or another country and then work within that viewpoint. Clients need to speak to counselors from the clients' own cultural experiences. Third, some individuals are more comfortable going beyond the limits of their culture than others—more willing to learn and try ways of living that are outside of their cultural experience—because of their personality or life experiences.

When working with culturally different individuals in counseling, then, the therapist must determine the clients' comfort levels for trying something different from what they have known. Initially, it may be more comfortable for clients to be exposed to counseling theories and techniques that fit well with their traditional cultures, but as they proceed in counseling, they may be willing to try something different. For example, a female client from an Asian culture may initially be most comfortable with client-centered counseling techniques in an individual setting, but as she progresses in counseling, she may become comfortable with joining a counseling group that is more confrontational in its style.

[Section taken from Miller (2010) pp. 273–274.]

SOCIAL-ENVIRONMENTAL ASPECTS

One approach to developing multicultural counseling methods is to develop a culturally sensitive environmental framework. Koss-Chioino and Vargas (1992) provide a framework of four environmental aspects that are important to take into account when working with individuals from different cultures: poverty, racism (or other *isms*) and prejudice, acculturation, and normative behavior. These aspects are reviewed in the following section, with some adaptations for working with addicted individuals. It is followed by a section on cultural diversity in America.

Poverty

Sometimes, different groups experience oppression along with their different cultural experiences. For example, women, people of color, and gays and lesbians may be oppressed as well as come from a different culture than that of the counselor. Women, for instance, who in their oppression have different cultural experience than that of men, often experience poverty as a part of their oppression. Ethnic minorities, the disabled, GLBT individuals, and older adults often live below the poverty line (American Psychological Association, 2006). Oppressed groups of individuals often experience different struggles in conjunction with their societal status, such as poverty. This experience of poverty may have a significant impact on their treatment. For example, for a recovering individual to be referred to self-help groups in the community, the issue of not having transportation to such groups because of a lack of money may arise. The reality of poverty may have a significant effect on the individual's treatment plan and recovery process.

A counselor needs to be aware of these social-environmental aspects and the impact they may place on counseling. When a client is from a different culture, the counselor needs to be careful not to assume that he or she has the same cultural advantages as the counselor. It is equally important for the counselor to avoid assuming that the client has had fewer cultural advantages than the counselor. Even when the counselor and client have similar cultural experiences, it is necessary for the counselor to maintain an open-minded approach, allowing the client's story to emerge rather than making assumptions about the client. For example, even if two women working together in therapy are the same ethnicity and age, if they were raised in different parts of the United States, their perspectives on how a person should live and act in the world are probably quite different. A counselor assuming almost complete sameness between them as counselor and client could miss ways in which they are different, which in turn could impact the therapeutic alliance. Extreme assumptions about clients must be avoided.

Isms *and Prejudice*

Individuals from different cultural groups may also experience an *ism* or prejudice about their status in the society. *Isms* is a term used here to summarize the prejudicial biases of individuals toward others. Oppressed individuals may be directly attacked physically or verbally for who they are, or they may experience systematic attacks by a system being organized around values that are unfamiliar to them. Experiencing these *isms* and prejudices may cause an individual to approach those who are considered mainstream with anger, bitterness, and distrust. If the counselor is considered mainstream by the client (e.g., by look, dress, or speech), then the counselor may need to stretch to assist the individual in trusting him or her. The same may be true if the client is the one who is considered mainstream and the counselor is of the oppressed group.

Acculturation

Individuals who are considered outside of the mainstream may also have difficulty adjusting to the predominant cultural values to which they are exposed. It may be helpful to ask these individuals whom they identify with in order to understand how they may be feeling alienated. Even individuals who have "made it" may struggle with these issues, because they may believe that somehow they have sold out and/or that they have missed specific things because of their standing outside of the mainstream culture.

Normative Behavior

Acculturation also brings up the issue of normative behavior. What is normal? What is typical for the environment in which an individual lives? How much of an adjustment should a person be required to make to fit in? These difficult questions need to be examined at the onset of counseling, yet easy answers may not emerge. However, counselors who examine these concepts increase their chances that they will be free of cultural biases about normative behavior. What are the differences between what the client and the counselor consider as normative behavior? The counselor needs to assist the client in being aware of these issues and then determine at what level the client wants or needs to adjust to these pressures. Some clients may be more flexible in terms of adjusting to different environments, whereas others will refuse to do so.

American History of Cultural Diversity

Murphy (1995) wrote a humorous article about the ease of forming opinions of others based on a lack of knowledge. He reports that the American Jewish Committee once included a group called Wisians (a nonexistent group) in an attitude survey. About 40 percent of survey respondents gave opinions on this nonexistent group. The author concludes that possibly what humans need is a nonexistent "scapegroup" for our negative projections on others—a scapegroup that could help meet our judgmental needs but not be harmful to any specific group.

Schwarz (1995) reports that the United States has a diversity myth that it promotes internationally. This is the myth that there is a long history of tolerance and harmony in the United States regarding different cultures. Schwarz attacks the myth with examples about race, ethnicity, and North–South differences. This history of oppression toward specific cultural groups, such as racial minorities and gay and lesbian populations (Vacc, DeVaney, & Wittmer, 1995), has resulted in negative experiences among specific U.S. cultural groups. Minority groups are discriminated against and then blamed for their social conditions that stem from the discrimination (e.g., victim blaming; Atkinson & Hackett, 2004). Therefore, counselors working with different cultural groups need to understand the history of that group's experience in the United States to provide some perspective for the struggles of different individuals in counseling.

BREAKDOWN OF COMMUNICATION

If an individual is from an oppressed group, it may be more difficult to establish sincere communication lines between the client and the counselor. The history of negative experiences may make it much easier to distrust than to work on a relationship with each other. This may be true regardless of whether the counselor or the client is from an oppressed group.

The breakdown of communication often seems to be based on schemata. *Schemata* means the systems of knowledge a person has about certain areas, such as types of people and situations (Mook, 1987). One type of schemata is person schemata, where the impressions of a group of people are overly simple, rigid, and generalized (e.g., stereotypes). Personal and social experiences are used as the sources of information about a group of individuals, and then that fixed knowledge of information is used to judge current experiences with individuals from that group (Fiske & Taylor, 1983). Simply stated, a person is caught in stereotypes of individuals from that group. There are numerous barriers to multicultural counseling that include differences between the counselor and clients (values, languages, worldviews); counselor stereotypes of clients as well as ethnocentrism, lack of own cultural awareness and conformity expectations of the counselor, and finally, client resistance.

Multicultural counseling requires the therapist to examine his or her perceptions of others and listen carefully to their stories to determine whether he or she is typecasting others. To prevent the limitation of stereotypes, therapists must accommodate their beliefs about an individual to new information received about the person.

MULTICULTURAL COMPETENCE

Atkinson, Morten, and Sue (1993) report that to develop cross-cultural competence, counselors must examine their own attitudes, beliefs, knowledge, and skills in terms of awareness of their own cultural values and biases, awareness of the client's worldview, and intervention strategies that fit the client's culture. Cross, Bazron, Dennis, and Isaacs (1989) developed a similar framework in which the counselor can be culturally incompetent, culturally sensitive, or culturally competent in terms of cognitive, affective, and skills dimensions, with overall effects ranging from destructive to neutral to constructive, respectively. In this latter framework, the culturally competent counselor is knowledgeable (cognitive), committed to change (affective), highly skilled (skill), and has a constructive effect on the counseling.

The Substance Abuse and Mental Health Services Administration (SAMHSA) (2000a) provides standards on providers of mental health counseling in terms of knowledge, understanding, skills, and attitudes, specifically with four underserved/underrepresented groups (African Americans, Hispanics, Native Americans/

Alaska Natives, Asian/Pacific Islander Americans). These ten competencies include knowledge and/or skills in these areas:

1. Client population background
2. Clinical issues
3. Appropriate treatment
4. Role of the agency/provider
5. Communication skills
6. Quality assessment
7. Quality care and treatment plan formulation and implementation
8. Quality treatment provision
9. Counselor use of self and knowledge in treatment
10. Counselor attitude that is respectful and open to working with others different from self

Whichever theoretical framework is adopted to encourage a multicultural counseling approach, the goal is for the counselor to develop a capacity to work with individuals who are different from him or her. The following section discusses some pragmatic approaches to facilitate multicultural counseling.

DIALOGUE

Friere (1989) describes dialogue as different from a communiqué, in which one person is above another without empathy; rather, dialogue is a horizontal relationship between two people who are empathically joined in a search. Burbules (1993) describes the necessary components of dialogues as respect, concern, interest, commitment, open participation (nonauthoritarian), continuous, developmentally sequenced, and exploratory and interrogative in nature. Oakeshott (1991) describes dialogue as conversation that lacks debate, does not attempt to discover the truth, is taken at face value, is unrehearsed, and is intellectual as well as rich in both seriousness and playfulness.

All of these definitions of dialogue combined indicate that it is a process in which two individuals are involved. A counselor attempting to work within a multicultural context needs to be able and willing to create a dialogue-friendly atmosphere so that schemata and stereotypes do not dominate the direction of the sessions.

How can a counselor create a dialogue-friendly atmosphere? Initially, it is helpful for the counselor to be aware of differences between himself or herself and the client. As stated previously, it is beneficial if the therapist has knowledge of the culture in which the client lives and the impact of that culture on the client's life. This awareness of potential or explicit differences will assist the counselor in maintaining an openness to learning about the client, rather than relying on stereotypes.

In addition, interpersonal factors such as genuineness, empathy, and unconditional positive regard (Rogers, 1987) can establish a solid baseline from which the therapist can work in counseling. If a client believes the counselor is genuine, empathic to the client's struggles, and holds a positive view of the client, many differences can be bridged. Chung and Bemak (2002) provide ten dimensions to developing cultural empathy with a client:

1. Being genuinely interested in the culture
2. Having some awareness of the client's culture
3. Appreciating cultural differences in the client
4. Including culture as a part of treatment
5. Understanding the dynamics of family and community
6. Including indigenous healing components in treatment
7. Knowing the history of the client's cultural group (including sociopolitical)
8. Knowing adjustments that had to be made psychologically in a move to another culture
9. Being sensitive to ongoing discrimination experienced by the client
10. Focusing on empowering the client

Another important factor is the role the counselor takes at a critical moment in therapy: Is the counselor a compassionate authority individual or a critical one? Multicultural counseling invariably includes places of conflict and differences. What is important is the approach taken by the counselor at those times. Rather than focusing the blame on someone for the event, which is the stance of the critical authority individual, it is more important that the counselor focus on what has occurred and its impact on the client and the counseling relationship. A sincere apology for the misunderstanding between the counselor and client can deeply facilitate the therapeutic relationship. In addition, a careful, thoughtful, respectful processing of the event can assist clients in trusting the counselor in therapy and learning about patterns of their own behavior.

So-called commonsense approaches are also helpful in therapy. Asking a client "What would you like to be called?" in terms of identification of ethnicity, or sexual orientation, or whatever, and then remembering to use that term is respectful. Also, gently and respectfully asking a client who is the only member of a specific group or culture, "What is it like to be the only ____ in this place?" is helpful. Finally, when there is a disagreement or conflict of some type, the counselor may not know what occurred that caused the client to withdraw; however, the counselor may feel a qualitative shift in the therapeutic relationship. This experience can be described as a glass wall that drops between the counselor and the client. The client may or may not appear engaged with the counselor, but it feels to the counselor that he or she has been shut out. At that point, it is necessary for the counselor to ask, "What happened here?" to learn what may have been offensive or alienating to the client. These general approaches can simply be invitations by the counselor.

The counselor can be responsible only for the effort, not the outcome. The client may have the understandable response of not wanting to educate the counselor about his or her opinions on how to be treated as part of his or her cultural group. However, many clients may respond to a sincere human outreach that is asking for assistance in how to treat a client with respect.

The danger for all counselors in multicultural counseling is experiencing a lack of compassion based on ignorance and fear. To operate out of ignorance and fear not only limits the counseling but also is hurtful to the client. When counseling struggles appear to be based in cultural differences, the counselor needs to process the struggle carefully with the client. It is helpful to take a deep breath and then proceed into the dialogue about the conflict with honesty, setting limits, and taking time to discuss the issues. The conflict and discussion need to be personal. At this point in the encounter, the counselor needs to show his or her humanness. The amount of disclosure required may vary from counselor to counselor, but what is most necessary is that the client feel the counselor's willingness to hear about the conflict and the counselor's commitment to attempt to work through it.

GENERAL COUNSELING SUGGESTIONS

Counselors who desire to be sensitive and effective with individuals from other cultures need to be aware of several areas. First, they must be aware of their own cultures and how those affect their life. Second, they need to be aware of the social-environmental aspects that may be experienced by some groups, including the history of treatment of these groups in the United States. Third, counselors need to work at continually creating a dialogue-friendly atmosphere to facilitate counseling across different cultures. As Edwards et al. (2003) state, counselors need to be respectful in differences and similarities, empathic to struggles, and patient with issues such as reimbursement, session limits, and speed of problem resolution. Some specific multicultural counseling suggestions follow:

1. Provide a respectful, open environment, particularly concerning cultural differences.
2. Be flexible.
3. Be an expert in the field of counseling, but not in the clients' lives.
4. Establish a relationship of trust with a client. Do not pretend you know what you do not know.
5. Remember that a person can be a part of several cultures at one time.
6. Say, "I do not know what it is like to be . . . ."
7. Ask clients to teach you what you do not know.
8. Do not create issues, but address them if they arise.
9. Do not fight with people, but respond to their statements; do not let things go by.
10. Share your own experience of a communication breakdown if it occurs.

11. Apologize when you are wrong.
12. Learn how to deal with people who do not like you.
13. Turn to other counselors for support.
14. Remember the commonalities among all people.

[Section taken from Miller (2010) pp. 274–280.]

Multicultural Counseling in the Context of Crisis Counseling

Beyond the general approaches regarding multicultural counseling as discussed previously, there is little written about applying this perspective to crisis counseling work (except, as stated previously, in some specific areas such as disaster mental health counseling). This section is a summary of some of the general approaches encouraged in practicing multicultural counseling within the context of a crisis.

Four characteristics are needed by counselors who are doing multicultural work (Kiselica, 1998 as summarized in James, 2008) are:

1. Know oneself (especially our own cultural biases).
2. Know the status and cultures of groups.
3. Have skills to intervene culturally at an appropriate place (and be flexible in terms of having and using alternative approaches).
4. Have experience working with culturally different people.

Crisis counselors can prepare for crisis multicultural counseling by addressing these four areas in training, counseling, and using colleagues, supervisors, and mentors to enhance these abilities. Such preparation prior to the crisis work can assist the counselor in best meeting the needs of the client in the crisis situation within the client's cultural context.

According to some authors, cultural awareness and sensitivity are more critical than cultural competence, because they do not view a counselor as ever being truly competent to understand a culture different from his or her own native culture (Hoff, Hallisey, & Hoff, 2009). There are two "truths" regarding multicultural counseling: We cannot ever understand or be as comfortable in another culture as we are in our own, and there are aspects of being human that we share across cultures. We need to find out what is unique to our clients regarding how they view and respond to the crisis and what they have in common with others who have experienced crises.

There is a paradox of crisis counseling work with regard to culture: To effectively assess and treat the client in a crisis, the counselor needs to slow down the process and take time to understand the crisis. This involves taking time to figure out what is happening, normalizing the process for the client, and encouraging the client's empowerment. These three important aspects of multicultural counseling in the context of crisis counseling work need to be done within the cultural world of the client. The counselor needs to assess, normalize, and encourage empowerment and resilience, all within an understanding of the client's culture. To understand the client's culture, the counselor needs to gather information on cultural background, including "ethnicity, language, assimilation, acculturation, spiritual beliefs" (Roberts, 2005, p. 154). While these multicultural approaches may require additional time for the crisis counselor, it is time well spent, because viewing the crisis through the cultural lens of the client will enhance the accuracy of the assessment and clarify the appropriate necessary interventions.

A multicultural approach is especially important in fieldwork/outreach work of a crisis nature. For example, in a disaster context, "culture" becomes a broad description that includes factors such as age and ethnicity. In such outreach work, the counselor needs to assess how to help (not help too much, but rather draw on the strengths of the community) and what type of help is needed within a cultural context—particularly with those individuals who are only marginally connected to the mainstream culture (e.g., the poor, older adults, ethnic minorities, and those individuals with limited education) (James, 2008). Also, collaborating with social support networks, which are especially important to some ethnic groups, and examining how client assistance is provided (for example, the language used by staff) can facilitate the effectiveness of this type of work (Shelby & Tredinnick, 1993). Crisis counseling services adapted to diverse needs in a particular location have greater community penetration in making mental health services more "user-friendly" (Rosen, Greene, Young, & Norris, 2010). Finally, three multicultural counseling suggestions to the disaster mental health counselor in a crisis situation are (Naturale, 2006):

1. Remember there is no single formula on how to work with culture.
2. Work with members of groups who can act as "cultural brokers in opening communication doors" (p. 371).
3. Be culturally competent in terms of being aware of problems (economic, social, historical) that can influence the crisis.

These general suggestions regarding the integration of multicultural counseling work are fused into suggestions for working with some specific populations in the next section. Some aspects of specific populations influence factors of the crisis in unique ways.

INFLUENCING FACTORS

Age

Overview
The focus in this section will be on older adults (individuals aged 65 and over), because while other age groups (children, adolescents) are also impacted by crises, they typically receive crisis counseling through adults or in specific contexts

discussed in Chapter 4. A few notations on working with children before focusing on older adults follow. Children commonly respond in two ways to crises (behavioral change, behavioral regression), and crises are especially challenging to them because they are forced to address issues that they are developmentally not equipped to address (Knapp, 2010). Specific crisis assessment and treatment issues related to children can be found in Knapp's chapter in Dass-Brailsford's book (2010) *Crisis and Disaster Counseling: Lessons Learned from Hurricane Katrina and Other Disasters*, referenced at the end of this chapter and a chapter in Greenstone and Leviton's book, *Elements of Crisis Intervention*, also referenced at the end of this chapter. Roberts and Yeager (2009) also have a section on working with abused children in their book, *Pocket Guide to Crisis Intervention*, that is referenced at the end of this chapter.

Older adults are a group whose vulnerability in a crisis may be magnified by their being on the margins of mainstream society due to economic, physical, psychological, or social limitations. In addition, they are subject to stereotypes and discrimination (Sue & Sue, 2008a), which also heightens their vulnerability. Depending on the extent of the disaster and the necessity of relocation, older adults may experience a decline in their independence as a result of the disaster (Cherry, Allen, & Galea, 2010). Such an enhancement of their vulnerability calls for a special emphasis on their issues in this section.

Older adults make up approximately 12 percent of the U.S. population and are the fastest-growing group in terms of age (Benshoff, Harrawood, & Koch, 2003; van Wormer and Davis, 2008). Counselors, then, will increasingly be working with this population. Crisis counselors can also expect to be treating them more in crisis counseling situations. However, mental health counselors have been shown to have biases against older adults by being reluctant to work with them, seeing them as being less interesting, rigid, and not benefiting from counseling (Sue & Sue, 2008a). Although our population is aging, we aren't equipped to handle either the current population of older adults or the expected increased population, and stereotypes and discrimination prevent older adults from accessing services. Specific issues that may impact this population are (Sue & Sue, 2008a; 2008b):

- Physical impairments
- Economic problems
- Mental health problems (often untreated due to stereotypes and discrimination)
- Mental deterioration
- Abuse and neglect
- Substance abuse
- Depression and suicide
- Sexuality issues

General Approaches
By being aware of these issues, the crisis counselor can assess whether he or she is having an impact on the current crisis situation. The crisis counselor needs to

avoid discrimination on either extreme of the assessment process with an older adult client: the counselor cannot assume issues to be present because the client is an older adult or assume that issues are not present for the client because he or she is an older adult. Rather, the counselor needs to be aware of his/her own biases toward the older adult population and must focus on doing a fair, balanced assessment of all the issues within the context of the crisis assessment in order to determine if they are influencing factors in the crisis situation. Influencing factors on the crisis that are related to aging then need to be addressed as a part of crisis counseling.

There are a couple of important, specific suggestions for counseling older adults in the context of disasters (Naturale, 2006). First, the counselor needs to be aware that physical restrictions may impact their reaching out for help and, as a result, may make their symptoms worse. Second, the counselor needs to alert primary care doctors, who are most likely to have contact with older adults, to watch for common disaster reactions in their older adult patients (difficulty sleeping, anxiety, depression).

Case Study 8.1 Age

Your client is in her 80s and she has just survived an earthquake. She is widowed, lives alone, and has a very limited income. She has lost her home and many of her worldly possessions. She has been taken in by some individuals in her church who are working with her to help her find resources to survive her significant losses. These individuals have brought her to you because in the past few weeks since the earthquake, she has increasingly talked in a despondent fashion about life, and this is very unusual for her (e.g., "What is the point of trying to make things better since I have lost everything that matters to me?"). As you talk with her, you realize that she is not suicidal, but she is grieving the loss of her husband who died four years ago, and that her significant losses in the earthquake were the collection of spoons he gathered for her in all his professional traveling over the years and the letters he wrote her daily. She is sending you verbal messages ("How can you understand in your youthfulness what I am going through?") and nonverbal messages during your initial contact that are communicating a significant lack of trust in your ability to be helpful to her.

1. What information about working with older adults would be helpful to you in developing a trusting relationship with her?
2. How would you use the information about her grief to help her through this crisis?
3. What aspects of yourself, personally and professionally, might limit your understanding of her crisis, and how would you address this in your session with her?

Exercise 8.1 Age

Make headings for children, adolescents, adults, and older adults and draw three columns next to the terms. Now spend a few moments writing in the first column the first words that come to mind regarding your views of children, adolescents, adults, and older adults. In the second column, jot down what would make it emotionally hard to work with them in a crisis situation. For example, if the words used for children are "innocent" or "untouched by the harsh reality of life," the second column might have a notation: "It would be sad to see them so mistreated by the world." In the third column, note how you might handle your reactions during the crisis situation. Again, staying with the previous example, you might note in the third column some form of self-talk: "There is nothing I can do to prevent the crisis from happening, but I can provide an opportunity for this child to experience some healing with me and I can help the child find inner and outer resources to respond to this situation."

Gender

Overview

As with older adults, women are focused on here because their vulnerability in a crisis may be magnified by being on the margins of mainstream society, due to oppression that plays out in negative stereotypes and social, financial, and other forms of discrimination. Sue and Sue (2008a) state that common problems that women face include economic status, career choice barriers, discrimination or victimization, unrealistic body standards, depression, and aging. These problems may be exacerbated in a crisis situation. For example, a woman may be having a crisis in relation to a discriminating work situation that is enhanced by her limited career opportunities and income, which in turn fuel her struggles with depression.

In terms of responding to the needs of women within a crisis counseling situation, it can be helpful to step back from the specific problems and look philosophically at how women tend to view themselves in the world. Women develop and have life experiences in relationship contexts (J. B. Miller, 1986); women come to understand themselves through the creation and maintenance of relationships (J. B. Miller, 1976). A woman needs to both be understood and to understand the significant others in her life; she needs to have mutuality in relationships in order to grow and be aware (Surry, 1985), and she defines power as being able to care for and give to others in her life (McClelland, 1975). How society views her is incorporated into this view of self (van der Walde, Urgenson, Weltz, & Hanna, 2002).

General Approaches

This relational focus can have a significant influence on a crisis situation. When assessing and treating a female client in a crisis, the counselor needs to focus on the impact of the crisis on her relationships and vice versa. Assessment and treatment need to especially consider the concepts of understanding/being understood with regard to others, the client's perception of power, and society's view of her. For example, a woman who is experiencing the breakup of an intimate relationship may have a heightened anguish of not understanding why the breakup is occurring, may see herself as less able to take care of the significant others in her life because of an anticipated drop in her income, and may have a negative view of herself based on what others around her (as well as the larger society) are saying about a woman in her situation (e.g., she is a failure because her relationship has failed). The counselor who considers the emphasis of such factors may be better able to intervene in the woman's crisis because of a heightened sensitivity to the import of these issues. Understanding the magnitude of the impact of such factors on the crisis situation can possibly decrease the intensity of the crisis and in itself become an effective intervention.

In addition, counselors need to examine themselves for diagnostic biases and sexism, and they should be aware of current information on psychological and physiological issues for women as well as violence and harassment issues and issues such as depression that may be related to factors such as limited economic means and negative self-image (Sue & Sue, 2008b). The crisis counselor who approaches a woman in crisis with a cultural sensitivity for the realities she faces as a member of an oppressed group, her worldview in terms of relationships, and her specific problems and needs, as well as an awareness of his or her (the counselor's) own countertransference, will be better able to assess and address the crisis situation.

Case Study 8.2 Gender

Your client is a different gender from you. During the crisis intake at your place of work, your client is intermittently acting very flirtatious with you (touching you, making suggestive eye contact, etc.). You are aware that you need to set limits with your client to adequately complete the intake assessment, but you also want to make sure that you do not alienate the client in setting boundaries and thereby lose the therapeutic connection.

1. Would you address the flirtatious behavior openly?
2. If so, what might you say to your client that would be limit-setting, but hopefully not hurtful to the therapeutic connection?
3. If you do not address the situation verbally and openly, how would you set limits with your client?

EXERCISE 8.2 GENDER

In the case study above, talk with a colleague about those aspects of the crisis situation that would be especially difficult for you and brainstorm different ways you might handle this situation.

Sexual Orientation

Overview

Sexual orientation is on a continuum that ranges from same-sex attraction to opposite-sex attraction (SAMHSA, 2003). The populations included in the discussion here are the gay, lesbian, bisexual, and transgender (GLBT) populations. Transgender individuals, who follow opposite sex gender roles or identify with the opposite sex, may find themselves attracted to males or females (either or both); typically, "transgender" is a term that is used for individuals who are about to have a sexual reassignment. Like the other groups discussed in this section, GLBT clients experience oppression and discrimination. They may also struggle with identity, coming out, aging, substance abuse, and HIV issues (Sue & Sue, 2008a).

SAMHSA (2003) summarizes some of the clinical issues experienced by the GLBT population that a counselor should consider. A counselor should be aware that:

- A client might require exploration of his/her circumstances and experiences.
- There are legal prohibitions against the client's behavior.
- The client may experience discrimination.
- The client may have internalized homophobia.
- The client may be a victim of violence and hate crimes.

Crisis counselors sensitive to these issues can better assess and treat the GLBT client in the crisis situation.

General Approaches

Again, first the crisis counselor needs to be sensitive to countertransference issues and problems related to oppression and discrimination (e.g., internalized homophobia, hate crimes/violence) that may be fueling the crisis situation. Second, counselors need to show an openness to discussing issues related to sexual orientation—discussions that may include the counselor answering questions about his/her own sexual orientation and speaking in an inclusive language that does not make assumptions about sexual orientation. Third, counselors need to form treatment plans in terms of common issues these clients may experience in terms of "life stage, coming-out process, support available, current and past relationships with significant others and family, comfort with sexuality, and issues related to career, finances, and health" (Miller, 2010, p. 301), as well as spiritual/religious needs (Sue & Sue, 2008a).

Case Study 8.3 Sexual Orientation

Use the same situation given in Case Study 8.2, only shift the perspective and say that you and your client are the same gender. How might this change the situation, and how might it change your responses?

EXERCISE 8.3 SEXUAL ORIENTATION

Again, use the Exercise 8.2, but change it so that you and your client are the same gender. Again, discuss with a colleague how this shifts the situation for you (if it does) and how you might change your approach.

Ethnicity

Overview

In counseling racial/ethnic minorities, it is important to remember that there is no evidence that they have more mental health issues than majority racial/ethnic groups (Atkinson, 2004). At the same time, counselors need to be aware that racial/ethnic minority clients may have been exposed to certain conditions (poverty, homelessness, incarceration, substance abuse, poor health care) at a disproportionately higher rate (Atkinson, 2004). The crisis counselor, then, can be aware that a racial/ethnic minority client in crisis may be experiencing heightened issues related to race that have resulted in a crisis situation.

An openness to discussing race and ethnicity in a counseling context can result in improvement of the therapeutic alliance and treatment outcome (Cardemil & Battle, 2003). The counselor, however, needs to approach such discussions with a great sensitivity toward possible transference and countertransference that can emerge simply based on the discussion of race/ethnicity in the session. Issues between counselor and client can be increased if one's projections onto the other's race/ethnicity are based on assumptions that are not first checked out. There may also be historical pain from one's racial/ethnic group that is brought to the sessions, by counselor, client, or both.

Because of the potential volatility of a discussion of race/ethnicity, the crisis counselor needs to assess the appropriateness and the timing of such a discussion carefully. Only if race/ethnicity is determined to be a possible influencing factor of significance may the counselor in a crisis counseling situation decide to bring up the concern. This is not advocating a stance of avoidance, but rather one of being practical in assessing whether race/ethnicity is contributing to the crisis and/or if the race/ethnicity of the client and/or the counselor is inhibiting the process of counseling. The degree to which race/ethnicity issues are openly addressed needs to be evaluated in terms of what is in the best interest of the client. A crisis counselor who finds a balance between ignoring racial/ethnic issues and addressing them by walking on eggshells can develop a therapeutic relationship with a client that allows for such a sensitive issue to be addressed in a thoughtful, caring, respectful, and humane manner that serves the best interest of the client.

General Approaches

While there is no one model for counseling racial/ethnic minority clients, different models can be used to facilitate the counselor's multicultural counseling approach

(Atkinson & Hackett, 2004). Various books, as listed in the suggested readings section of this chapter, summarize different theoretical and identity development models that the reader may find helpful to use in the assessment and treatment of racial/ethnic minority clients.

Essentially, each client needs to be seen as an individual who has his/her own unique identification with his/her own racial/ethnic group. The counselor needs to ask the client about his/her unique identification as well as how this identification plays out in terms of social and community support networking regarding race/ethnicity. Basically, the counselor needs to learn to see the client's worldview through the lens of his/her race/ethnicity, which includes, but is not limited to: (a) the label, as chosen by the client, of his/her ethnic group; (b) the identity development stage with which the client identifies; (c) social and community supports; and (d) networking on a regular basis. The counselor needs to learn the racial/ethnic "root system" of the client.

Six suggestions to counselors doing multicultural work with regard to race/ethnicity are (Cardemil & Battle, 2003):

1. Avoid making assumptions about the client and his/her family about race/ethnicity.
2. Understand that in relation to identity development and acculturation, the client may be different from other members of his/her racial/ethnic group.
3. Determine how differences between counselor and client regarding race/ethnicity might affect counseling.
4. Have awareness of the possible influence on counselor/client relations of power, privilege, and racist dynamics.
5. Be willing to take risks to talk with clients about race.
6. Be willing to learn about race and diversity.

Case Study 8.4 Ethnicity

Your client is of the same ethnic group as you, but you have very different life experiences in terms of class as it relates to income. Both you and your client are aware of these differences, as you have gathered information about the external resources available to your client in this crisis situation. You are concerned that the significant differences might impact the amount, type, and accuracy of information you receive from your client and the degree to which the client trusts you.

1. How might you address these differences in the crisis situation? As in the section on gender, would you address these directly and if so, how?
2. How would it change the dynamics if prior to the crisis the client had more money than you?
3. How would it change the dynamics if the client had less money than you prior to the crisis?

EXERCISE 8.4 ETHNICITY

Write down a few paragraphs on how you view your ethnicity and how you believe it impacts you both personally and professionally. As a result of your ethnic experiences, do you believe there are some populations you might work better with in a crisis situation when your ethnicity is similar? When it is different? Process your comments with a trusted mentor, supervisor, or colleague.

SUMMARY

This chapter addressed general approaches in multicultural counseling that can be useful in crisis counseling work. Specific populations were examined (age, gender, sexual orientation, ethnicity), with the goal of providing a brief overview of general counseling information and suggesting some specific approaches for working with that population in a crisis setting. To assist the reader in applying this information professionally, a case study and exercise was provided for each of the specific populations.

QUESTIONS

1. What are some common multicultural approaches that may be helpful in crisis counseling?
2. How might I use these approaches and the information presented in this chapter in my clinical work?
3. While working with the case studies and exercises, which populations do I believe I can work with comfortably? Which ones would feel like a stretch for me? How might I enhance my strengths in this work and diminish my weaknesses?

SUGGESTED READINGS

Overall

Sue, D. W., & Sue, D. (2008a). *Counseling the culturally diverse: Theory and practice* (5th ed.). Hoboken, NJ: Wiley.

This book is divided into two sections (multiple dimensions of multicultural counseling and therapy; multicultural counseling and specific populations) that are divided into nine parts and 26 chapters. Specific counseling populations discussed include various ethnic groups, sexual minorities, women, and disabled individuals.

Children

Dass-Brailsford, P. (Ed.) (2010). *Crisis and disaster counseling: Lessons learned from Hurricane Katrina and other disasters.* Los Angeles, CA: Sage.

This 258-page book has 15 chapters that provide an overview of disaster and crisis counseling, specific disasters, interventions, and populations impacted by disasters (families, children, older adults, rural and diverse communities) as well as the impact on workers and specific topics (spirituality, federal government involvement).

Greenstone, J.L., & Leviton, S.C. (2002). *Elements of crisis intervention* (3rd ed.). Belmont, CA: Brooks/Cole.

This short book has 11 chapters that briefly cover basic approaches and strategies in crisis work with focused chapters on children, families, hotline workers, loss, legal implications, and disasters.

Roberts, A.R., & Yeager, K.R. (2009). *Pocket guide to crisis intervention*. New York, NY: Oxford University Press.

This brief book has 33 chapters. Each of them covers, in a few pages, the major topics of crisis work. It may be thought of as a "CliffsNotes" or a primer of crisis work. It has a specific, concise chapter on "do's and don'ts."

Older Adults

Moody, H. R. (2010). *Aging* (6th ed.). Thousand Oaks, CA: Pine Forge.

This 503-page book is divided into three basic concepts (life perspective on aging; aging, health care, and society; and social and economic outlook for an aging society), with each section addressing 3–4 controversial areas related to aging.

Professional

Substance Abuse and Mental Health Services Administration (SAMHSA) (1998a). *Substance abuse among older adults*. Rockville, MD: Author.

This 173-page manual provides an excellent overview of the issues of substance abuse, providing general information, specifics on assessment, treatment, legal/ethnical concerns, and assessment tools.

Gender

Professional

Brady, K. T., Back, S. E., & Greenfield, S. F. (2009). *Women & addiction*. New York, NY: Guilford.

This book has seven sections (overview, biological issues, co-occurring psychiatric disorders, treatment outcome, specific substances, special populations, and social policy issues) and 30 chapters.

Center for Substance Abuse Treatment (CSAT). (1994). *Practical approaches in the treatment of women who abuse alcohol and other drugs* (DHHS Publication No. 94–3006). Rockville, MD: Author.

This 275-page publication provides general information on addiction in women as well as specific suggestions for assessment, treatment, and aftercare issues.

Straussner, S. L. A., & Brown, S. (Eds.). (2002). *The handbook of addiction treatment for women: Theory and practice*. San Francisco, CA: Jossey-Bass.

This 620-page book has eight sections: understanding addicted women, major addictions, life cycle issues, ethnically diverse issues, special populations, treatment approaches, an epilogue, and resources.

Personal

Miller, B. (2005). *The woman's book of resilience: 12 qualities to cultivate*. York Beach, ME: Conari Press.

This book has 12 chapters: vulnerability, connection, personal management, meeting of needs, recognition of gifts/talents, limit setting, resentment/forgiveness, use of humor, adaptive responses, endurance of suffering, finding meaning, and balancing self- and other-dependence. There are stories and exercises throughout the text to encourage the reader to develop resilient qualities.

Sexual Orientation

Barret, B., & Logan, C. (2002). *Counseling gay men and lesbians*. Pacific Grove, CA: Brooks/Cole.

This book is a general counseling book for working with the GLBT population. It includes chapters on identity development, couples counseling, youth, spiritual, parenting, and health issues.

Savin-Williams, R. C. (2001). *Mom, Dad. I'm gay*. Washington, DC: American Psychological Association.

This book has nine chapters that discuss GLBT concerns within the context of the family. Especially helpful are the chapters that examine the relationship between different family members (e.g., daughters and fathers).

Substance Abuse and Mental Health Services Administration (SAMHSA). (2003). *A provider's introduction to substance abuse treatment for lesbian, gay, bisexual, and transgender individuals*. Rockville, MD: Author.

This publication is an excellent resource for working with the GLBT population in terms of substance abuse treatment. It is divided into three main sections: an overview, a clinician's guide (the coming-out process; health issues; and clinical issues with lesbians, gay males, bisexuals, transgender individuals, youth, and families), and a program administrator's guide.

Race/Ethnicity

Substance Abuse and Mental Health Services Administration (SAMHSA). (2000a). *Cultural competence standards*. Rockville, MD: Author.

This 68-page booklet describes the standards for four underserved and underrepresented racial/ethnic groups in an easy-to-read, understandable format.

212

VIDEOTAPES/DVDs

Gender

New Day Films (Producer). (1996). *Stories of change* [VHS]. Available from www.newday.com
This 58-minute film tells the stories of four women who struggle with alcoholism/drug abuse, racism, sexism, and classism.

Sexual Orientation

Buendia Productions (Producer). (2005). *Psychotherapy with gay, lesbian, & bisexual clients* [DVD]. Available from www.buendiaproductions.com
This two-part DVD has a section on assessment and psychotherapy (48 minutes), and a section on relationships, families, and couples (40 minutes).

Race/Ethnicity

Mystic Fire Video (Producer). (1991). *Circle of recovery* [Video]. Available through Amazon.com
This hour-long video portrays seven African-American men who have weekly meetings to help each other live with being addicts.

WEB SITES

General

National Institutes of Mental Health. www.nimh.nih.gov
This Web site provides information on understanding and treating mental illness.

Substance Abuse and Mental Health Services Administration (SAMHSA). www.samhsa.gov
This Web site provides a variety of information and resources on substance abuse and mental health.

Professional Organizations

The reader is also encouraged to check with the national professional organization with which he/she is affiliated in order to obtain current guidelines relating to the practice of multicultural counseling.

American Association for Marital and Family Therapy. www.aamft.org
American Counseling Association. www.counseling.org
American Psychiatric Association. www.psych.org
American Psychological Association. www.apa.org
National Association of Social Workers. www.naswdc.org

Specific Populations

Older Adults

American Psychological Association Office on Aging. www.apa.org/pi/aging
   This Web site has general (research, intervention), publication, and referral information about older adults.

Eldercare Locator. www.eldercare.gov
   This service provides information on resources available to older adults.

Gender

National Advocates for Pregnant Women. www.advocatesforpregnantwomen.org
   The Web site for National Advocates for Pregnant Women is in Spanish as well as English. It has publications, events, and a blog.

National Women's Health Resource Center. www.healthywomen.org
   This Web site for the National Women's Health Resource Center has health topics, centers, and publications/resources.

Sexual Orientation

National Association of Lesbian, Gay, Bisexual, and Transgender Addiction
   Professionals and their Allies. www.nalgap.org
   The Web site for this group has a section on services, resources, and news/articles.

Parents, Families, and Friends of Lesbians and Gays (PFLAG). www.pflag.org
   The PFLAG Web site has information for families and friends of gay, lesbian, bisexual, and transgender individuals.

Pride Institute. www.pride-institute.com
   This Web site has information on substance abuse treatment for GLBT individuals, including general information, admissions information, and treatment center listings.

Southern Poverty Law Center. www.splcenter.org
   In addition to other things, this organization files lawsuits against hate groups. It also publishes the magazine *Teaching Tolerance* and has free resources for teachers. The group's Web site has information about U.S. hate groups, as well as a newsletter and a blog.

Race/Ethnicity

American Indian Health Resources. www.ldb.org/vl/geo/america/indi_hn.htm
   This Web site for American Indian Health Resources is a listing of national public health networks, nongovernmental organizations, and private associations.

National Society for Hispanic Professionals. network.nshp.org
   This Web site provides information on mental health counseling with the Hispanic population. Do a search on the Web site for specific areas of mental health

counseling by entering "Mental health" in the search engine on that Web site to obtain information on contacts, literature, research, etc.

National Association for Advancement of Colored People. www.naacp.org

This Web site provides information on the civil rights of African Americans and minority group members. It has general information as well as a legal section and a blog.

Self-Care

LEARNING OBJECTIVES

1. Learn what can contribute to burnout.
2. Understand specific stress coping techniques.
3. Comprehend the five fundamental lessons of self-care.

> If your face is swollen from the severe beatings of life,
> smile and pretend to be a fat man.
>
> —*Nigerian Proverb, Little Bee*

Most professionals begin their careers with little or no information about what they will really experience as practitioners or academicians in a particular field. Building on childhood and adolescent ambitions, they careen from their years in undergraduate programs directly into their graduate training with little time for thought or preparation. The graduate years consist of anxiety-ridden rituals of hard work and dedication. There is practically no time to reflect on the wisdom of the commitment to join a particular profession, since all of the student's energy is taken up with the tasks of gaining entry in the first place. It is only years later, after graduating, passing the licensure examinations, and engaging in the first job or two in the field, that the average individual begins to recognize the tremendous effects that the decade of hard work has had on his or her life.

(Kilburg, Nathan, & Thoreson, 1989, pp. 15–16)

The above quote points out the tendency of the mental health professional to neglect self-examination—of which self-care is a component—throughout the professional development journey until there comes a point when he/she begins to consider the existential professional questions of "What is it all about?" and "What price am I willing to pay for this profession?" In the formal education and training of mental health professionals who will work in high-stress situations, self-care is rarely discussed (Christopher, 2006). We are typically trained to overlook our needs as mental health professionals and to focus on the care of others (O'Halloran & Linton, 2000). That is why this chapter is included in this book. It is important for those of us in the mental health professions (students and experienced professionals alike) to reflect throughout our professional development on our self-care and commit ourselves to this practice throughout our careers. Every mental health professional is vulnerable to the possibility of impairment (Norcross & Barnett, 2008). A commitment to self-care can simply help us be the best mental health professionals we can be and can prevent possible impairment in our therapeutic work. We need to practice self-care from the beginning of our work (Bein, 2008). It can help us listen to the difficult stories our clients tell. Self-care can promote resiliency that can prevent the fatigue described as "empathy fatigue"—when the mental health professional's wounds are stirred by the life stories of clients (Stebnicki, 2007). Self-care can also help us with our psychological, spiritual, and emotional vulnerabilities, so we can be the best wounded healers we can be, bridging the world of wellness and the world of illness. Practicing self-care can strengthen our vulnerability so we can: (a) effectively draw on the suffering we experience in the world (Bein, 2008), and (b) make choices, provide empathy, and experience stamina in therapy that benefits the welfare of the client (Mander, 2009). If we do not develop coping strategies, we may leave the mental health profession, act dysfunctionally at work—perhaps by not setting appropriate boundaries—or practice while impaired. We must renew ourselves and nurture our happiness (Willer, 2009). For example, leisure impacts the work and personal lives of mental health professionals by encouraging balance and integration, improving coping abilities and work performance, and creating meaningful connections (Grafanaki et al., 2005).

This chapter on self-care will attempt to avoid "should-ing" the reader with pat formulas of self-care and instead will encourage the mental health professional to practice self-care in a humane, self-respecting, realistic manner. It is anchored in the belief that all of us deserve compassion, including ourselves (Neff, 2008). It means that we attempt to find the precarious balance between being aware of the storyline of our lives and not becoming lost in it. That means we have reactions in response to what happens to us (we are not in denial about them), but we do not become lost in those reactions, lost in the storyline. Self-care assists us in experiencing this balance, because through self-care we are compassionately attending to ourselves. This chapter begins with a philosophical discussion of self-care followed by discussions of the basic hazards of crisis intervention work (burnout and related issues), which underscore the importance of self-care, self-care approaches, the application of a self-care philosophy, and approaches to a case example.

SELF-CARE IN THE CONTEXT OF THE MENTAL HEALTH PROFESSION

Most ethical codes of the mental health professions have sections on professional self-care, but because we come into these professions to learn to help others, this very focus makes self-care a complicated process of practicing self-care while we are caring for others (Norcross & Barnett, 2008). Because the therapeutic relationship is core to the therapeutic process, and the mental health professional invites the quality of the therapeutic relationship, self-care of the mental health professional has an important influence on therapy (Norcross & Barnett, 2008). Therefore, mental health professionals have both an ethical and moral responsibility to be committed to self-care.

Those of us who work in the mental health field as professionals know the importance of self-care. How can we avoid viewing self-care from an idealized ethical imperative and instead use that ethical imperative as more of a guide? This is where our philosophical view of self-care is critical. We can read about self-care and become frustrated or discouraged because of the "messiness" of being human. We may want to practice better self-care, but life may have given us personal or professional stressors over which we have no control and that, in effect, limit our self-care practices in terms of time, energy, or money.

We need to first look at what or who in our lives gives us a sense of hope and helps us face the day. What provides us with hope and meaning in our lives? The positive impact of being connected with these resources can have a positive contagion effect on our clients. By nurturing ourselves, we can nurture our clients (Hood & Ersever, 2009). Exercises are provided at the end of this chapter to help the reader clarify these resources. However, it is the underpinnings of the self-care perspective that are so critical in our approaches to self-care. If we take information on self-care and apply it to ourselves in an idealistic, rigid, formula-based manner, we can end up with a high degree of negative self-criticism. Paradoxically, we have increased the very stress we are trying to reduce. We can also practice self-care so "perfectly" that it essentially backfires: we are stressed out from how much we attempt to care for ourselves.

The resolution to such binds and paradoxes concerning self-care is to hold two opposing truths as both being true: We do need to practice self-care in order to be the best mental health professionals we can be; and we need to acknowledge up front that this is an ideal that we cannot achieve, because we are human beings working with human beings in an imperfect world. As hard as we try, we will make mistakes and not be able to reach the ideal. We need to avoid catastrophizing our failures and our inability to reach ideal self-care standards. The reality is that we have difficulties and stressors beyond our control, as do our clients, and we work in an imperfect world that does not always provide enough or the right resources for ourselves or for our clients.

We step outside the paradox by holding the ethical imperative—the ideal of self-care—as a guide, while being flexible in the application of the ideal to our lives.

While we need to follow the maxim "Do no harm," we also need to keep in mind some others, such as the presented Self-Care Tips.

We need to practice "self-care on the run," meaning we need to personalize and individualize our self-care practice with consideration of the realistic limits facing us in terms of time, energy, and money. We need to be flexible and adaptable to fit our changing needs and the changing contexts of our lives. We need to make a commitment to practice self-care through the integration of our self-care activities into our daily lives, by listening to our stress levels and responding to them. We need to address our whole being (mind, body, emotions, and spirit) through practices such as meditation, self-talk, and physical exercise.

A part of this approach is the inclusion, then, of self-forgiveness for when we do not reach our ideals of self-care. Smedes (1984) provides a self-forgiveness model with four stages:

1. *Hurt*: We hurt ourselves through our mistakes and vices.
2. *Hate*: We hate ourselves for having done wrong.
3. *Heal*: We write our own script; we allow others to love us.
4. *Home*: Our split within ourselves is healed.

The practice of self-forgiveness applies to those self-care practices that we deeply wish we did better. For example, it may be very important to us to lose weight, but as hard as we try, we continue to struggle with a sensible weight-loss plan. This is where the axioms listed above and a self-forgiveness model are so important. They can help us develop a realistic self-care plan in the context of our present situation and avoid the harsh self-criticism that can so easily evolve from not being able to

---

Self-Care Tips

- "*Progress, not perfection.*" One can work at achieving progress and not be discouraged or overwhelmed by flaws or limitations, even though perfection cannot be reached.
- "*Don't compare your insides with other people's outsides.*" We tend to compare how we feel with how others look and thus may underestimate their struggles in life, which actually might be similar to ours.
- "*Run interference with yourself.*" We may need to do the opposite behavior of our tendency in order to act our way into a new way of thinking or feeling.
- "*Be responsible for the effort, not the outcome.*" We are only responsible for making the best effort we can make, but we must recognize that we cannot control the outcome of our efforts.

meet our ideals. Connected with the concept of self-forgiveness is self-compassion. Self-compassion means that we are kind to ourselves and show understanding for ourselves when we experience failure, inadequacy, and misfortune; we respond to our human suffering in a balanced way (Neff, 2008). To respond in a balanced way, we need to practice self-care as we are aware of our pain.

It is from this philosophical view of self-care that some of the hazards of crisis intervention work are explored. The hazards presented here are: burnout, secondary traumatic stress disorder, vicarious traumatization, and compassion fatigue.

BURNOUT AND ITS CAUSES

Originally the term *burnout* came from the psychiatric view of patients being "burned out" from a holistic perspective where they were completely exhausted (Paine, 1982, p. 16), and then the term began to be applied to work situations where health care volunteers showed signs of having more problems than their clients (Freudenberger, 1974, 1975). Freudenberger's writings were based on experiences at a New York City drug abuse community agency. While drug abusers were labeled "burnouts" (i.e., they only cared about drugs and slowly had become unmotivated and incompetent), Freudenberger used the term "burnout" to describe the workers in his 1974 article, "Staff Burnout." While that article seemed to kick off a collective, intuitive understanding of the term, we still seem to have difficulty defining it with clarity (Skovholt, 2001). There are numerous definitions of burnout as described by *symptoms* (negativism, exhaustion, cynicism, etc.; Leviton, 1993) or *dimensions* ("lack of personal accomplishment, emotional exhaustion, and depersonalization and deindividuation of clients"; Maslach & Jackson, 1986, as described in Kanel, 2007, p. 32).

The definition of burnout used in this text is:

> . . . a state of physical, mental, and emotional exhaustion caused by long-term involvement in emotionally demanding situations. It is accompanied by an array of symptoms including physical depletion, feelings of helplessness and hopelessness, disillusionment, negative self-concept, and negative attitudes toward work, people, and life itself.
>
> **(James, 2008, p. 531)**

In addition to the term *burnout*, other terms have emerged to describe what happens to crisis intervention workers that can lead to burnout. These terms include *secondary traumatic stress disorder* (STSD) (James, 2008). STSD has also been called *vicarious traumatization* (VT) (McCann & Pearlman, 1990), *compassion fatigue* (CF) (Danieli & Dingman, 2005; Figley, 1995), and *negative countertransference* (Greene, Kane, Christ, Lynch, & Corrigan, 2006). Specifically, *vicarious traumatization* is what happens when the mental health professional adopts the trauma-related symptoms of the client (Halpern & Tramontin, 2007; Hoff, Hallisey, & Hoff, 2009; James, 2008). *Compassion fatigue* is ongoing severe compassion stress in which one feels helpless, confused, and isolated; it is similar to posttraumatic stress disorder (PTSD), but different in that the reaction is not to the event, as in PTSD, but to the person telling about the event.

Although the different terms can be confusing, at their essence, these interchangeable terms describe an out-of-balance relationship between the mental health professional and the client; they provide mental health professionals with a framework to understand some of the dangers of crisis work. When the mental health professional intervenes in a crisis, there may be a temptation toward heroic action that minimizes one's own needs. Personal needs, physical health, nutrition, safety, and self-direction may fall by the wayside for the mental health professional as he/she is drawn into responding to the crisis (Leviton, 1993). Such "other direction" can lead to burnout, in which the mental health professional is negative, cynical, and less supportive toward clients (Vettor & Kosinski, 2000).

The danger of burnout and STSD is that they can endanger the welfare of both the client and the mental health professional. This danger, then, underscores the importance of the self-care of the mental health professional. Workers in crisis situations need to know how to identify this state so they can respond to it effectively (Kanel, 2007). Approaches to self-care can assist in the prevention or intervention of burnout and STSD. The more coping strategies possessed by the mental health professional, the less burnout experienced. Coping strategies that are inadequate increase stress and burnout, while constructive ones decrease them (Wilkerson, 2009).

SELF-CARE APPROACHES

> There may be times when people need to limit doing new things, such as forming new relationships and terminating old ones, and simply rest as much as they can, eat nutritious food, be with friends who are accepting and nurturing, care for their own bodies, love themselves as much as they can, and keep things as predictable as possible until they are in a better place to again risk change, and reach out to others.
>
> **(Schneider, 1984, p. 20)**

The above description of a strategic retreat is an example of how self-care can be used in a self-respecting, compassionate manner. Sometimes life simply gives us too much, and we need to simply do the best we can to catch our breath, to regroup.

General Techniques

There are numerous techniques available for self-care. Some of these are outlined in the additional readings section at the end of this chapter. A few are highlighted here.

A Substance Abuse and Mental Health Services Administration (SAMHSA) (2005a) brochure provides ten tips for effective stress management:

1. Familiarize yourself with signs of stress.
2. Get enough rest, exercise regularly, and maintain a healthy diet.

3. Have a life outside of your job.
4. Avoid tobacco, alcohol, drugs, and excessive caffeine.
5. Draw strength from faith, friends, and family.
6. Maintain your sense of humor.
7. Have a personal preparedness plan.
8. Participate in training offered at your workplace.
9. Get a regular physical checkup.
10. Ask for help if you need it.

Some additional basic techniques are to make a daily plan and follow it; to reduce the changes in one's life (if possible); to handle one situation at a time; to have realistic self-goals; and to manage fear/anger. The management of fear and anger can be done by avoiding extreme reactions, practicing reassuring, comforting rituals, doing something for someone else, getting out of the stressful situation as quickly as possible, and talking with a professional counselor.

Effective stress management includes the concept of resilience. Resilience is ordinary and can help us cope with the difficulties and adversities of life. We can learn resilience in our own unique ways through the personal application of time and effort; however, resilience is not a guarantee against difficult times (Masten, 2001).

The Discovery Health Channel and the American Psychological Association's packet, *Aftermath: The Road to Resilience*, outlines ten ways to build resilience (2002):

1. Making connections
2. Avoiding seeing crises as insurmountable
3. Accepting change as a part of living
4. Moving toward one's goals
5. Taking decisive actions
6. Looking for self-discovery opportunities
7. Nurturing a positive view of self
8. Keeping things in perspective
9. Maintaining a hopeful outlook
10. Taking care of self

Item 8, keeping things in perspective, can include examination of the organization's dynamics as well as the individual's dynamics (SAMSHA, 2006). The organization is examined on the dimensions of: (a) effective management structure and leadership, (b) clear purpose and goals, (c) functionally defined roles, (d) team support, and (e) plan for stress management. Individual dimensions include: (a) management of workload, (b) balanced lifestyle, (c) stress reduction strategies, and (d) self-awareness. The mental health professional can use these dimensions as an evaluation assessment of organizational and individual dynamics that are contributing to the stress of the individual. Item 10, taking care of self, which is the focus of this chapter, underscores the importance of the development of resilience in a mental health professional's life.

Specific Techniques

Specific individual stress management strategies include educative, relaxation, and related techniques, and cognitive-behavioral models (Kilburg, Nathan, & Thoreson, 1989). The *educative strategies* are those connected with workshops that typically involve information and experiential activities regarding stress management. For example, a workshop may have a component on body awareness using the acronym HALT. HALT is like a temperature gauge: It can remind the mental health professional not to become too Hungry, Angry, Lonely, or Tired, and to address each area as necessary for self-care. The *relaxation techniques* are those involving the areas of yoga, meditation, relaxation training, biofeedback, and the like. *Cognitive-behavioral models* are those that examine the person's ideas that encourage the disturbance.

One example of a cognitive-behavioral model is *mindfulness*: "observing, seeing one thing in the moment" (Marra, 2004, p. 100). Mindfulness is one of the three components of self-compassion; the other two components are *self-kindness* and a *recognition of common human struggles* (Neff, 2008). Note that mindfulness has a positive impact on the counseling skills and therapeutic relationships of counseling graduate students (Schure & Christopher, 2008).

Mindfulness strategies include being nonjudgmental and active, being mindful of one thing at a time and of the moment, and being focused on our senses (sound, smell, touch, visual, body, thought, feeling, taste) as well as descriptive of our experience (Marra, 2004). In emotional mindfulness, we specifically identify the emotion, examine how it is expressed in the body, determine thoughts about the emotion, track down environmental triggers, document our own behavior, and document our (and possibly others') follow-up reactions to our behavior (Marra, 2004).

Another technique that crosses both relaxation and cognitive-behavioral approaches is the use of *humor*. Humor may help us in four ways (Martin, 2007). First, humor may have stress-buffering effects. In part, this may be a result of our being able to change our perspective on a situation in terms of reference frame, a positive challenge, and having a sense of control. Second, humor may help us in terms of "enhancing social support, denying reality, venting aggressive feelings, and providing distraction" (Martin, 2007, p. 285). Third, if we have a humorous perspective, we tend to be more realistic and flexible, have more and various coping strategies and defenses (e.g., cognitive reframes and management of emotions), and view stress as less threatening cognitively. Fourth, humor may also be helpful emotionally in times of extreme and uncontrollable stress.

Humor, then, can be very helpful to the mental health professional in crisis situations. For example, when I was doing 9/11 disaster mental health work in New York, I had a client who was frustrated with a copy machine yell at me, "I'm not always this difficult!" This seemed like such an understatement in the context of the extreme disaster he was facing in his life that both he and I burst into laughter. Following the laughter I said to the client, "It only seems reasonable that you are frustrated with everything happening to you," and we both smiled. An exchange of humor between the mental health professional and the client needs to be very sensitively done. For example, it may be prudent to let the client introduce the humor. In the previous story, the client laughed first and I followed his lead with my laughter.

While humor may help *during* the crisis situation, it may also help both *before* and *after* the crisis situation. Humor can be useful prior to a situation, when the mental health professional intentionally brings some elements of humor (for oneself) into the crisis situation in an appropriate way (carrying around a humorous quote or silly cartoon in a billfold or purse) or uses the humorous element following the crisis situation (doing something silly or lighthearted after heavy emotional work).

The use of general or specific techniques for stress management and self-care in a crisis situation requires that we be realistic about our work within the current situation and specifically what we can do in the specific crisis situation being faced.

Fundamental Lessons and Strategies

Although techniques for self-care can be helpful, five fundamental lessons regarding self-care can also benefit us as mental health professionals (Norcross & Barnett, 2008). First, having guiding principles rather than techniques allows us to have broad strategies that can be adjusted to fit our situations and personal preferences. Second, we need to have a broad variety of strategies to draw on for self-care. Third, we need to remember that self-care is an interactive process between the person and the environment. Fourth, our self-care must fit us in terms of our unique emotional resources and vulnerabilities. Fifth, we must practice self-care both at work and away from work. Twelve strategies (Norcross & Barnett, 2008) that we can use as a guiding framework are:

1. *Valuing the person of the psychotherapist:* Make self-care a priority.
2. *Refocusing on the rewards:* Look at what is rewarding about being a mental health professional.
3. *Recognizing the hazards:* Remember that the profession has inherent stressors and work within that reality.
4. *Minding the body:* Meet the needs of the body.
5. *Nurturing relationships:* Ask ourselves: "Who has my back?"
6. *Setting boundaries:* Establish boundaries between ourselves and others as well as between professional and personal lives (with a transition ritual between them).

7. *Reconstructing cognitions:* Monitor internal dialogue and countertransference, with the adage of "Be gentle with yourself."

8. *Sustaining healthy escapes:* Ask ourselves, "How do I play?" and "How can I structure in that time?"

9. *Creating a flourishing environment:* Examine our work environment in terms of specific dimensions (workload, control, reward, sense of community, respect, similar values) and the comfort of work (safety, privacy, lighting, ventilation, furniture, aesthetics) and positively change that which we can.

10. *Undergoing personal therapy:* Use therapy as a way to examine and heal ourselves.

11. *Cultivating spirituality and mission:* Be able to "pull hope from heal" (p. 26).

12. *Fostering creativity and growth:* Have diverse activities as a part of our job; go to conferences, read, and have study groups.

See Exercise 9.5 for personal application of these strategies.

COMMUNITY OF SUPPORT

To be resilient, we need to have a community of support (Discovery Health Channel & APA, 2002). Nurturing relationships and flourishing environments that include a sense of community help us cope with stress personally and professionally. Being resilient and able to face adversity is fused with the quality of one's social networks (Hoff et al., 2009). We need, then, as mental health professionals, to examine our support networks to determine whether they have enough to help sustain us in the work we are facing. Some specific types of support are discussed here to assist

---

Top 10 Practical Suggestions for Self-Care

1. Be flexible with your self-care plan.
2. Practice self-care on the run.
3. Listen to your body.
4. Care for your body.
5. Feed your "spirit": Do what helps you feel alive.
6. Be gentle with yourself, kind to yourself, and forgiving toward yourself.
7. Practice reassuring, comforting rituals.
8. Practice mindfulness.
9. Maintain a sense of humor.
10. Play whenever possible.

in the mental health professional's self-assessment: defusing, debriefing, "having a buddy," and consultation with a supervisor, mentor, or colleague.

Defusing is the process of talking out the crisis-related experience (Weaver, 1995). This is often informal and unplanned. It needs to be positive, supportive, and without criticism; it must involve individuals who have experienced the crisis intensely, and it must encourage as few war stories as possible (Hartsough & Myers, 1985). Mental health professionals can find it very helpful to have someone with whom they can quickly process a crisis situation that they handled.

Debriefing is a formal meeting that usually occurs somewhere between 24 and 72 hours after the crisis, with the focus being on addressing any of the emotional experiences left over from the event (Weaver, 1995). It may be helpful for the mental health professional to check in with other professionals regarding the current strains being experienced in handling the crisis situations.

Simply *"having a buddy"* in high-stress situations helps one cope. Norcross and Barnett (2008) exemplify the importance of this concept when they ask in their strategy of nurturing relationships, "Who has my back?" It is much easier to cope with stress when one has a buddy, personally or professionally, and when we can view another person as "on our side." This perspective, this sense of not being alone, can provide an oasis of support and nurturance even in the face of the greatest stressors. Mutual aid self-help groups can also be resources of support.

Consultation with a supervisor, mentor, or colleague can also reduce one's sense of aloneness and increase one's sense of support. Supervision can reduce the stress of a job (Kilburg, Nathan, & Thoreson, 1989). The mental health professional with a trusted supervisor, mentor, or colleague may feel deeply supported in addressing stress experienced with regard to personal or professional crises.

Top 10 Practical Suggestions for Building a Community of Support

1. Develop nurturing relationships.
2. Develop supportive communities.
3. Develop relationships and communities both personally and professionally.
4. Defuse when necessary.
5. Build debriefing into one's professional/personal life.
6. Find a buddy in one's professional arena.
7. Find a buddy in one's personal life.
8. Find a supervisor who can be trusted.
9. Develop a mentoring relationship.
10. Find a colleague who will be supportive.

CASE EXAMPLE

The following true-life case of self-care in response to personal and professional stress is punctuated in bold where sections of the text on self-care are reflected.

For three years a mental health professional in her 50s experienced a great amount of personal and professional stress. Three crises occurred during an eight-month period of time, and in response to this stress, the mental health professional began working from 4:30 a.m. to 10 p.m. Monday through Friday for five months, and then added the same work schedule to a Saturday or Sunday for two years. These were responsibilities that could not be avoided or delegated because of the nature of the crises.

During this time, many people told her she would collapse mentally and/or physically under the stress, or that she would collapse once it was over. The mental health professional was determined to discover ways to live with the personal and professional pressure, which she had not experienced before in her life.

Although she had never been an athlete, in response to the stress she began working out at a wellness center every day (except Sundays) from one and a quarter hours to one and a half hours and working out with a personal trainer three times a week **(community support; personal life away from stressors)**. At the suggestion of her trainer, she, who had never boxed before, began boxing to cope with stress. She found that even though she could not hit anyone, she loved the motion she experienced when hitting a bag and hitting pads held by her trainer. She boxed for two years **(physical activity)**. When an additional stressor was experienced at her workplace after two years, and her trainer asked her if she wanted to try hula hooping, she, who had never been able to hula hoop, began hula hooping to cope with the stress **(physical activity)**.

Because she had never been able to hula hoop, the encouragement of the young people at the local wellness center meant a lot to her **(community support)**. They said things such as, "You can do this," and "You have to practice to get better." It took her three months to learn to hula hoop **("Progress, not perfection"; "Responsible for the effort, not the outcome")**. During that time, many strangers gave her advice on how to hula hoop, because she was so bad at it **(community support)**. It also became a bridge between herself and others where, again, total strangers would tell her stories when they saw her hula hooping at the wellness center: "I used to be good at that," "I had a hula hoop that looked like . . .," or "I was a teenager when the hula hoop was invented" **(community support)**.

So what does this story have to do with self-care? The mental health professional found that it was hard to take herself too seriously on a day that she had started by hula hooping **(play; running interference with self; humor)**. She also found that she was so bad at hula hooping that she could not do anything or think about anything else when hula hooping other than hula hooping itself **(mindfulness)**.

After three months, she learned to hula hoop—and two weeks later she broke her wrist badly and had to have surgery. One week after surgery, she discovered she could hula hoop with one hand and began practicing hula hooping daily, since it was one of the few forms of exercise she could still do with a broken wrist **(physical exercise)**. Hula hooping gave her hope for recovery during the pain of the break, surgery, and rehabilitation **(play; running interference with self; humor)**.

She began to take hula hooping into her professional presentations and her trainings of graduate students and mental health professionals over the next four months (during which her wrist was in a cast), using hula hooping as a metaphor for self-care. For example, during breaks in a summer class, she invited the students to hula hoop with her in the grassy area outside of the building in which she taught. She found that it invited in everyone a playfulness that she believed is critical to self-care. Because it was so out of the ordinary for typical discussions on self-care, it freed both her and participants to talk about self-care in a more realistic, fun perspective.

The professional in this case example is me, the author of this text. So much healing and so many delightful discussions on self-care resulted in my decision to include this personal disclosure in this text. It is an excellent example (but not ideal by any means) of self-care practiced in the face of significant stressors. A more detailed description of my journey is outlined in the article "Cultivating the Capacity for Joy through Therapists' Self-Care: Examples of Daily Practices" (Ersever, Atkins, & Miller, 2009).

SUMMARY

This chapter summarized a philosophical and practical approach to self-care. Specific hazards of crisis work for the mental health professional were addressed. Both general and specific approaches to self-care were explored.

QUESTIONS

1. What are the interchangeable terms that can lead to burnout?
2. What role can humor play in coping with stress?
3. What are five fundamental lessons of self-care?

Case Study 9.1

Bob is a new mental health professional at a mental health center, and he has been picking up on-call responsibilities at his work in the last six months. The center requires mental health professionals to be on-call for a week once every four weeks. Bob has a lot of responsibilities personally, with a new family (a second child born in the last four months) and a new house, and he felt overwhelmed when his employer announced two months into his job that all mental health professionals would now

---

be required to take rotating on-call shifts in their area of expertise. Bob had not done any crisis intervention work prior to this job, and found that being on-call was generally stressful, and the phone calls and interventions were quite demanding in terms of their emotional urgency and the time they required.

1. How would you suggest that Bob generally approach his situation in terms of self-care?
2. In the event he needs to stay at his job, how would you suggest he practice self-care at work?
3. How might Bob practice self-care in his personal life, particularly during the week that he is on call?

Case Study 9.2

Brenda has been a disaster mental health professional for a number of years and has volunteered in response to local, state, and federal disasters. She came into the most recent disaster volunteer work with a lot of confidence because of her good experiences as a worker in previous settings. At this disaster, however, some different dynamics were in place. First, her supervisor was encouraging the mental health professionals to work almost nonstop during their 12-hour shifts (e.g., verbally positively reinforcing mental health professionals who skipped their lunches and 15-minute breaks). Second, her team consisted of four people who typically taught at universities and had never worked full-time as mental health professionals; at most, some had worked part-time in private practices away from their university settings. Third, she was worried about her marriage of 25 years because of her husband's ongoing resentment of her volunteer disaster mental health work, which resulted in one of the most vicious marital arguments they had ever had prior to her leaving for this last disaster. After one week at the site, Brenda was finding it difficult to concentrate when clients were telling her stories, she was having a hard time sleeping, and she was experiencing increasing difficulties with her ulcer.

1. What does Brenda need to do regarding self-care from an ethical perspective (i.e., for the welfare of the client)?
2. From the top 10 suggestions for self-care, which two would you strongly recommend she implement? How would you encourage her to implement them?
3. From the top 10 suggestions for community support, which two would you strongly recommend she implement? How would you encourage her to implement them?

EXERCISES

Exercise 9.1 Resilience

In this exercise, you will examine the past, present, and future. First, note at least one past time of difficulty where you overcame obstacles. Then answer these questions:

1. What strengths did I find in myself that helped me overcome the obstacles and survive the difficulties?

    _____

2. What strengths did I find outside myself (people and resources) that helped me survive that difficult time?

    _____

3. Which of those internal and external strengths are currently active in my life?

    _____

4. What have been two or three of the greatest joys I have experienced in my life?

    _____

5. What are current joys in my life?

    _____

6. What are one or two dreams/hopes I have for my future?

    _____

Exercise 9.2 Self-Care Through the Senses

Choose someone with whom you feel comfortable for this exercise. Then briefly answer each of the three items under the main heading being discussed (from Miller, 2010, pp. 382–383).

1. Hearing
    One of my favorite *sounds* is: _____
    My strongest positive memory of this *sound* is: _____
    I promise you I will include this *sound* more in my life by:

    _____

2. Touching
    One of my favorite *things to touch* is: _____
    My strongest positive memory of this *body experience* is: _____
    I promise you I will include this *body experience* more in my life by:

    _____

3. Seeing
    One of my favorite *sights* is: _____
    My strongest positive memory of this *sight* is: _____
    I promise you I will include this *sight* more in my life by: _____

4. Smelling
   One of my favorite *smells* is: _____
   My strongest positive memory of this *smell* is: _____
   I promise you I will include this *smell* more in my life by: _____
5. Tasting
   One of my favorite *tastes* is: _____
   My strongest positive memory of this *taste* is: _____
   I promise you I will include this *taste* more in my life by: _____

Exercise 9.3 Examination of Self-Care

Complete the following questions:

1. Who are people in my life who encourage me to care for myself?
   _____

2. What are self-care activities I have done/would like to do that do not take much time, energy, or money?
   _____

3. What are self-care activities I have done that would require more time, energy, or money?
   _____

4. What are three barriers I experience when I try to practice self-care?
   _____

   Now in a dyad or small group, respond to the following questions:

1. What are three barriers I experience when I try to practice self-care?
   _____

2. What are three ways I can work around those barriers?
   _____

Exercise 9.4 Further Examination of Self-Care

Answer these questions:

1. What are three of my main current stressors?
2. What are stressful messages I am receiving right now from others in my life?
3. What are three of my major wants in my life, and are they being met or not being met at this time?
4. What is one of my overall life goals?
5. How are current stressors and current stressful messages keeping me from my major wants and/or my overall life goal?
6. What are some small changes I can make toward obtaining those unmet wants and overall life goal?
7. Who does *not* criticize me that I can turn to for support?
8. Where are healing places I can go to for refuge?

Exercise 9.5 Further Examination of 12 Self-Care Strategies

Rate yourself on a scale of 1 to 10 for each of these strategies where 1 = poorest ever done in this area in one's professional life, and 10 = best one has ever done in one's professional life. Then after each section, write one small thing you can do in this area to enhance this strategy in your current work life.

1. Valuing the person of the psychotherapist

      1   2   3   4   5   6   7   8   9   10

2. Refocusing on the rewards

      1   2   3   4   5   6   7   8   9   10

3. Recognizing the hazards

      1   2   3   4   5   6   7   8   9   10

4. Minding the body

      1   2   3   4   5   6   7   8   9   10

5. Nurturing relationships

      1   2   3   4   5   6   7   8   9   10

6. Setting boundaries

      1   2   3   4   5   6   7   8   9   10

7. Reconstructing cognitions

      1   2   3   4   5   6   7   8   9   10

8. Sustaining healthy escapes

      1   2   3   4   5   6   7   8   9   10

9. Creating a flourishing environment

      1   2   3   4   5   6   7   8   9   10

10. Undergoing personal therapy

      1   2   3   4   5   6   7   8   9   10

11. Cultivating spirituality and mission

      1   2   3   4   5   6   7   8   9   10

12. Fostering creativity and growth

      1   2   3   4   5   6   7   8   9   10

SUGGESTED READINGS

Bein, A. W. (2008). *The Zen of helping*. Hoboken, NJ: Wiley.

    This book has ten chapters that address a mindfulness approach in counseling clients in general.

Domar, A. D. (2000). *Self-nurture: Learning to care for yourself as effectively as you care for everyone else*. New York, NY: Penguin.

    The entire book is filled with general suggestions and exercises for self-care from a cognitive-behavioral perspective.

Germer, C. K. (2009). *The mindful path to self-compassion*. New York: Guilford.

The entire book has suggestions and exercises for self-compassion that come from a mindfulness perspective.

Greenstone, J. L., & Leviton, S. C. (2002). *Elements of crisis intervention*. Pacific Grove, CA: Brooks/Cole.

Chapter 5 of this book is short, but offers specific suggestions on counselor self-care.

Kilburg, R. R., Nathan, P. E., & Thoreson, R. W. (1989). *Professionals in distress: Issues, syndromes, and solutions in psychology*. Washington, DC: American Psychological Association.

Chapter 13 in this text addresses the prevention and management of work-related stress within the context of individual, group, and organizational strategies.

Norcross, J. C., & Barnett, J. E. (2008, Spring). Self-care as ethical imperative. *The Register Report*, 20–27.

This short article provides information on 12 evidence-based methods for therapists to practice self-care.

Roberts, A. R., & Yeager, K. R. (2009). *Pocket guide to crisis intervention*. New York, NY: Oxford University Press.

This brief book has 33 chapters. Each of them covers, in a few pages, the major topics of crisis work. It may be thought of as a "CliffsNotes" or a primer of crisis work. It has two chapters that relate to self-care: Signs and Symptoms of Stress and Burnout; and Stress Reduction and Coping Skills.

Skovholt, T. M. (2001). *The resilient practitioner*. Boston, MA: Allyn & Bacon.

Part 2 of this book has four chapters on self-care (Chapters 9–12) and a specific chapter (Chapter 14) on a self-care action plan.

Substance Abuse and Mental Health Services Administration (SAMHSA). (2005a). *A guide to managing stress in crisis response professions*. Bethesda, MD: Author.

This 25-page guide is an excellent condensed summary that summarizes the dynamics of stress, how to prevent and manage it, and specific self-care strategies.

Substance Abuse and Mental Health Services Administration (SAMHSA). (2006). *Field manual for mental health and human service workers in major disasters*. Bethesda, MD: Author.

This 29-page guide provides overall information on disaster mental health counseling with a short section of basic information on individual and organizational stress management. It has two excellent charts at the end of the brochure on dimensions and responses in terms of organizational and individual approaches for stress prevention and management.

WEB SITES

General Information

Substance Abuse & Mental Health Services Administration (SAHMSA). www .samhsa.gov

This Web site contains information on self-care as it relates to the mental health professional.

Professional Organizational Affiliations

American Psychological Association. http://search.apa.org/search?query=self-care

This Web site provides information and access to articles and presentations specific to counselor self-care.

In addition to this Web site, readers can contact the following Web sites for information on mental health professional self-care as it relates to their professional organizational affiliation.

American Association for Marital and Family Therapy. www.aamft.org

American Counseling Association. www.counseling.org

American Psychiatric Association. www.psych.org

National Association of Social Workers. www.naswdc.org

References

Adams, J. B., & Madson, M. B. (2006). Reflection and outlook for the future of addictions treatment and training: An interview with William R. Miller. *Journal of Teaching in the Addictions, 5*, 95–109.

American Psychiatric Association (2000). *Diagnostic and statistical manual of mental disorders* (4th ed., text rev.). Washington, DC: Author.

American Psychological Association (1996). *Research agenda for psychosocial and behavioral factors in women's health.* Washington, DC: Author.

American Psychological Association (2006). *Report of the APA task force on socioeconomic status.* Washington, DC: Author.

Amodeo, M., & Jones, L. K. (1997). Viewing alcohol and other drug use cross culturally: A cultural framework for clinical practice. *Families in Society: Journal of Contemporary Human Services, 78*, 240–253.

Anderson, B. S. (1996). *The counselor and the law* (4th ed.). Alexandria, VA: American Counseling Association.

Araoz, D. L., & Carrese, M. A. (1996). *Solution-oriented brief therapy for adjustment disorders: A guide for providers under managed care.* New York, NY: Brunner/Mazel.

Arkowitz, H., Westra, H. A., Miller, W. R., & Rollnick, S. (2008). *Motivational interviewing in the treatment of psychological problems.* New York, NY: Guilford.

Association for Religious and Value Issues in Counseling (ARVIC) (n.d.). *A position paper of the Association for Spiritual, Ethical, and Religious Values in Counseling.* Retrieved November 20, 2001 from www.counseling.org/aservic/Spirituality. html. (As of this printing, article no longer accessible at this site.).

Aspinwall, L. G., & Staudinger, U. M. (2003). *A psychology of human strengths: Fundamental questions and future directions for a positive psychology.* Washington, DC: American Psychological Association.

Atkinson, D. R. (2004). *Counseling American minorities* (6th ed.). Boston, MA: McGraw-Hill.

Atkinson, D. R., & Hackett, G. (2004). *Counseling diverse populations* (3rd ed.). Boston, MA: McGraw-Hill.

Atkinson, D. R., Morten, G., & Sue, D. W. (1993). *Counseling American minorities: A crosscultural perspective* (4th ed.). Madison, WI: Brown & Benchmark.

Babor & Higgins (2002). *AUDIT: The Alcohol Use Disorders Identificaton Test: Guidelines for use in primary care* (2nd ed.). World Health Organization: Geneva, Switzerland.

Barret, B., & Logan, C. (2002). *Counseling gay men and lesbians*. Pacific Grove, CA: Brooks/Cole.

Bass, E. (Ed.) (1983). *I never told anyone: Writings by women survivors of child sexual abuse*. New York, NY: Harper Perennial.

Bass, E., & Davis, L. (1988). *The courage to heal*. New York, NY: Harper & Row.

Baum, N. (2010). Shared traumatic reality in communal disasters: Toward a conceptualization. *Psychotherapy Theory, Research, Practice, Training, 47*, 249–259.

Beck, A. T. (1976). *Cognitive therapy and the emotional disorders*. New York, NY: International Universities Press.

Bein, A. (2008). *The Zen of helping: Spiritual principles for mindful and open-hearted practice*. Hoboken, NJ: Wiley.

Belkin, G. S. (1984). *Introduction to counseling* (2nd ed.). Dubuque, IA: William C. Brown.

Benshoff, J. J., Harrawood, L. K., & Koch, D. S. (2003). Substance abuse and the elderly: Unique issues and concerns. *Journal of Rehabilitation, 69*, 43–48.

Berg, I. K. (1995). Solution-focused brief therapy with substance abusers. In A. M. Washton (Ed.), *Psychotherapy and substance abuse: A practitioner's handbook* (pp. 223–242). New York, NY: Guilford Press.

Berg, I. K. (2000). *Building solutions with mandated clients* [workshop handout]. Milwaukee, WI: Brief Focused Therapy Center.

Berghuis, D. J., & Jongsma, A. E. (2002). *The addiction progress notes planner*. Hoboken, NJ: Wiley.

Bersoff, D. N. (1976). Therapists as protectors and policemen: New roles as a result of Tarasoff. *Professional Psychology, 7*, 267–273.

Bloom, B. L. (1997). *Planned short-term psychotherapy: A clinical handbook* (2nd ed.). Boston, MA: Allyn & Bacon.

Bowlby, J. (1977). The making and breaking of affectional bonds, I and II. *British Journal of Psychiatry, 130*, 201–210, 421–431.

Bozarth, A. R. (1990). *A journey through grief*. Center City, MN: Hazelden.

Brady, K. T., Back, S. E., & Greenfield, S. F. (2009). *Women & addiction*. New York, NY: Guilford.

Brammer, L.M. (1985). *The helping relationship: Process and skills* (3rd ed.). Upper Saddle River, NJ: Prentice Hall.

Briere, J. (1989). *Therapy for adults molested as children: Beyond survival*. New York, NY: Springer.

Briere, J., & Scott, C. (2006). *Principles of trauma therapy*. Thousand Oaks, CA: Sage.

Bryant, R. A., & Harvey, A. G. (2000). Telephone crisis intervention skills: A simulated caller paradigm. *Crisis: The Journal of Crisis Intervention and Suicide Prevention, 21*, 90–94.

Buelow, G. D., & Buelow, S. A. (1998). *Psychotherapy in chemical dependence treatment: A practical and integrative approach.* Pacific Grove, CA: Brooks/Cole.

Burbules, N. C. (1993). *Dialogue in teaching.* New York, NY: Teachers College Press.

Bureau of Justice Statistics (FBJ) (2004). *National crime victimization survey, criminal victimization, 2003.* Retrieved October 6, 2006, from http://www.ojp.usdoj.gov/bjs/pub/pdf/cv03.pdf#search=22%National%20Crime% (no longer accessible at this site).

Bureau of Justice Statistics (FBJ) (2005). *Family Violence Statistics, 2004.* Retrieved October 6, 2009, from http://www.ojp.usdoj.gov/bjs/pub/pdf/cv03.pdf#search=22%National%20Crime% (no longer accessible at this site).

Cade, B., & O'Hanlon, W. H. (1993). *A brief guide to brief therapy.* New York, NY: W. W. Norton.

Campbell, L., Vasquez, M., Behnke, S., & Kinscherff, R. (2010). *APA ethics code commentary and case illustrations.* Washington, DC: American Psychological Association.

Caplan, G. (1961). *An approach to community mental health.* New York, NY: Grune & Stratton.

Caprara, G. V., & Cervone, D. (2003). A conception of personality for a psychology of human strengths: Personality as an agentic, self-regulating system. In L. G. Aspinwall & U. M. Staudinger (Eds.), *A psychology of human strengths: Fundamental questions and future directions for a positive psychology* (pp. 61–74). Washington, DC: American Psychological Association.

Cardemil, E. V., & Battle, C. L. (2003). Guess who's coming to therapy? Getting comfortable with conversations about race and ethnicity in psychotherapy. *Professional Psychology: Research and Practice, 34*, 278–286.

Carter, W. L. (2002). *It happened to me: A teen's guide to overcoming sexual abuse.* Oakland, CA: New Harbinger.

Carver, C. S., & Scheier, M. F. (2003). Three human strengths. In L. G. Aspinwall & U. M. Staudinger (Eds.), *A psychology of human strengths: Fundamental questions and future directions for a positive psychology* (pp. 87–102). Washington, DC: American Psychological Association.

Cashwell, C. S., & Young, J. S. (2005). *Integrating spirituality and religion into counseling: A guide to competent practice.* Alexandria, VA: American Counseling Association.

Center for Substance Abuse Treatment (CSAT) (1994). *Practical approaches in the treatment of women who abuse alcohol and other drugs* (DHHS Publication No. 94-3006). Rockville, MD: Author.

Center for Substance Abuse Treatment (CSAT) (2003). *Co-occurring disorders: Integrated dual disorders treatment: Implementation resource kit.* Rockville, MD.

Center for Substance Abuse Treatment (CSAT) (2005). *Substance abuse treatment for persons with co-occurring disorders.* Treatment Improvement Protocol (TIP) Series,

No. 42. DHHS Publication No. (SMA) 05-3922. Rockville, MD: Substance Abuse and Mental Health Services Administration.

Center for Substance Abuse Treatment (CSAT) (2008). *Managing depressive symptoms in substance abuse clients during early recovery.* Treatment Improvement Protocol (TIP) Series, No. 48. DHHS Publication No. (SMA) 05-3922. Rockville, MD: Substance Abuse and Mental Health Services Administration.

Cherry, K. E., Allen, P. D., & Galea, S. (2010). Older adults and natural disasters: Lessons learned from Hurricanes Katrina and Rita. In P. Dass-Brailsford (Ed.), *Crisis and disaster counseling: Lessons learned from Hurricane Katrina and other disasters.* (pp. 115–130). Los Angeles: Sage.

Christopher, J. C. (2006). Teaching self-care through mindfulness practices: The application of yoga, meditation and Qigong to counselor training. *Journal of Humanistic Psychology, 46,* 494–509.

Chung, R. C.-Y., & Bemak, F. (2002). The relationship of culture and empathy in cross-cultural counseling. *Journal of Counseling and Development, 80,* 154–159.

Cohen, J. A., Berliner, L., & Mannarino, A. P. (2010). Trauma focused CBT for children with co-occurring trauma and behavior problems. *Child Abuse & Neglect: The International Journal, 34,* 215–224.

Cohen, J. A., Mannarino, A. P., Gibson, L. E., Cozza, S. J., Brymer, M. J., & Murray, L. (2006). Interventions for children and adolescents following disasters. In E. C. Ritchie, P. J. Watson, & M. J. Friedman (Eds.), *Interventions following mass violence and disasters* (pp. 227–256). New York, NY: Guilford.

Cohen-Posey, K. (2000). *Brief therapy client handouts.* New York, NY: Wiley.

Collins, B. G., & Collins, T. M. (2005). *Crisis and trauma: Developmental-ecological intervention.* Lahaska, PA: Lahaska Press.

Connors, G. J., Donovan, D. M., & DiClemente, C. C. (2001). *Substance abuse treatment and the stages of change.* New York, NY: Guilford Press.

Connors, G. J., & Tarbox, A. R. (1985). Michigan Alcoholism Screening Test. In D. J. Keyer & R. C. Sweetland (Eds.), *Test critiques* (vol. 3, pp. 439–446). Kansas City, MO: Westport.

Coombs, R. H. (Ed.) (2005). *Addiction counseling review: Preparing for comprehensive, certification, and licensing examination.* Mahwah, NJ: Lawrence Erlbaum Associates.

Corey, G. (1995). *Theory and practice of group counseling* (4th ed.). Pacific Grove, CA: Brooks/Cole.

Corey, G. (2009). *Theories and practice of counseling and psychotherapy* (8th ed.). Belmont, CA: Wadsworth.

Corey, G., Corey, M. S., Callanan, P., & Russell, J. M. (2004). *Group techniques* (3rd ed.). Pacific Grove, CA: Brooks/Cole.

Cross, T. L., Bazron, B. J., Dennis, K. W., & Isaacs, M. R. (1989). *Towards a culturally competent system of care: A monograph on effective services for minority children who are severely emotionally disturbed.* Washington, DC: Georgetown University Child

Development Center, Child and Adolescent Service System Program Technical Assistance Center.

Csikszentmihalyi, M. (1990). *Flow*. New York, NY: Harper Perennial.

Cunningham, C., & MacFarlane, K. (1991). *When children molest children: Group treatment strategies for young sexual abusers*. Orwell, VT: The Safer Society Press.

Danieli, Y., & Dingman, R. L. (2005). Introduction. In Y. Danieli & R. L. Dingman (Eds.), *On the ground after September 11* (pp. 1–15). Binghamton, NY: Haworth Press.

Dass-Brailsford, P. (Ed.) (2010). *Crisis and disaster counseling: Lessons learned from Hurricane Katrina and other disasters*. Los Angeles: Sage.

Dattilio, F. M., & Freeman, A. (Eds.) (2007). *Cognitive-behavioral strategies in crisis intervention* (3rd ed.). New York, NY: Guilford.

Dattilio F. M. & van Hout G. C. M. (2006). The problem-solving component in cognitive-behavioral couples' therapy. *Journal of Family Psychotherapy, 17*, 1–19.

Davanloo, H. (1980). A method of short-term dynamic psychotherapy. In H. Davanloo (Ed.), *Short-term dynamic psychotherapy* (pp. 75–91). Northvale, NJ: Aronson.

Davis, L. (1990). *The courage to heal workbook*. New York, NY: Harper & Row.

De Shazer, S. (1985). *Keys to solution in brief therapy*. New York, NY: Norton.

DeWolfe, D. J. (2000). *Training manual for mental health and human service workers in major disasters*. U.S. Department of Health and Human Services: Center for Mental Health Services (Publication No. ADM 90-538). Washington, DC: Government Printing Office.

DiClemente, C. C. (2003). *Addiction and change*. New York, NY: Guilford Press.

DiClemente, C. C., Garay, M., & Gemmell, L. (2008). Motivational enhancement. In M. Galanter & H. D. Kleber (Eds.), *Substance abuse treatment* (4th ed., pp. 361–371). Washington, DC: American Psychiatric Publishing.

Dilsaver, S. C. (1990). The mental status examination. *American Family Physician, 41*, 1489–1497.

Dimeff, L. A., Comtois, K. A., & Linehan, M. M. (2009). Co-occurring addiction and borderline personality disorder. In R. K. Ries, D. A. Fiellin, S. C. Miller, & R. Saitz (Eds.), *Principles of addiction medicine* (4th ed., pp. 1227–1237). Philadelphia: Wolters Kluwer/Lippincott Williams & Wilkins.

Dimeff, L. A., & Linehan, M. M. (2008). Dialectical behavior therapy for substance abusers. *Addiction Science & Clinical Practice, 4*, 39–47.

Dingman, R. L., & Weaver, J. D. (2003). *Days in the lives of counselors*. Boston, MA: Allyn & Bacon.

Discovery Health Channel & American Psychological Association (2002). *Aftermath: The road to resilience* [Packet]. Washington, DC: American Psychological Association.

Domar, A. D. (2000). *Self-nurture: Learning to care for yourself as effectively as you care for everyone else*. New York, NY: Penguin.

Domestic Abuse Intervention Project (2002). *A guide for conducting domestic violence assessments*. Duluth, MN: Author.

Downs, W. R., & Harrison, L. (1998). Childhood maltreatment and the risk of substance abuse problems in later life. *Health and School Care in the Community, 6*, 35–36.

Dziegielewski, S. F., & Sumner, K. (2005). An examination of the U.S. response to bioterrorism: Handling the threat and aftermath through crisis intervention In A. R. Roberts (Ed.), *Crisis intervention handbook* (3rd ed., pp. 262–278). New York, NY: Oxford.

Edelson, J. L., & Tolman, R. M. (1992). *Intervention for men who batter: An ecological approach*. Newbury Park, CA: Sage.

Edwards, C. L., Johnson, S., & Feliu, M. (2003, November/December). Diversity and cultural competence: Part 2. Issues of practical conceptualization and implementation. *North Carolina Psychologist, 55*, 1–13.

Eisenberg, N., & Wang, V. O. (2003). Toward a positive psychology: Social developmental and cultural contributions. In L. G. Aspinwall & U. M. Staudinger (Eds.), *A psychology of human strengths: Fundamental questions and future directions for a positive psychology* (pp. 61–74). Washington, DC: American Psychological Association.

el-Guebaly, N. (2008). Cross-cultural aspects of addiction. In M. Galanter & H. D. Kleber (Eds.), *Substance abuse treatment* (4th ed., pp. 45–52). Washington, DC: American Psychiatric Publishing.

Ellis, A. (1962). *Reason and emotion in psychotherapy*. New York, NY: Stuart.

Engel, G. L. (1961). Is grief a disease? A challenge for medical research. *Psychosomatic Medicine, 23*, 18–22.

Erbele, P. (1982). Alcohol abusers and non-users: A discriminant analysis of differences between two subgroups of batterers. *Journal of Health and Social Behavior, 23*, 260–271.

Ersever, O. H., Atkins, S., & Miller, G. (2009, Winter). Cultivating the capacity for joy through therapist's self-care: Examples of daily practices. *Spectrum, 70*, 15–21.

Evans, K., & Sullivan, J. M. (2001). *Dual diagnosis: Counseling the mentally ill substance abuser* (2nd ed.). New York, NY: Guilford Press.

Everly, G. S., & Flynn, B. W. (2006). Principles and practical procedures for acute psychological first aid training for personnel without mental health experience. *International Journal of Emergency Mental Health, 8*, 93–100.

Everly, G. S., Lating, J. M., & Mitchell, J. T. (2005). Innovations in group crisis intervention. In A. R. Roberts (Ed.), *Crisis intervention handbook* (3rd ed., pp. 221–245). New York, NY: Oxford.

Ewing, J. A. (1984). Detecting alcoholism: The CAGE questionnaire. *Journal of the American Medical Association, 252*, 1905–1907.

Fall, K. A., & Howard, S. (2004). *Alternatives to domestic violence* (2nd ed.). New York, NY: Brunner/Routledge.

Fallot, R. D. (1998). *Spirituality and religion in recovery from mental illness*. New York, NY: Jossey-Bass.

Figley, C. R. (Ed.) (1995). *Compassion fatigue: Coping with secondary traumatic stress disorder in those who treat the traumatized*. New York, NY: Brunner-Mazel.

Finkelhor, D. (1986). *A sourcebook on child sexual abuse*. Beverly Hills, CA: Sage.

References

Finley, J. R., & Lenz, B. S. (1999a). *The chemical dependence treatment documentation sourcebook*. New York, NY: Wiley.

Finley, J. R., & Lenz, B. S. (1999b). *Chemical dependence treatment homework planner*. New York, NY: Wiley.

Finley, J. R., & Lenz, B. S. (2003). *Addiction treatment homework planner* (2nd ed.). Hoboken, NJ: Wiley.

Fiske, S. T., & Taylor, S. E. (1983). *Social cognition*. Reading, MA: Addison-Wesley.

Fleming, M. F. (2003). Screening for at-risk, problem, and dependent alcohol use. In R. K. Hester & W. R. Miller (Eds.), *Handbook of alcoholism treatment approaches: Effective alternatives* (3rd ed., pp. 64–77). Boston, MA: Allyn & Bacon.

Foa, E. B., Keane, T. M., Friedman, M. J., & Cohen, J. A. (2009). *Effective treatments for PTSD: Practice guidelines from the International Society for Traumatic Stress Studies* (2nd ed.). New York, NY: Guilford.

Freudenberger, H. J. (1974). Staff burn-out. *Journal of Social Issues, 30*, 159–165.

Freudenberger, H. J. (1975). The staff burnout syndrome in alternative institutions. *Psychotherapy: Theory, Research, and Practice, 12*, 73–82.

Friedman, R., & James, J. W. (2009). The myth of the stages of dying, death and grief. *Counseling Today, 51*, 48–52.

Friere, P. (1989). *Pedagogy of the oppressed*. New York, NY: Continuum International.

Gelso, C. J., & Woodhouse, S. (2003). Toward a positive psychotherapy: Focus on human strength. In W. B. Walsh (Ed.), *Counseling psychology and optimal human functioning* (pp. 171–197). Mahwah, NJ: Erlbaum.

Gilbert, K. (2001). *From grief to memories: A workbook on life's significant losses*. Silver Spring, MD: Soras Corporation.

Goldsmith, S., Pellmar, T., Kleinman, A., & Bunney, W. (2002). *Reducing suicide: A national imperative*. Washington, DC: National Academies Press.

Goldstein, E. G. (2004). Substance abusers with borderline disorders. In S. L. A. Straussner (Ed.), *Clinical work with substance-abusing clients* (2nd ed., pp. 370–391). New York, NY: Guilford.

Gomberg, E., & Nirenberg, T. (1991). Commentary: Women and substance abuse. *Journal of Substance Abuse, 3*, 255–267.

Gonsiorek, J. C., Bera, W. H., & LeTourneau, D. (1994). *Male sexual abuse*. Thousand Oaks, CA: Sage.

Goodman, M. S., & Fallon, B. C. (1995). *Pattern changing for abused women*. Thousand Oaks, CA: Sage.

Gould, M. S., Greenberg, T., Munfakh, J. L. H., Kleinman, M., & Lubell, K. (2006). Teenagers' attitudes about seeking help from telephone crisis services (hotlines). *Suicide & Life-Threatening Behavior, 36*, 601–613.

Grafanaki, S., Pearson, D., Cini, F., Godula, D., McKenzie, B., Nason, S., & Anderegg, M. (2005). Sources of renewal: A qualitative study on the experience and role of leisure in the life of counselors and psychologists. *Counseling Psychology Quarterly, 18*, 31–40.

Graham-Bermann, S. A., & Edleson, J. L. (Eds.) (2001). *Domestic violence in the lives of children*. Washington, DC: American Psychological Association.

Granvold, D. K. (2005). The crisis of divorce: Cognitive-behavioral and constructivist assessment and treatment. In A. R. Roberts (Ed.), *Crisis intervention handbook* (3rd ed., pp. 650–681). New York, NY: Oxford University Press.

Greene, K., & Bogo, M. (2002). The different faces of intimate violence: Implications for assessment and treatment. *Journal of Marital and Family Therapy, 28*(4), 455–466.

Greene, P., Kane, D., Christ, G., Lynch, S., & Corrigan, M. (2006). FDNY crisis counseling: Innovative responses to 9/11 firefighters, families, and communities. Hoboken, NJ: Wiley.

Greenstone, J. L., & Leviton, S. C. (2002). *Elements of crisis intervention* (3rd ed.). Belmont, CA: Brooks/Cole.

Griffin, R. E. (1991). Assessing the drug involved client. *Families in Society: The Journal of Contemporary Human Services, 72*, 87–94.

Griffith, J. L., & Griffith, M. E. (2002). *Encountering the sacred in psychotherapy: How to talk with people about their spiritual lives*. New York, NY: Guilford.

Haen, C. (2005). Rebuilding security: Group therapy with children affected by September 11. *International Journal of Group Psychotherapy, 55*, 391–414.

Haley, M. (2008). Professional issues. In D. Capuzzi & M. D. Stauffer (Eds.), *Foundations of addictions counseling* (pp. 46–75). Boston, MA: Allyn & Bacon.

Halford, W. K. (2001). *Brief therapy for couples*. New York, NY: Guilford.

Halpern, J., & Tramontin, M. (2007). *Disaster mental health: Theory and practice*. Belmont, CA: Thomson Brooks/Cole.

Hamilton, T., & Samples, P. (1994). *The twelve steps and dual disorders*. Center City, MN: Hazelden.

Harris, A. H. S., Thoresen, C. E., & Lopez, S. J. (2007). Integrating positive psychology into counseling: Why and (when appropriate) how. *Journal of Counseling & Development, 85*, 3–13.

Hartsough, D.M., & Myers, D. G. (1985). Stress and mental health interventions in three major disasters. In D. M. Hartsough & D. G. Myers (Eds.), *Disaster work and mental health: Prevention and control of stress among workers* (DHHS Publication No. ADM 85-1422, pp. 1–44). Rockville, MD: U.S. Department of Health and Human Services, Public Health Service, Alcohol, Drug Abuse, and Mental Health Administration, National Institute of Mental Health.

Harvard Health Publications (2008a). *Alcohol use and abuse*. Boston, MA: Harvard University.

Harvard Health Publications (2008b). *Overcoming addiction*. Boston, MA: Harvard University.

Harvard Health Publications (2010). *Coping with grief and loss*. Boston, MA: Harvard University.

Harvard Mental Health Letter (March 2006). First aid for emotional trauma. *Harvard Mental Health Letter, 22*, 1–3.

Harvard Mental Health Letter (May 2008). Positive psychology in practice. *Harvard Mental Health Letter, 24*, 1–3.

Harvard Mental Health Letter (February 2011). Motivating behavior change. *Harvard Mental Health Letter, 27*, 1–2.

Hazelden (1993). *The dual disorders recovery book*. Center City, MN: Hazelden.

Hazelden (2005a). *Client recovery workbook*. Center City, MN: Author.

Hazelden (2005b). *Client cognitive skills workbook*. Center City, MN: Author.

Hazelden (2005c). *Client life skills workbook*. Center City, MN: Author.

Hien, D., Litt, L. C., Cohen, L. R., Miele, G. M., & Campbell, A. (2009). *Trauma services for women in substance abuse treatment*. Washington, DC: American Psychological Association.

Hilton, N. Z., Harris, G. T., & Rice, M. E. (2010). *Risk assessment for domestically violent men*. Washington, DC: American Psychological Association.

Hines, D. A., & Malley-Morrison, K. M. (2005). *Family violence in the United States*. Thousand Oaks, CA: Sage.

Hoff, L. A., Hallisey, B. J., & Hoff, M. (2009). *People in crisis: Clinical and diversity perspectives* (6th ed.). New York, NY: Routledge.

Holden, G. W., Geffner, R., & Jouriles, E. N. (Eds.) (1998). *Children exposed to marital violence*. Washington, DC: American Psychological Association.

Hood, R., & Ersever, H. (2009, June). *Ethics*. Workshop presented at the annual Al Greene Addictions Institute, Boone, NC.

Housley, J., & Beutler, L. E. (2007). *Treating victims of mass disaster and terrorism*. Cambridge, MA: Hogrefe & Huber.

Huber, C. H., & Backlund, B. A. (1992). *The twenty minute counselor*. New York, NY: Continuum International.

Ingersoll, K. S., Wagner, C. C., & Gharib, S. (2002). *Motivational groups for community substance abuse programs*. Richmond, VA: Mid-Atlantic ATTC (804-828-9910). E-mail: mid-attc@mindspring.com

Jacobs, G. A., & Meyer, D. L. (2006). Psychological first aid: Clarifying the concept. In L. Barbanel & R. J. Sternberg (Eds.), *Psychological interventions in times of crisis* (pp. 55–71). New York, NY: Springer.

Jacobson, N., & Gottman, J. (1998). *When men batter women: New insights into ending abusive relationships*. New York, NY: Simon & Schuster.

James, R. K. (2008). *Crisis intervention strategies* (6th ed.). Belmont, CA: Thomson Brooks/Cole.

Janosik, E. H. (1984). *Crisis counseling: A contemporary approach*. Monterey, CA: Wadsworth Health Sciences Division.

Johnson, J. L. (2004). *Fundamentals of substance abuse practice*. Belmont, CA: Brooks/Cole.

Jongsma, A. E., & Peterson, L. M. (2003). *The complete adult psychotherapy treatment planner*. Hoboken, NJ: Wiley.

Juhnke, G. A., Granello, D. H., & Granello, P. F. (Eds.) (2011). *Suicide, self-injury, and violence in the schools*. Hoboken, NJ: Wiley.

Kafrissen, S. R., Heffron, E. F., & Zusman, J. (1975). Mental health problems in environmental disaster. In H. L. P. Resnik, H. L. Ruben, & D. D. Ruben (Eds.), *Emergency psychiatric care: The management of mental health crises* (pp. 157–170). Bowie, MD: Charles Press.

Kalafat, J., Gould, M. S., Munfakh, J. L. H., & Kleinman, M. (2007). An evaluation of crisis hotline outcomes. Part 1: Nonsuicidal crisis callers. *Suicide & Life-Threatening Behavior, 37,* 322–337.

Kanel, K. (2007). *A guide to crisis intervention* (4th ed.). Belmont, CA: Thomson.

Kasper, L. B., Hill, C. E., & Kivlighan, D. M. (2008). Therapist immediacy in brief psychotherapy: Case study I. *Psychotherapy Theory, Research, Practice, Training, 45,* 281–297.

Kauffman, C. (2006). Positive psychology: The science at the heart of coaching. In D. R. Stober & A. M. Grant (Eds.), *Evidence-based coaching handbook: Putting best practices to work for your clients* (pp. 219–253). Hoboken, NJ: Wiley.

Kelin, R. H., & Schermer, V. L. (Eds.) (2000). *Group psychotherapy for psychological trauma.* New York, NY: Guilford.

Kemp, C. O. (2000). *A book of hope for the storms of life: Healing words for troubled times.* Franklin, TN: The Wisdom Company.

Keyes, C. L. M., & Haidt, J. (2003). Introduction: Human flourishing—The study of that which makes life worthwhile. In C. L. M. Keyes & J. Haidt (Eds.), *Flourishing: Positive psychology and the life well-lived* (pp. 3–12). Washington, DC: American Psychological Association.

Kilburg, R. R., Nathan, P. E., & Thoreson, R. W. (1989). *Professionals in distress: Issues, syndromes, and solutions in psychology.* Washington, DC: American Psychological Association.

Kingsbury, S. J. (1997, April). What is solution-focused therapy? *Harvard Mental Health Letter, 8.*

Kinney, J. (2003). *Loosening the grip.* Boston, MA: McGraw-Hill.

Kiselica, M. S. (1998). Preparing Anglos for the challenges and joys of multiculturalism. *The Counseling Psychologist, 26,* 5–21.

Klingman (1988), as referenced in Newgass, S., & Schonfeld, D. J. (2005). School crisis intervention, crisis prevention, and crisis response. In A. R. Roberts (Ed.), *Crisis intervention handbook* (3rd ed, pp. 499–518). New York, NY: Oxford.

Knapp, K.C. (2010). Children and crisis. In P. Dass-Brailsford (Ed.), *Crisis and disaster counseling: Lessons learned from Hurricane Katrina and other disasters.* (pp. 83–97). Los Angeles: Sage.

Knapp, S. J., & VandeCreek, L. (1997). *Treating patients with memories of abuse: Legal risk management.* Washington, DC: American Psychological Association.

Kogan, M. (2001). Where happiness lies. *Monitor on Psychology, 32,* 74–76.

Koss, M. P., & Shiang, J. (1994). Research on brief psychotherapy. In A. E. Bergin & S. L. Garfield (Eds.), *Handbook of psychotherapy and behavior change* (pp. 664–700). New York, NY: Wiley.

Koss-Chioino, J. D., & Vargas, L. A. (1992). Through the cultural looking glass: A model for understanding culturally responsive psychotherapies. In L. A. Vargas &

J. D. Koss-Chioino (Eds.), *Working with culture* (pp. 1–22). San Francisco, CA: Jossey-Bass.

Kubler-Ross, E. (1968). *On death and dying.* New York, NY: MacMillan.

Kuczmarski, R. J., Ogden, C. L., Guo, S. S., Grummer-Strawn, L. M., Flegal, K. M., Mei, Z., . . . Johnson, C. L. (2002). 2000 CDC growth charts for the United States: Methods and development. Hyattsville, MD: Department of Health and Human Services, Centers for Disease Control and Prevention.

L'Abate, L. L., Farrar, J. E., & Serritella, D. A. (1992). *Handbook of differential treatments for addictions.* Boston, MA: Allyn & Bacon.

Lawrence, E. C., & Sovik-Johnston, A. F. (2010). A competence approach to therapy with families with multiple problems. In D. A. Crenshaw (Ed.), *In reverence in healing: Honoring strengths without trivializing suffering* (pp. 137–149). Lanham, MD: Jason Aronson.

Lazarus, A. (Ed.) (1976). *Multimodal behavior therapy.* New York, NY: Springer.

Lazarus, A. (1981). *The practice of multimodal therapy.* New York, NY: McGraw-Hill.

Leadbeater, B., Dodgen, D., & Solarz, A. (2005). The resilience revolution: A paradigm shift for research and policy? In R. D. Peters, B. Leadbeater, & R. J. McMahon (Eds.), *Resilience in children, families, and communities: Linking context to practice and policy* (pp. 47–61). New York, NY: Kluwer Academic/Plenum.

Lee, C. C. (2003, Fall). Counseling in a changing world. *Chi Sigma Iota Exemplar,* 1–3, 6, 7.

Leitner, L. A. (1974). Crisis counseling may save a life. *Journal of Rehabilitation, 40,* 19–20.

Leming, M. R., & Dickinson, G. E. (1998). The grieving process. In M. R. Leming and G. E. Dickinson (Eds.), *Dying, death, and bereavement* (pp. 476–487). Fort Worth, TX: Holt, Rinehart, & Winston.

Leventhal, B., & Lundy, S. E. (1999). *Same-sex domestic violence.* Thousand Oaks, CA: Sage.

Leviton, G. (1993). *Elements of crisis intervention.* Pacific Grove, CA: Brooks/Cole.

Lew, M. (1988). *Victims no longer: Men recovering from incest and other sexual child abuse.* New York, NY: Harper & Row.

Lew, M. (2004). *Victims no longer: The classic guide for men recovering from sexual child abuse.* New York, NY: Harper Paperbacks.

Ligon, J. (2005). Mobile crisis units: Frontline community mental health services. In A. R. Roberts (Ed.), *Crisis intervention handbook* (3rd ed., pp. 602–618). New York, NY: Oxford.

Lindemann, E. (1944). Symptomatology and management of acute grief. *American Journal of Psychiatry, 101,* 141–148.

Linehan, M. M. (1993a). *Cognitive-behavioral treatment of borderline personality disorder.* New York, NY: Guilford.

Linehan, M. M. (1993b). *Skills training manual for treating borderline personality disorder.* New York, NY: Guilford.

Linehan, M. M. (in press). *Skills training manual for disordered emotional regulation.* New York, NY: Guilford.

Littrell, J. M. (1998). *Brief counseling in action*. New York, NY: Norton.

Lopez, S. R., Grover, K. P., Holland, D., Johnson, M. J., Kain, C. D., Kanel, K., . . . Rhyne, M. C. (1989). Development of culturally sensitive psychotherapists. *Professional Psychology: Research and Practice, 20*, 369–376.

MacDonald, K., Lambie, I., & Simmonds, L. (1995). *Counseling for sexual abuse: A therapist's guide to working with adults, children, and families*. Melbourne, Australia: Oxford University Press.

MacKinnon, C. (1998). Empowered consumers and telephone hotlines. *Crisis: The Journal of Crisis Intervention and Suicide Prevention, 19*, 21–23.

Malchiodi, C. A. (Ed.) (2008). *Creative interventions with traumatized children*. New York, NY: Guilford.

Malekoff, A. (2004). *Group work with adolescents: Principles and practice* (2nd ed.). New York, NY: Guilford.

Mander, G. (2009). *Diversity, discipline, and devotion in psychoanalytic psychotherapy: Clinical and training perspectives*. London, England: Karmac Books.

Margolis, R. D., & Zweben, J. E. (1998). *Treating patients with alcohol and other drug problems: An integrated approach*. Washington, DC: American Psychological Association.

Marmor, J. (1968). New directions in psychoanalytic theory and therapy. In J. Marmor (Ed.), *Modern psychoanalysis: New directions and perspectives* (pp. 237–243). Northvale, NJ: Aronson.

Marra, T. (2004). *Depressed & anxious: The dialectical behavior therapy workbook for overcoming depression & anxiety*. Oakland, CA: New Harbinger.

Martin, R. A. (2007). *The psychology of humor: An integrative approach*. Amsterdam: Elsevier.

Maslach, C., & Jackson, S. E. (1986). *Maslach burnout inventory: Manual* (2nd ed.). Palo Alto, CA: Consulting Psychologists Press.

Masten, A. S. (2001). Ordinary magic: Resilience processes in development. *American Psychologist, 56*, 227–238.

Mathias, R. (2003, June). Joint treatment of PTSD and cocaine abuse may reduce severity of both disorders. *NIDA Notes, 18*(1), 6, 14.

McCann, I. L., & Pearlman, L. A. (1990). Vicarious traumatization: A framework for understanding the psychological effects of working with victims. *Journal of Traumatic Stress, 3*(1), 131–149.

McClelland, D. (1975). *Power: The inner experience*. New York, NY: Irvington.

McFadden, J. (1999). Historical approaches in trans-cultural counseling. In J. McFadden (Ed.), *Trans-cultural counseling* (2nd ed., pp. 3–22). Alexandria, VA: American Counseling Association.

McKeon, R. (2009). *Suicidal behavior*. Cambridge, MA: Hogrefe & Huber.

McMullin, D., & White, J. W. (2006). Long-term effects of labeling a rape experience. *Psychology of Women Quarterly, 30*, 96–105.

Mendel, M. P. (1995). *The male survivor*. Thousand Oaks, CA: Sage.

Metcalf, L. (1998). *Solution focused group therapy*. New York, NY: Free Press.

Miller, B. (2005). *The woman's book of resilience: 12 qualities to cultivate.* York Beach, ME: Conari Press.

Miller, G. A. (2003). *Incorporating spirituality in counseling and psychotherapy: Theory and techniques.* Hoboken, NJ: Wiley.

Miller, G. A. (2010). *Learning the language of addiction counseling* (3rd ed.). Hoboken, NJ: Wiley.

Miller, G., Clark, C., & Herman, J. (2007). Domestic violence in a rural setting. *Journal of Rural Mental Health, 31,* 28–42.

Miller, G. A., & Hood, R. (2005). *American Red Cross Disaster Mental Health Services I Training.* September 29, 2005, Boone, NC.

Miller, G., & Hood, R. (2009). Mental health intervention in disasters: Application in the American Red Cross. Presentation to the NASW Local Program Unit, Boone, NC.

Miller, J. B. (1976). *Toward a new psychology of women.* Boston, MA: Beacon Press.

Miller, J. B. (1986). *Toward a new psychology of women* (2nd ed.). Boston, MA: Beacon Press.

Miller, W. R., & Rollnick, S. (2002). *Motivational interviewing* (2nd ed.). New York, NY: Guilford Press.

Miller, W. R., & Rollnick, S. (2009). Ten things that motivational interviewing is not. *Behavioral and Cognitive Psychotherapy, 37,* 129–140.

Miller, W. R., & Rose, G. S. (2009). Toward a theory of motivational interviewing. *American Psychologist, 64,* 527–537.

Miller, W. R., & Sanchez, V. C. (1994). Motivating young adults for treatment and lifestyle change. In G. Howard (Ed.), *Issues in alcohol use and misuse by young adults* (pp. 55–81). Notre Dame, IN: University of Notre Dame Press.

Minnesota Coalition for Battered Women (1992). *Safety first: A guide for battered women.* St. Paul, MN: Author.

Mishara, B. L., Chagnon, F., Daigle, M., Balan, B., Raymond, S., Marcoux, I., . . . Berman, A. (2007). Comparing models of helper behavior to actual practice in telephone crisis intervention: A silent monitoring of calls to the U.S. 1-800-SUICIDE Network. *Suicide & Life-Threatening Behavior, 37,* 291–307.

Mitchell, J. T. (1983). When disaster strikes: The critical incident stress debriefing process. *Journal of Emergency Medical Services, 8,* 36–39.

Mitchell, J. T., & Everly, G. S. (1999). Critical incident stress management: A new era in crisis intervention. *Traumatic Stress Points, 1* (Fall), 6–7, 10–11.

Mitchell, J. T., & Everly, G. S. (2001). *Critical incident stress debriefing: An operations manual.* Ellicott City: MD: Chevron.

Moleski, S. M., & Kiselica, M. S. (2005). Dual relationships: A continuum ranging from the destructive to the therapeutic. *Journal of Counseling and Development, 83,* 3–11.

Mook, D. G. (1987). *Motivation: The organization of action.* New York, NY: Norton.

Mueser, K. T., Noordsy, D. L., Drake, R. E., & Fox, L. (2003). *Integrated treatment for dual disorders.* New York, NY: Guilford Press.

Murphy, C. (1995). Scapegroup. *Atlantic Monthly, 275,* 22–24.

Myer, R. A., & Moore, H. (2006). Crisis in context theory: An ecological model. *Journal of Counseling & Development, 84,* 139–147.

Myers, D. G. (1985). Helping the helpers: A training manual. In D. M. Hartsough & D. G. Myers (Eds.), *Disaster work and mental health: Prevention and control of stress among workers* (DHHS Publication No. ADM 85-1422, pp. 45–149). Rockville, MD: U.S. Department of Health and Human Services, Public Health Service, Alcohol, Drug Abuse, and Mental Health Administration, National Institute of Mental Health.

Myers, P. L., & Salt, N. R. (2007). *Becoming an addictions counselor: A comprehensive text* (2nd ed.). Sudbury, MA: Jones and Bartlett.

Nadeau, J. W. (2006). Metaphorically speaking: The use of metaphors in grief therapy. *Illness, Crisis, & Loss, 14,* 201–221.

Najavits, L. M. (2002). *Seeking safety: A treatment manual for PTSD and substance abuse.* New York, NY: Guilford.

National Child Traumatic Stress Network and National Center for PTSD (2005). *Psychological first aid: Field operations guide.* Available online at http://www.ptsd.va.gov/professional/manuals/psych-first-aid.asp

National Institute of Mental Health (2002). *Mental health and mass violence: Evidence-based early psychological intervention for victims/survivors of mass violence: A workshop to reach consensus on best practices.* Washington, DC: U.S. Department of Defense; U.S. Department of Health and Human Services; the National Institute of Mental Health; the Substance Abuse and Mental Health Services Administration; Center for Mental Health Services; U. S. Department of Justice; Office of Victims of Crime; U.S. Department of Veteran Affairs; National Center for PTSD; and the American Red Cross.

National Institute on Alcohol Abuse and Alcoholism (1995). *Assessing alcohol problems: A guide for clinicians and researchers* (NIH Publication No. 95-3745). Rockville, MD: Author.

National Institute on Drug Abuse (NIDA) (2003). *Family therapy. Addiction alternatives.* Retrieved July 14, 2003, from www.aa2.org/philosophy/brieffamily.htm

National Institute of Drug Abuse (NIDA) (2006) *Stress and substance abuse.* Community Drug Alert Bulletin. Rockville, MD: NIDA.

National Institute on Drug Abuse (NIDA) (2008a). Comorbidity: Addiction and other mental illnesses. *Research Report Series.* Rockville, MD: NIDA.

National Institute on Drug Abuse (NIDA) (2008b). High-risk drug offenders do better with close judicial supervision. NIDA Notes, 22, 9–10. Rockville, MD: NIDA.

Naturale, A. (2006). Outreach strategies: An experiential description of the outreach methodologies used in the September 11, 2001, disaster response in New York. In E. C. Ritchie, P. J. Watson, & M. J. Friedman (Eds.), *Interventions following mass violence and disasters* (pp. 365–383). New York, NY: Guilford.

Neff, K. D. (2008). Self-compassion: Moving beyond the pitfalls of a separate self-concept. In H. A. Wayment & J. J. Bauer (Eds.), *Transcending self-interest* (pp. 95–105). Washington, DC: American Psychological Association.

Neimeyer, R. A. (2002). The language of loss: Grief therapy as a process of meaning reconstruction. In R. A. Neimeyer (Ed.), *Meaning reconstruction & the experience of loss*. Washington, DC: American Psychological Association.

Neimeyer, R. A., & Wogrin, C. (2008). Complicated bereavement: A meaning-oriented approach. *Illness, Crisis, & Loss, 16*, 1–20.

Newgass, S., & Schonfeld, D. (2005). School crisis intervention, crisis prevention, and crisis response. In A. R. Roberts (Ed.), *Crisis intervention handbook* (3rd ed., pp. 499–518). New York, NY: Oxford University Press.

NiCarthy, G. (1987). *The ones who got away: Women who left abusive partners*. Seattle, WA: Seal Press.

NiCarthy, G. (1997). *Getting free: You can end abuse and take back your life*. Seattle, WA: Seal Press.

Norcross, J. C., & Barnett, J. E. (2008, Spring). Self-care as ethical imperative. *The Register Report, 34*, 20–27.

Nugent, F. A. (1994). *An introduction to the profession of counseling* (2nd ed.). New York, NY: Macmillan.

Oakeshott, M. (1991). *Rationalism in politics and other essays*. Indianapolis, IN: Liberty Press.

Ogden, P., Minton, K., & Pain, C. (2006). *Trauma and the body: A sensorimotor approach to psychotherapy*. New York, NY: Norton.

O'Halloran, T. M., & Linton, J. M. (2000). Stress on the job: Self-care resources for counselors. *Journal of Mental Health Counseling, 22*, 354–364.

Paine, W. S. (1982). Overview of burnout stress syndromes and the 1980s. In W. S. Paine (Ed.), *Job stress and burnout* (pp. 11–25). Newbury Park, CA: Sage.

Patterson, J., Williams, L., Edwards, T., Chamow, L., & Grauf-Grounds, C. (2009). *Essential skills in family therapy* (2nd ed.). New York, NY: Guilford.

Pence, E., & Paymar, M. (1993). *Education groups for men who batter: The Duluth model*. New York, NY: Springer.

Perkinson, R. R., & Jongsma, A. E. (1998). *The chemical dependence treatment planner*. New York, NY: Wiley.

Pfeiffer, E. (1975). A short portable mental status questionnaire for the assessment of organic brain deficit in elderly patients. *Journal of American Geriatrics Society, 23*, 433–441.

Pichot, T., & Smock, S. A. (2009). *Solution-focused substance abuse treatment*. New York, NY: Routledge.

Pokorny, A. D., Miller, B. A., & Kaplan, H. B. (1972). The brief MAST: A shortened version of the Michigan Alcoholism Screening Test. *American Journal of Psychiatry, 129*, 342–345.

Preston, J. (1998). *Integrative brief therapy*. San Luis Obispo, CA: Impact.

Prochaska, J. O., DiClemente, C. C., & Norcross, J. C. (1992). In search of how people change. *American Psychologist, 47*, 1102–1114.

Prochaska, J. O., & Norcross, J. C. (2001). Stages of change. *Psychotherapy: Theory/Research/Practice/Training, 38*, 443–448.

Prochaska, J. O., & Norcross, J. C. (2002). Stages of change. In J. C. Norcross (Ed.), *Psychotherapy relationships that work: Therapist contributions and responsiveness to patients* (pp. 303–313). New York, NY: Oxford University Press.

Raphael, B. (1977). Preventive intervention with the recently bereaved. *Archives of General Psychology, 34*(12), 1450–1454.

Raphael, B. (1986). *When disaster strikes: How individuals and communities cope with catastrophe.* New York, NY: Basic Books.

Rapoport, L. (1967). Crisis-oriented short-term casework. *Social Service Review, 41,* 31–43.

Reid, C., & Kampfe, C. (2000). *Multicultural issues.* (ERIC Document Reproduction Service No. ED440351).

Rich, P. (2001). *Grief counseling homework planner.* Hoboken, NJ: Wiley.

Richards, P. S., & Bergin, A. E. (1997). *A spiritual strategy for counseling and psychotherapy.* Washington, DC: American Psychological Association.

Robbins, B. D. (2008). What is the good life? Positive psychology and the renaissance of humanistic psychology. *The Humanistic Psychologist, 36,* 96–112.

Roberts, A. R. (2005). *Crisis intervention handbook* (3rd ed.). New York, NY: Oxford University Press.

Roberts, A. R., & Yeager, K. R. (2009). *Pocket guide to crisis intervention.* New York, NY: Oxford University Press.

Rogers, C. (1970). *Carl Rogers on encounter groups.* New York, NY: Perennial.

Rogers, C. R. (1951). *Client-centered therapy.* Boston, MA: Houghton Mifflin.

Rogers, C. R. (1987). The underlying theory: Drawn from experiences with individuals and groups. *Counseling and Values, 32,* 38–45.

Rosen, C. S., Greene, C. J., Young, H. E., & Norris, F. H. (2010). Tailoring disaster mental health services to diverse needs: An analysis of 36 Crisis Counseling Projects. *Social Work, 35,* 211–220.

Rosenbloom, D., & Williams, M. B. (1999). *Life after trauma: A workbook for healing.* New York, NY: Guilford Press.

Rosengren, D. B. (2009). *Building motivational interviewing skills: A practitioner workbook.* New York, NY: Guilford Press.

Rothschild, B. (2000). *The body remembers.* New York, NY: Norton.

Ruzek, J. I., Brymer, M. J., Jacobs, A.K., Layne, C. M., Vernberg, E. M., & Watson, P. J. (2007). Psychological first aid. *Journal of Mental Health Counseling, 29,* 17–49.

Ryff, C. D., & Singer, B. (2003). Flourishing under fire: Resilience as a prototype of challenged thriving. In C. L. M. Keyes & J. Haidt (Eds.), *Flourishing: Positive psychology and the life well-lived.* Washington, DC: American Psychological Association.

Saladin, M. E., Back, S. E., & Payne, R. A. (2009). Posttraumatic stress disorder and substance use disorder comorbidity. In R. K. Ries, D. A. Fiellin, S. C. Miller, & R. Saitz (Eds.), *Principles of addiction medicine* (pp. 1249–1262). Philadelphia: Wolters Kluwer.

Sandovai, J., Scott, A. N., & Padilla, I. (2009). Crisis counseling: An overview. *Psychology in the Schools, 46,* 246–256.

Sattler, J. M. (1992). *Assessment of children* (3rd ed.). San Diego, CA: Author.

Saunders, J. B., Aasland, O. G., Babor, T. F., de la Fuente, J. R., & Grant, M. (1993). Development of the Alcohol Use Disorders Identification Test (AUDIT): WHO collaborative project on early detection of persons with harmful alcohol consumption-II. *Addiction, 88*, 791–804.

Savin-Williams, R. C. (2001). *Mom, Dad. I'm gay.* Washington, DC: American Psychological Association.

Schechter, N. E., & Barnett, J. E. (2010). Psychotherapy and the suicidal client: A brief introduction. *Psychotherapy Bulletin, 45*, 11–15.

Schechter, S. (1987). *Guidelines for mental health practitioners in domestic violence cases.* Washington, DC: National Coalition Against Domestic Violence.

Schenker, M. D. (2009). *A clinician's guide to 12 step recovery: Integrating 12 step programs into psychotherapy.* New York, NY: Norton.

Schlesinger, S. E., & Epstein, N. B. (2007). Couple problems. In F. M. Dattilio & A. Freeman (Eds.), *Cognitive-behavioral strategies in crisis intervention* (3rd ed., pp. 300–326). New York, NY: Guilford.

Schneider, J. (1984). *Stress, loss, & grief.* Baltimore: University Park Press.

Schure, M., & Christopher, J. (2008). Mind-body medicine and the art of self-care: Teaching mindfulness to counseling students through yoga, meditation, and Qigong. *Journal of Counseling & Development, 86*, 47–56.

Schwartz, M. F., & Cohn, L. (Eds.) (1996). *Sexual abuse and eating disorders.* New York, NY: Brunner/Mazel.

Schwarz, B. (1995). The diversity myth: America's leading export. *Atlantic Monthly, 275*, 57–67.

Seligman, M. E. P. (2002). *Authentic happiness.* New York, NY: Free Press.

Seligman, M. E. P., & Csikszentmihalyi, M. (2000). Positive psychology: An introduction. *American Psychologist, 55*, 5–14.

Seligman, M. E. P., Steen, T. A., Park, N., & Peterson, C. (2005). Positive psychology progress: Empirical validation of interventions. *American Psychologist, 60*, 410–421.

Selzer, M. L. (1971). The Michigan Alcohol Screening Test: The quest for a new diagnostic instrument. *American Journal of Psychiatry, 127*, 1653–1658.

Selzer, M. L., Vinokur, A., & van Rooijen, L. (1975). A self-administered Short Michigan Alcoholism Screening Tests (SMAST). *Journal of Studies on Alcohol, 36*, 117–126.

Shallcross, L. (2009). Rewriting the "rules" of grief. *Counseling Today, 52*, 28–33.

Shaw, B. F., Ritvo, P., & Irvine, J. (2005). *Addiction & recovery for dummies.* Hoboken, NY: Wiley.

Shea, S. C. (2002). *The practical art of suicide assessment: A guide for mental health professionals and substance abuse counselors.* Hoboken, NJ: Wiley.

Shelby, J. S., & Tredinnick, M. J. (1993). Crisis intervention with survivors of natural disaster: Lessons from Hurricane Andrew. *Journal of Counseling & Development, 73*, 491–497.

Skovholt, T. M. (2001). *The resilient practitioner.* Boston, MA: Allyn & Bacon.

Slaikeu, K. A. (1990). *Crisis intervention: A handbook for practice and research* (2nd ed.). Boston, MA: Allyn & Bacon.

Smedes, L. B. (1984). *Forgive and forget: Healing the hurts we don't deserve.* San Francisco, CA: Harper & Row.

Smith, T. (2008). *A balanced life: 9 strategies for coping with the mental health problems of a loved one.* Center City, MN: Hazelden.

Smith, P. H., Earp, J. A., & DeVellis, R. (1995). Measuring battering: Development of the Women's Experience with Battering (WEB) scale. *Women's Health. Winter 1*(4), 273–288.

Snyder, D. K., & Mitchell, A. E. (2008). Affective-reconstructive couple therapy: A pluralistic, developmental approach. In A. S. Gurman (Ed.), *Clinical handbook of couple therapy* (4th ed., pp. 353–382). New York, NY: Guilford.

Solomon, J., Zimberg, S., & Shollar, E. (Eds.) (1993). *Dual diagnosis: Evaluation, treatment, training, and program development.* New York, NY: Plenum Press.

Sorbell, L. (August 2009). *Motivational interviewing: Common currency among health and mental health care practitioners for treating risky problem behaviors.* Paper session presented at the meeting of the American Psychological Association, Toronto.

Staudinger, U. M., Marsiske, M., & Baltes, P. B. (1995). Resilience and reserve capacity in later adulthood: Potentials and limits of development across the life span. In D. Cicchitti & D. J. Cohen (Eds.), *Developmental psychopathology* (Vol. 2: *Risk, disorder, and adaptation*, pp. 801–847). New York, NY: Wiley.

Stebnicki, M. A. (2007). Empathy fatigue: Healing the mind, body, and spirit of professional counselors. *American Journal of Psychiatric Rehabilitation, 10*, 317–338.

Stewart, C., & MacNeil, G. (2005). Crisis intervention with chronic school violence and volatile situations. In A. R. Roberts (Ed.), *Crisis intervention handbook* (3rd ed., pp. 519–540). New York, NY: Oxford.

Straussner, S. L. A., & Brown, S. (Eds.) (2002). *The handbook of addiction treatment for women: Theory and practice.* San Francisco, CA: Jossey-Bass.

Stroebe, M. S., Hansson, R. O., Stroebe, W., & Schut, H. (2001). Introduction: Concepts and issues in contemporary research on bereavement. In H. Schut (Ed.), *Handbook of bereavement research: Consequences, coping, and care* (pp. 3–22). Washington, DC: American Psychological Association.

Stromberg, G., & Merrill, J. (2006). *Feeding the fame.* Center City, MN: Hazelden.

Sturza, M. L., & Campbell, R. (December 2005). An exploratory study of rape survivors' prescription drug use as a means of coping with sexual assault. *Psychology of Women Quarterly, 29*, 253–263.

Substance Abuse and Mental Health Services Administration (1994). *Assessment and treatment of patients with coexisting mental illness and alcohol and other drug abuse* (DHHS Publication No. 94-2078). Rockville, MD: Author.

Substance Abuse and Mental Health Services Administration (1996). *Counselor's manual for relapse prevention with chemically dependent criminal offenders* (Technical Assistance Publication Series 19; DHHS Publication No. SMA 96-3115). Rockville, MD: Author.

Substance Abuse and Mental Health Services Administration (1997). *Substance abuse treatment and domestic violence*. Treatment Improvement Protocol (TIP 25) Series. (DHHS Publication No. SMA 97-3163). Rockville, MD: Author.

Substance Abuse and Mental Health Services Administration (1998a). *Substance abuse among older adults*. Rockville, MD: Author.

Substance Abuse and Mental Health Services Administration (1998b). *Substance abuse disorder treatment for people with physical and cognitive disabilities*. Rockville, MD: Author.

Substance Abuse and Mental Health Services Administration (2000a). *Cultural competence standards*. Rockville, MD: Author.

Substance Abuse and Mental Health Services Administration (2000b). *Substance abuse treatment for persons with child abuse and neglect issues*. Treatment Improvement Protocol (TIP 36) Series (DHHS Publication No. SMA 00-3357). Rockville, MD: Author.

Substance Abuse and Mental Health Services Administration (2002a). *Domestic violence and the new Americans: Directory of programs and resources for battered refugee women* (CMHS-SVP-0061). Rockville, MD: Author.

Substance Abuse and Mental Health Services Administration (2002b, November). *Report to Congress on the prevention and treatment of co-occurring substance abuse disorders and mental disorders*. Rockville, MD: Author.

Substance Abuse and Mental Health Services Administration (2003). *A provider's introduction to substance abuse treatment for lesbian, gay, bisexual, and transgender individuals*. Rockville, MD: Author.

Substance Abuse and Mental Health Services Administration (2005a). *A guide to managing stress in crisis response professions*. Bethesda, MD: Author.

Substance Abuse and Mental Health Services Administration (2005b). *Substance abuse relapse prevention for older adults: A group treatment approach* (DHHS Publication No. SMA 05-4053). Rockville, MD: Author.

Substance Abuse and Mental Health Services Administration (2006). *Field manual for mental health and human service workers in major disasters*. Bethesda, MD: Author.

Substance Abuse and Mental Health Services Administration (2008a). *Addiction counseling competencies: The knowledge, skills, and attitudes of professional practice* (Technical Assistance Publication Series 21; DHHS Publication No. SMA 08-3171). Author.

Substance Abuse and Mental Health Services Administration, Office of Applied Studies (2008b). *Results from the 2008 National Survey on drug use and health: National findings*. Retrieved October 16, 2009, from www.oas.samhsa.gov/NSDUH/2k8NSDUH/2k8results.htm

Sue, D. W., & Sue, D. (2008a). *Counseling the culturally diverse: Theory and practice* (5th ed.). Hoboken, NJ: Wiley.

Sue, D., & Sue, D. M. (2008b). *Foundations of counseling and psychotherapy: Evidence-based practices for a diverse society*. Hoboken, NJ: Wiley.

Surry, J. (1985). *The "self-in-relation": A theory of women's development*. Work in progress (No. 13).

Talmon, M. (1990). *Single session therapy*. San Francisco, CA: Jossey-Bass.

Taylor, E. (2001). Positive psychology and humanistic psychology: A reply to Seligman. *Journal of Humanistic Psychology, 41*, 13–29.

Tedeschi, R. G., & Calhoun, L. G. (1995). *Trauma and transformation: Growing in the aftermath of suffering*. Thousand Oaks, CA: Sage.

Thompson, J. K., Heinberg, L. J., Altable, M., & Tantleff-Dunn, S. (1999). *Exacting beauty: Theory, assessment, and treatment of body image disturbance*. Washington, DC: American Psychological Association.

Tisdell, E. J. (2003). *Exploring spirituality and culture in adult and higher education*. San Francisco, CA: Jossey-Bass.

Tober, G., & Raistrick, D. (2007). What is motivational dialogue? In G. Tober & D. Raistrick (Eds.), *Motivational dialogue* (pp. 3–15). New York, NY: Routledge.

Trickett, P. K., & Schellenbach, C. J. (1998). *Violence against children in the family and the community*. Washington, DC: American Psychological Association.

Vacc, N. A., DeVaney, S. B., & Wittmer, J. (1995). Introduction. In N. A. Vacc, S. B. DeVaney, & J. Wittmer (Eds.), *Experiencing and counseling multicultural and diverse populations* (pp. 1–8). Bristol, PA: Accelerated Development.

Van der Walde, H., Urgenson, F. T., Weltz, S. H., & Hanna, F. J. (2002). Women and alcoholism: A biopsychosocial perspective and treatment approaches. *Journal of Counseling and Development, 80*, 145–153.

Van Wormer, K., & Davis, D. (2008). *Addiction treatment: A strengths perspective* (2nd ed.). Belmont, CA: Thomson.

Velasquez, M. M., Maurer, G. G., Crouch, V., & DiClemente, C. C. (2001). *Group treatment for substance abuse: A stages-of-change therapy manual*. New York, NY: Guilford.

Vettor, S. M., & Kosinski, F. A., Jr. (2000). Work-stress burnout in emergency medical technicians and the use of early recollections. *Journal of Employment Counseling, 37*, 216.

Walsh, F. (2006). *Strengthening family resilience* (2nd ed.). New York, NY: Guilford.

Washton, A. M., & Zweben, J. E. (2006). *Treating alcohol and drug problems in psychotherapy practice*. New York, NY: Guilford.

Watkins, T. R., Lewellen, A., & Barrett, M. C. (2001). *Dual diagnosis: An integrated approach to treatment*. Thousand Oaks, CA: Sage.

Weaver, J. D. (1995). *Disasters: Mental health interventions*. Sarasota, FL: Professional Resource.

Weaver, J. D., Dingman, R. L., Morgan, J., Hong, B. A., & North, C. S. (2000). The American Red Cross Disaster Mental Health Services: Development of a cooperative, single function, multidisciplinary service model. *Journal of Behavioral Health Services & Research, 27*, 314–322.

Webb, P. (2001). Play therapy with traumatized children: A crisis response. In G. L. Landreth (Ed.), *Innovations in play therapy: Issues, process, and special populations* (pp. 289–302). New York, NY: Brunner-Routledge.

Webber, J., Bass, D. D., & Yep, R. (Eds.) (2005). *Terrorism, trauma, and tragedies: A counselor's guide to preparing and responding* (2nd ed.). Alexandria, VA: American Counseling Association.

West, W. (2000). *Psychotherapy & spirituality: Crossing the line between therapy and religion*. Thousand Oaks, CA: Sage.

White, E. C. (1994). *Chain, chain, change: For black women in abusive relationships*. Seattle, WA: Seal Press.

White, J. R., & Freeman, A. S. (2000). *Cognitive-behavioral group therapy for specific problems and populations*. Washington, DC: American Psychological Association.

Wilkerson, K. (2009). An examination of burnout among school counselors guided by stress-strain-coping theory. *Journal of Counseling & Development, 87*, 428–437.

Willer, J. (2009). *The beginning psychotherapist's companion*. Lanham, MD: Rowman & Littlefield.

Williams, L., Edwards, T. M., Patterson, J., & Chamow, L. (2011). *Essential assessment skills for couple and family therapists*. New York, NY: Guilford.

Williams, M. B., & Poijula, S. (2002). *The PTSD workbook*. Oakland, CA: New Harbinger.

Winek, J. (2009). *Systemic family therapy: From theory to practice*. Thousand Oaks, CA: Sage.

Wise, E. A. (2000). Mental health intensive outpatient programming: An outcome and satisfaction evaluation of a private practice model. *Professional Psychology: Research and Practice, 31*, 412–417.

Wise, L. (2001). *Inside grief*. Incline Village, NV: Wise Press.

Worden, W. (1991). *Grief counseling & grief therapy*. New York, NY: Springer.

Worden, W. (2009). *Grief counseling & grief therapy: A handbook for the mental health practitioner* (4th ed.). New York, NY: Springer.

Yalom, I. D. (1985). *The theory and practice of group psychotherapy* (4th ed.). New York, NY: Basic Books.

York, S. (2000). *Remembering well: Rituals for celebrating life and mourning death*. San Francisco, CA: Jossey-Bass.

Zealberg, J. J., Santos, A. B., & Fisher, R. K. (1993). Emergency psychiatry: Benefits of mobile crisis programs. *Hospital and Community Psychiatry, 44*(1): 16.

Zonnebelt-Smeenge, S. J., & DeVries, R. C. (2001a). *The empty chair*. Grand Rapids, MI: Baker Books.

Zonnebelt-Smeenge, S. J., & DeVries, R. C. (2001b). *Getting to the other side of grief: Overcoming the loss of a spouse*. Grand Rapids, MI: Baker Books.

Author Index

Aasland, O. G., 102
Adams, J. B., 158
Allen, P. D., 203
American Counseling Association, 87
American Psychiatric Association, 99
American Psychological Association, 52, 87, 112, 170, 171, 172, 176, 195, 223, 226
Amodeo, M., 173
Anderegg, M., 218
Anderson, B. S., 89
APA. *See* American Psychological Association
Arkowitz, H., 158
Atkins, S. A., 229
Atkinson, D. R., 196, 197, 208, 209

Babor, T. F., 102
Back, S. E., 173
Backlund, B. A., 156
Balan, B., 43
Baltes, P. B., 170, 174
Bardon, C., 43
Barnett, J. E., 126, 218, 219, 225, 227
Bass, D. D., 47
Battle, C. L., 208, 209
Baum, N., 35
Bazron, B. J., 197
Beck, A. T., 155
Behnke, S., 87
Bein, A., 218
Belkin, G. S., 23
Bemak, F., 199
Benshoff, J. J., 203
Berg, I. K., 157
Bergin, A. E., 174

Berliner, L., 76
Berman, A., 44
Bersoff, D. N., 130
Beutler, L. E., 20, 32, 33, 34
Bloom, B. L., 150, 151, 152, 153, 154, 155, 156
Bogo, M., 108
Bowlby, J., 167
Brammer, L. M., 18
Briere, J., 112
Bryant, B. A., 43
Brymer, M. J., 20, 44
Buelow, N. C., 126
Buelow, S. A., 126
Bunney, W., 126
Burbules, N. C., 198
Bureau of Justice, 50, 108
Bureau of Justice Statistics, 111

Calhoun, L. G., 170, 174
Campbell, J. K., 43
Campbell, L., 87
Campbell, R., 50, 51, 111
Caplan, G., 5, 16
Caprara, G. V., 172
Cardemil, E. V., 208, 209
Carver, C. S., 172
Cervone, D., 172
Chagnon, F., 43
Chamow, L., 83, 87, 99
Cherry, K. E., 203
Christ, G., 221
Christopher, J. C., 218, 224
Chung, R. C.-Y., 199
Cini, F., 218

259

Cohen, J. A., 44, 76
Collins, B. G., 23
Collins, T. M., 23
Connors, G. J., 105
Coombs, R. H., 86
Corey, G., 16, 80
Corrigan, M., 221
Cozza, S. J., 44
Cross, T. L., 197
Csikszentmihalyi, M., 163, 164

Daigle, M., 43
Danieli, Y., 221
Dass-Brailsford, P., 28, 34, 203
Dattilio, F. M., 77, 83
Davanloo, H., 154
Davis, D., 50, 111, 158, 173, 203
de la Fuente, J. R., 102
Dennis, K. W., 197
De Shazer, S., 156
DeVaney, S. B., 196
DeVellis, R., 109
DeWolfe, D. J., 32
Dickinson, G. E., 167
DiClemente, C. C., 76, 107, 157, 158, 161, 162
Dilsaver, S. C., 99
Dingman, R. L., 29, 42, 47, 221
Discovery Health Channel, 170, 171, 172, 176, 223, 226
Dodgen, D., 171
Domestic Abuse Intervention Project, 108
Downs, W. R., 111
Duluth Intervention Project, 108
Dziegielewski, S. F., 77

Earp, J. A., 109
Eberle, 50, 108
Edwards, C. L., 193, 200
Edwards, T. M., 83, 99
Eisenberg, N., 172
el-Guebaly, N., 193
Ellis, A., 155
Engel, G. L., 167
Epstein, N. B., 83
Ersever, O. H., 219, 229
Everly, G. S., 20, 80
Ewing, J. A., 104

Feliu, M., 193, 200
Figley, C. R., 221
Finkelhor, D., 51
Fisher, R. K., 46
Fiske, S. T., 197

Flegal, K. M., 120
Fleming, M. F., 104
Flynn, B. W., 20
Freeman, A., 77
Freudenberger, H. J., 221
Friedman, R., 168
Friere, P., 198

Galea, S., 203
Garay, M., 157, 158
Garner, D. M., 116
Gelso, C. J., 165
Gemmell, L., 157, 158
Gibson, L. E., 44
Gilliland, 18
Godula, D., 218
Goldsmith, S., 126
Gomberg, E., 50, 108
Gottman, J., 50, 108
Gould, M. S., 43, 44
Grafanaki, S., 218
Grant, M., 102
Granvold, D. K., 47, 83
Grauf-Grounds, C., 83, 87, 99
Greenberg, T., 44
Greene, C. J., 202
Greene, K., 108
Greene, P., 221
Greenstone, J. L., 203
Grover, K. P., 193
Grummer-Strawn, L. M., 120
Guo, S. S., 120

Hackett, G., 196, 209
Haen, C., 79
Haidt, J., 163
Haley, M., 87
Halford, W. K., 83, 87
Hallisey, B. J., 3, 4, 14, 18, 45–46, 77, 78, 80, 82, 87, 127, 129, 201, 221
Halpern, J., 18, 28–30, 31, 32, 35, 221
Hanna, F. J., 205
Hansson, R. O., 167
Harrawood, L. K., 203
Harris, A. H. S., 165
Harris, G. T., 110
Harrison, L., 111
Hartsough, D. M., 227
Harvard Mental Health Letter, 34, 100, 158, 163, 164
Harvey, A. G., 43
Heath, 82
Heffron, E. F., 28

Hill, C. E., 152
Hilton, N. Z., 110
Hoff, L. A., 3, 4, 14, 18, 45–46, 77, 78, 80, 82, 87, 127, 129, 201, 221
Hoff, M., 4, 14, 18, 77, 78, 80, 82, 87, 127, 129, 201, 221
Holland, D., 193
Hong, B. A., 29
Hood, R., 30, 33, 35, 219
Housley, J., 20, 32, 33, 34
Huber, C. H., 156

Irvine, J., 158
Isaacs, M. R., 197

Jackson, S. E., 221
Jacobs, A. K., 20
Jacobson, N., 50, 108
James, J. W., 168
James, R. K., 3, 5, 14, 18, 20, 43, 44, 75, 76, 83, 85, 89, 97, 127, 202, 221
Janosik, E. H., 14, 15(f)
Johnson, C. L., 120
Johnson, J. L., 14, 75
Johnson, M. J., 193, 200
Johnson, S., 193, 200
Jones, L. K., 173

Kafrissen, S. R., 28
Kain, C. D., 193
Kalafat, J., 43
Kampfe, C., 193
Kane, D., 221
Kanel, K., 3, 5, 6, 16, 86, 87, 127, 129, 193, 221, 222
Kasper, L. B., 152
Kauffman, C., 164–65
Keyes, C. L. M., 163
Kilburg, R. R., 217, 224
Kingsbury, S. J., 156, 227
Kinney, J., 126
Kinscherff, R., 87
Kiselica, M. S., 86
Kivlighan, D. M., 152
Kleinman, A., 126
Kleinman, M., 43, 44
Klingman,, 44
Knapp, K. C., 203
Koch, D. S., 203
Kogan, M., 163
Kosinski, F. A., Jr., 222
Koss, M. P., 150
Kubler-Ross, E., 168
Kuczmarski, R. J., 120

Lambie, I., 51, 113
Lating, J. M., 80
Lawrence, E. C., 83
Layne, C. M., 20
Lazarus, A., 21, 76
Leadbeater, B., 171
Leitner, L. A., 23
Leming, M. R., 167
Leviton, G., 221, 222
Leviton, S. C., 203
Ligon, J., 46
Lindemann, E., 4, 5, 16
Linton, J. M., 218
Littrell, J. M., 150, 157
Lopez, S. J., 165
Lopez, S. R., 193
Lubell, K., 44, 151
Lynch, S., 221

MacDonald, K., 51, 113
MacKinnon, C., 43
MacNeil, G., 44
Madson, M. B., 158
Malchiodi, C. A., 76
Mander, G., 218
Mannarino, A. P., 44, 76
Marcoux, I., 43
Marmor, J., 153
Marra, T., 224
Marsiske, M., 170, 174
Martin, R. A., 224
Maslach, C., 221
Maslow, A., 163
Masten, A. S., 170, 223
McCann, I. L., 221
McClelland, D., 205
McFadden, J., 193
McKenzie, B., 218
McKeon, R., 127
McMullin, D., 50, 111
Mei, Z., 120
Meyer, D. L., 20
Miller, G., 229
Miller, G. A., 4, 30, 33, 35, 86, 87, 88, 98, 111, 129, 149, 150, 151, 153, 165, 170, 172, 193–94
Miller, J. B., 205
Miller, W. R., 76, 157, 158, 159, 160, 161, 162, 200–201
Mishara, B. L., 43
Mitchell, A. E., 83
Mitchell, J. T., 34, 80

Moleski, S. M., 86
Mook, D. G., 197
Moore, H., 23
Morgan, J., 29
Morten, G., 197
Munfakh, J. L. H., 43, 44
Murphy, C., 196
Murray, L., 44
Myer, R. A., 23
Myers, D. G., 227
Myers, P. L., 87

Nadeau, J. W., 169
Nason, S., 218
Nathan, P. E., 217, 224, 227
National Child Traumatic Stress Network and
   National Center for PTSD, 33
National Institute of Mental Health, 3, 20
National Institute on Alcohol Abuse and
   Alcoholism, 98, 104
National Institute on Drug Abuse, 83, 107, 171
National Survey on Drug Use and Health, 101–2
Naturale, A., 202
Neff, K. D., 218, 221, 224
Neimeyer, R. A., 166, 168, 170, 204
Newgass, S., 44
NIAAA. See National Institute on Alcohol Abuse
   and Alcoholism
NIDA. See National Institute on Drug Abuse
Nirenberg, T., 50, 108
Norcross, J. C., 76, 161, 162, 218, 219, 225, 227
Norris, F. H., 202
North, C. S., 29
Nugent, F. A., 150, 151

Oakeshott, M., 198
Ogden, C. L., 120
O'Halloran, T. M., 218

Padilla, I., 169
Paine, W. S., 221
Park, N., 163, 165
Patterson, J., 83, 87, 99
Payne, R. A., 173
Pearlman, L. A., 221
Pearson, D., 218
Pellmar, T., 126
Peterson, C., 163, 165
Preston, 151, 156
Prochaska, J. O., 76, 161, 162

Raistrick, D., 158
Raphael, B., 3, 20, 28

Rapoport, L., 5
Raymond, S., 43
Reid, C., 193
Rice, M. E., 110
Richards, P. S., 174
Ritvo, P., 158
Robbins, B. D., 163, 164
Roberts, A. R., 3, 4, 5, 43, 47, 75, 82, 85,
   202, 203
Rogers, C., 158, 163–64, 199
Rollnick, S., 76, 157, 158, 159, 160, 161, 162
Rose, G. S., 158
Rosen, C. S., 202
Ruzek, J. I., 20
Ryff, C. D., 170, 171, 174

Saladin, M. E., 173
Salt, N. R., 87
SAMHSA. See Substance Abuse and Mental
   Health Services Administration
Sandovai, J., 169
Santos, A. B., 46, 108
Sattler, J. M., 98
Saunders, J. B., 102
Schechter, N. E., 126
Scheier, M. F., 172
Schlesinger, S. E., 83
Schneider, J., 222
Schonfeld, D., 44
Schure, M., 224
Schut, H., 167
Schwarz, B., 196
Scott, A. N., 169
Seligman, M. E. P., 163, 164, 165
Selzer, M. L., 104
Shallcross, L., 169
Shaw, B. F., 158
Shea, S. C., 126
Shelby, J. S., 202
Shiang, J., 150
Simmonds, L., 51, 113
Singer, B., 170, 171, 174
Skovholt, T. M., 221
Slaikeu, K. A., 3, 4, 19, 20, 97, 98
Smedes, L. B., 220
Smith, P. H., 109
Snyder, D. K., 83
Solarz, A., 171
Sommers-Flanagan & Sommers-Flanagan, 87
Sorbell, L., 158
Sovik-Johnston, A. F., 83
Stanton, 82
Staudinger, U. M., 170, 174

Author Index

Stebnicki, M. A., 218
Steen, T. A., 163, 165
Stewart, C., 44
Stroebe, M. S., 167
Stroebe, W., 167
Sturza, M. L., 50, 51, 111
Substance Abuse and Mental Health Services Administration, 48, 51, 100, 101–2, 106, 108, 111, 197–98, 207, 222–23
Sue, D., 203, 205, 206, 207
Sue, D. W., 197, 203, 205, 206, 207
Sumner, K., 77
Surry, J., 205

Talmon, M., 151
Tarbox, A. R., 105
Taylor, E., 163
Taylor, S. E., 197
Tedeschi, R. G., 170, 174
Thoresen, C. E., 165
Thoreson, R. W., 217, 224, 227
Tisdell, E. J., 173, 175
Tober, G., 158
Tramontin, M., 18, 28–30, 31, 32, 35, 221
Tredinnick, M. J., 202

Urgenson, F. T., 205

Vacc, N. A., 196
Van der Walde, H., 205
van Hout, 83
Van Wormer, K., 50, 111, 158, 173, 203

Vasquez, M., 87
Vernberg, E. M., 20
Vettor, S. M., 222

Walsh, F., 83
Wang, V. O., 172
Washton, A. M., 163
Watson, P. J., 20
Weaver, J. D., 29, 31, 42, 227
Webb, P., 166
Webber, J., 47
Weltz, S. H., 205
Westra, H. A., 158
White, J. W., 50, 111
Wilkerson, K., 222
Willer, J., 218
Williams, L., 83, 84, 87, 99
Winek, J., 82, 87
Wise, E. A., 47
Wittmer, J., 196
Wogrin, C., 166, 178
Woodhouse, S., 165
Worden, W., 167, 169

Yalom, I. D., 78, 79
Yeager, K. R., 203
Yep, R., 47
Young, H. E., 202

Zealberg, J. J., 46
Zusman, J., 28
Zweben, J. E., 163

Subject Index

Note: Page numbers followed by (t) indicate tables.

abused children. *See* child abuse
acculturation, 194, 196, 202, 209
action
  beliefs link, 155–56
  as change stage, 76, 162, 163
acute stress disorder, 32, 34
acute support (treatment model Stage I), 20, 33
adaptational theory, 17(t)
addiction, 42, 47–52
  assessment, 31, 101–6
  case study, 48, 106
  co-occurring disorders, 49–50, 106–7
  eating disorder components, 51–52, 113
  exercise, 48, 106
  hot lines, 43
  motivational interviewing, 157
  suicide rate, 126
  See also substance use/abuse/dependence
adolescent counseling, 85
Adult Suicidal Ideation Questionnaire, 128
affective processes, 21
affective profile (BASIC personality), 4
African Americans. *See* race/ethnicity
age, 195, 202–5
agency setting, 42, 45–46
Alcoholics Anonymous, 5
alcohol use. *See* substance use/abuse/dependence
Alcohol Use Disorders Identification Test, 102–3,
  103–4(t)
American diversity myth, 196
American Red Cross, 29
anger, 167, 223

anorexia nervosa, 51
  definition of, 113
anxiety, 154, 167, 204
anxiety disorder, 127
anxiety management, 33
apology, counselor, 201
applied crisis theory (domains), 18–19, 19(t)
ASD (acute stress disorder), 32, 34
ASIQ (Adult Suicidal Ideation
  Questionnaire), 128
assessment, 4, 5, 95–130
  brief therapy, 151, 152
  commonly occurring diagnoses, 41–53
  disaster mental health, 31–32, 34, 99–101
  instruments, 96, 98–101
    Adult Suicidal Ideation Questionnaire, 128
    alcohol use tests, 102–4
    BASIC personality profiles, 4, 21–22, 76,
      97–98
    Beck Depression Inventory, 128
    Childhood Trauma Questionnaire, 111–12
    Domestic Violence Wheel/Risk Appraisal
      Guide, 108, 109–10
    DSM-IV-TR, 51, 99, 107, 113
    eating attitudes questionnaires/BMI indexes,
      113–24
    Eight Cs for Couple Functioning and
      Assessment, 83
    Hare Psychopathy Checklist, 110
    OARS+ strategies, 160
    short portable mental status
      questionnaire, 100

265

assessment (*Continued*)
    trauma symptom inventory, 101
    Women's Experience with Battering (WEB)
        scale, 109–10
    instrument selection guidelines, 98–99, 101
    overview, 97–98
    positive psychology, 164–65
assimilation, 202
attachment, 167
AUDIT. *See* Alcohol Use Disorders Identification
    Test
Australian railway disaster, 3, 20
automatic-responding thought, 156
avoidance, 51, 99–100, 113

basic crisis theory, 16
BASIC ID (seven modalities of personality), 4,
    21–22, 76
    case study, 22
BASIC personality profile (Behavioral, Affective,
    Somatic, Interpersonal, Cognitive), 97–98
battered women, 108, 109
Beck Depression Inventory (BDI), 128
behavior
    changes from brief therapy, 151, 152
    child crisis reaction, 203
    emotions affecting, 155
    motivation for, 153, 158
    normative, 194, 196
    as personality module, 21
    values conflict, 159
behavioral therapy. *See* cognitive-behavioral
    strategies
beliefs-actions link, 155–56
bereavement. *See* grief therapy
bibliotherapy, 155, 162
binge eating, 113
biofeedback, 224
biomedical model, 77
bisexuals, 195, 207–8
body awareness, 35, 224, 226
body mass index (BMI), 118–25
    calculation, 123–24(t)
    norms variance, 121
    3rd/5th/10th percentiles, 125(t)
    underweight, 119(t)
    underweight/very underweight, 122(t)
borderline personality disorder, 127
brief therapy, 32, 149, 150–57, 176
    advantages, 152
    assessment, 152
    case study, 177
    components, 151

exercise, 179
focus, 150
techniques, 153–57
    cognitive-behavioral, 155–56
    solution-based, 156–57
theoretical perspectives, 153
treatment, 152–53
    FRAMES components, 152–53
bulimia nervosa, 51
    definition of, 113
bullying, 44
burnout, 76, 221–26
    definitions of, 221
    self-care approaches, 222–25

CAGE (alcohol use test), 104
calm, counselor, 6, 8, 31
"catastrophic outbursts," 44
cathartic ventilation, 81
CF. *See* compassion fatigue
change
    grief reaction to, 167
    motivational interviewing, 157–61
    motivation/readiness, 76–77
    post-trauma growth, 174–75
    See also stages of change model
change talk, eliciting, 160–61, 179
chaos theory, 16, 17(t)
character strengths, 165
child abuse, 5, 108, 203
    assessment/trauma screening, 111–12
    counselor duty to report, 87, 112
    sexual, 50–51
Childhood Trauma Questionnaire, 111–12
children
    crisis assessment/counseling, 203, 205
    disaster-response group counseling, 79
    trauma treatment techniques, 76, 166
CISD. *See* critical incident stress debriefing
Civil Rights Act (1964), 193
client
    coping methods failure, 3
    crisis situation behavior, 6–7
    culturally different, 191–210
    difficult, 43, 82
    distorted schema, 155–56
    informed consent, 86, 87
    motivation to change, 76
    patterns of crisis, 96
    perception of crisis, 3
    resistant, 29, 34
    strengths-weaknesses assessment, 165
    suicidal, 126–28

triangle of person, 154
See also counselor-client connection
client assessment. *See* assessment
client-centered approach, 31, 157
client resilience, 149, 170–72, 177
   main concepts, 170
   spiritual perspective, 175–76
   techniques, 171–72
Cocoanut Grove nightclub fire
      (Boston, 1944), 4
cognitive-behavioral strategies, 16, 33, 75, 85,
      153, 157
   brief therapy, 155–56
   counselor self-care, 224
   focus of, 155
cognitive crisis intervention model, 23, 23(t)
cognitive restructuring therapy, 155–56, 169
commitment, 163, 198
commonly occurring diagnoses, 47–53
   addiction, 42, 47–50
   eating disorders, 42, 51–52, 112–26
   intimate partner violence, 42, 49–51
   sexual abuse, 42, 44, 50–51, 111–12
commonly occurring diagnoses settings, 41–47
   agency, 42, 45–46
   private practice, 42, 47
   school, 42, 44–45
   telephone, 42, 43–44
commonsense approaches, 199
communication breakdown, 197
communication skills, 176
community mental health, 5, 47, 151
   resilience development, 172, 176
   spirituality, 176
   trauma response, 44–46
   See also mental health/general trauma
      assessment
Community Mental Health Centers Act
      (1963), 45
community of support. *See* support networks
comorbidity. *See* co-occurring disorders
compassion fatigue (counselor), 218, 221–22
compulsiveness, 51, 113
confidentiality, 85, 86–88
   exceptions, 87–88, 130
consciousness raising techniques, 162
consultation, 85, 227
contemplation (change stage), 76, 77, 162, 163
co-occurring disorders, 33, 42, 49–50
   assessment, 106–7
   case study, 49, 107
   exercise, 49, 107
   settings, 41–47

suicide risk, 126–28
   See also substance use/abuse/dependence
coping strategies
   as brief therapy focus, 150, 155
   counselor burnout prevention, 222–25
   crisis counseling groups, 80
   cycle of normalcy, 74
   failure of, 3, 28
   reduction of negative, 33, 34
   resilience development, 171
   stages of change, 77
   See also self-care
counselor. *See* mental health professional
counselor-client connection
   bridge building, 192, 193–94
   calmness and compassion, 2, 8
   commitment to client's welfare, 166
   communication breakdown, 197, 200
   countertransference, 30, 86, 151, 174, 192, 206,
      207, 208, 221
   cross-cultural dialogue, 197–98, 201, 202, 209
   cultural/normative behavior differences, 195,
      196, 197
   dual instances, 86
   goal focus, 150, 151, 157, 162, 164
   here-and-now approach, 151–52
   legal/ethical concerns, 86–89
   motivational interaction, 158–59
   motivational traps to avoid, 159–60
   out-of-balance, 222
   race/ethnicity issues, 208
   rapport establishment, 20, 29, 30, 36, 77
   resilience development, 171, 172, 175–76
   spirituality integration, 173, 174–75
   therapeutic relationship, 33, 47, 151, 152, 192,
      208, 219, 224
   transference, 151, 154, 208
   trust establishment, 76, 200
   See also therapy types and techniques
counterconditioning, 163
countertransference, 30, 86, 151, 174, 192, 206,
      207, 208
   negative, 221
couples counseling, 82–85
   case study, 88, 89–90
   exercise, 84–85
   problem-solving approach, 83, 156, 157
   top 10 practical suggestions, 84
crisis
   client patterns of, 96
   complex elements of, 97
   counselor poise during, 6
   as danger and opportunity, 4

crisis (*Continued*)
  definition of, 3
  disaster vs., 28
  existential issues, 172–73
  factors in, 77
  as isolating experience, 75
  spiritual development from, 175
  stages theory, 5
  two types of, 28
  See also crisis theories
crisis hotlines, 5, 43–44
crisis intervention and counseling, 3–8, 13–24
  agency counseling teams, 45
  case study, 9, 24
  components, 3, 4, 19, 20
  continuum, 4
  core of crisis, 42
    addiction, 47–50
    eating disorders, 51–52
    intimate partner violence, 49–51
    sexual abuse, 50–51
  definition of, 3
  defusing/debriefing, 227
  disaster mental health counseling vs., 28–29
  ethical/legal issues, 85–90
  exercise, 8–9, 24
  general interventions
    multimodal therapy, 19, 21–22
    psychological first aid, 3, 4, 19–21, 33
  handling violent situations, 87–89
  hazards of, 21–25
    burnout, 76, 221–26
  history of, 4–6, 16
  interactive approach, 3
  interagency cooperation, 7–8
  intervention models, 22–23, 23(t)
  layers of crisis, 49, 50
  research-based approaches, 5
  settings, 41–53
    agency, 42, 44–45
    private practice, 47
    school, 42, 44–45
    telephone, 42, 43–44
  short-term techniques, 16
  specific populations, 73–90
    couples/family therapy, 82–85
    group therapy, 78–82
    individual therapy, 75–78
    multicultural counseling, 191–210
  theory flexibility, 15–18
  timing of, 4
  See also assessment; therapy types and
    techniques

crisis theories, 13–24
  applied theory (domains), 14, 18–19, 19(t)
    four areas, 18
  case study, 17–18
  choice of, 14–16
    basic, 16
    expanded, 16–18, 16–17(t)
  as counselor's metaphorical rudder, 14
  eclectic sources, 16
  exercises, 18, 19, 22, 24
  learning objectives, 13
  overall framework, 14, 15
critical incident stress debriefing, 33, 34, 80
  cautions on use, 34
critical incident stress management, 80
Crombach's coefficient alpha (reliability), 98
"cultural brokers," 202
cultural differences, 77
  acculturation/normative behavior, 196
  cross-cultural competence, 197–98, 202
  grief processing, 169
  respect for, 200, 201, 206
  sensitivity development, 193–94
  See also multicultural counseling
culture, definition of, 193

DARN-C (change talk components), 161
DBT (dialectical behavior therapy), 34
death
  grief reaction, 167–68
  lethality potential, 31, 44, 127
  school setting, 44
  See also homicide; suicide risk
debriefing, definition of, 227
debriefing model, 34
defensive reaction, 154
defusing, definition of, 227
denial, 7, 108, 167
depersonalization, 166
depression, 32, 33, 34, 51
  Beck Depression Inventory, 128
  childhood sexual abuse victims, 111
  diagnosis of cause, 166
  distorted schemata, 155–56
  grief-related, 167
  hot lines, 43
  older adults, 203, 204
  trauma screening, 111
  women, 205, 206
developmental crisis, definition of, 28
developmental/ecological crisis intervention
    model, 23, 23(t)
developmental theory, 16, 17(t), 18, 19(t)

diagnosis. *See* assessment
dialectical behavior therapy, 34
dialogue, components of, 198
dialogue letter, 169
differential diagnoses, 96
directive counseling, 158
disabled people, 195
disaster mental health counseling, 6, 20, 27–36, 47
  assessment, 31–32, 34, 99–100
  case study, 36
  cultural factors, 202–5
    children, 203, 205
    gender, 205–6
    older adults, 203–5
  exercises, 36
  group format, 79
  hazards of, 30–31
  learning objective, 27
  legislation, 45
  overview, 28–30
  self-care suggestions, 34–35
  techniques and treatment, 30–35
  three stages, 33–34
  traditional clinical work vs., 29
disasters, 5, 28–32
  emotional intensity range, 31
  four time frames for, 32
  natural or human-caused, 28
  seven stages of, 28, 31
  situational intensity of, 30–31
discrepancy (motivational interviewing component), 158, 159
discrimination, 203, 204, 205, 207
disillusionment phase (disaster), 32
distorted schema, 155–56
distress reduction, 20, 33
diversity, American myth of, 196. *See also* multicultural counseling
divorce counseling, 47
documentation, 85
domains. *See* applied crisis theory
domestic violence. *See* intimate partner violence
Domestic Violence Risk Appraisal Guide, 109, 110
Domestic Violence Wheel, 108
drug abuse. *See* substance use/abuse/dependence
DSM-IV-TR, 51, 99, 107, 113
dual diagnosis, 31
dual relationship (counselor-client), 86
Duluth Intervention Project, 108
duty to report, 87–88, 112
duty to warn, 87, 88–89

DVRAG (Domestic Violence Risk Appraisal Guide), 109, 110

Eating Attitudes Test (Eat-26©), 113–25, 113–117(t)
  behavioral questions form, 120–121(t)
  interpretation, 116–25
  scoring system, 118
eating disorders, 42, 51–52, 112–26
  assessment, 31, 112–25
  case study, 52, 126
  exercise, 52, 126
ecosystems theory, 17(t), 18, 19(t)
Eight Cs for Couple Functioning and Assessment, 83
emotional maturity, 6
emotions
  as behavior effect, 155
  disaster-reaction intensity, 31
  grief-linked, 167
  management of, 171, 172, 176
  mindfulness, 224, 226, 228
  negative, 86
  positive, 163
empathy (brief therapy FRAMES component), 152, 153
empathy (motivational interviewing component), 158–59
empathy, cultural, 198, 199
empathy fatigue (counselor), 218, 221–22
empty chair technique, 169
environmental stress management, 8
equilibrium crisis intervention model, 23, 23(t)
ethical/legal issues, 85–90
  duty to report, 87–88, 112
  homicide potential, 130
  professional self-care, 219
ethnicity. *See* race/ethnicity
ethnocentrism, 197, 200
evolutionary epistemology, 168, 169
exercise. *See* physical exercise
existential theory, 16, 18, 19(t)
expanded crisis theory, 16–18, 16–17(t)

families
  brief therapy for, 155, 156
  of disaster victim, 4, 31
  group therapy re-creation of, 78
  high-functioning vs. poorly-functioning, 83
  See also child abuse; intimate partner violence
family counseling, 82–85
  case study, 88, 89–90
  confidentiality, 87

family counseling (*Continued*)
   exercise, 85
   problem-solving approach, 83
   top 10 practical suggestions, 84
fatigue, 167, 218, 221–22
fear, 1, 2, 86
   counselor management of, 223
feedback (brief therapy FRAMES component), 152, 153
feedback loops, 171, 176
feelings. *See* emotions
flexibility
   client self-concept, 171
   counselor, 6–7, 29, 30, 42, 127, 200
   counselor self-care plan, 226
   crisis assessment, 97
flow, 163, 164
focused single-session therapy, 153
FRAMES (brief therapy aspects), 152–53

gays, 195, 196, 207–8
gender, 205–6
   case study, 206
   exercise, 206
   homicidal tendency, 129
   intimate family violence, 108–10
   rape victims, 111
   See also sexual orientation; women
general systems theory, 16
genograms, three-generation, 160
GLBT individuals, 195, 207–8
goals, 164, 223
   brief therapy focus, 150, 151, 157
   stages of change, 162
gratitude visit (positive psychology technique), 165
grief
   complicated, 32, 34
   definition of, 167
   symptoms of, 167
   unresolved, 4
grief exercises, 162
grief therapy, 32, 149, 165–70, 176
   case study, 178
   exercise, 179
   main concepts, 167–69
   techniques, 169–70
group counseling, 78–82
   case study, 88, 89–90
   confidentiality, 87
   crises within group, 79–80, 82
   developmental structure of group, 79–80
   exercise, 81–82

practical suggestions, 81
   specific crisis types, 80–81
   training for, 79, 80

HALT (Hungry, Angry, Lonely, Tired), 35, 224
happiness, 163, 164
Hare Psychopathy Checklist, 110
hate crimes, 207
health insurance, 45, 46, 150
helplessness, feelings of, 167
here-and-now approach (brief therapy), 151–52
heroic phase (disaster), 32
Hispanics. *See* race/ethnicity
HIV/AIDS, 89, 207
homelessness, 208
homework, 33, 51, 155, 156, 165
homicide, 4, 126, 129–30
   assessment instrument, 130
   case study, 129
   exercise, 130
homophobia, 207
homosexuals. *See* sexual orientation
honeymoon phase (disaster), 32
hope, 163, 164, 165, 172
   counselor, 219
hopelessness, 127, 155–56
hotlines, 5, 41, 43–44
human-caused disasters, 28
humanistic psychology, 16, 163
humor, 35, 224–25, 226, 228
Hurricane Katrina, 5
hypervigilence, 100

identity development, 209
impulse, 127, 154
impulse control, 176
incarceration, 208
individual counseling, 75–78
   case study, 88, 89–90
   exercise, 78
   top 10 practical suggestions, 77
informed consent, 86, 87
interagency collaboration, 7–8
   case study, 9
inter-feedback loops, 171, 176
intermediate support (Stage 2), 33
Internet, 5
   counseling, 85
interpersonal relationships, 21, 82
   BASIC personality profile, 4
   bridges, 192, 193–94
   brief therapy re-enactment of, 152
   deepened, 174, 175

developing quality of, 171
loss effects, 167–68
of mental health professional, 225, 226–27
supportive, 172, 175
as women's focus, 205–6
See also support network
interpersonal theory, 16, 17(t)
intervention. *See* crisis intervention and
    counseling
intimate partner violence, 5, 42, 49–51, 85
assessment, 31, 108–10
case study, 50, 110
counselor duty to report, 87–88
definition of, 49–50, 108
different settings, 42
exercise, 110
hot lines, 43
overview, 108
recidivism prediction, 110
intimidation, 108
intra-feedback loop, 171, 176
IPV. *See* intimate partner violence
irrational beliefs, 155
isms, 194, 195

journal keeping, 156, 169

Kuder-Richardson formula 20 coefficient
    (reliability), 98

language, 202
grief expression, 168–69
legal issues. *See* ethical/legal issues
lesbians, 196, 207–8
lethality potential, 31, 44, 127
life transitions, 173, 179
looking back/forward, 161
loss, 167–68, 169, 204

maintenance (change stage), 76, 162, 163
male privilege, 108
managed health care, 45, 46, 150
marginality, 173, 205
marriage. *See* couples counseling; family
    counseling; intimate partner violence
Massachusetts General Hospital, 4
MAST (Michigan Alcohol Screening Test), 104–6
maturational/developmental theory, 18
meaning, 219
reconstruction of, 168–69
means (brief therapy FRAMES component), 152
medical emergencies, 44
meditation, 220, 224

meltdown, 7
memories, intrusive, 99
memory book, 169
memory problems, 167
mental health/general trauma assessment, 31–32,
    34, 99–101
alcohol/drug problem, 107, 172–73
case study, 101
exercise, 101
older adults, 203–4
school response, 44
suicide overlap, 126, 127
See also community mental health; disaster
    mental health counseling
mental health professional
brief therapy attitudes, 151, 152
budget constraints, 152
burnout, 221–26
common diagnoses, 41–53
crisis-context multicultural counseling, 201–2
crisis intervention model choice, 22–24
crisis problem layers, 49, 50
cross-cultural competence, 197–98, 202
cultural sensitivity development, 193–94
diagnostic bias, 194, 195, 197, 200, 204, 206
disaster situation, 28–35, 204
economy-motivated cutback effects, 42, 45
ethical concerns, 86–89
fundamental lessons/strategies, 225–26
helpful characteristics, 2, 6–8, 75, 199, 201
    flexibility, 6–7, 29, 30, 127, 194, 200
    humor, 35, 224–25
    other awareness, 192
    resilience, 6, 7, 218, 223, 224, 226, 229–30
    sensitivity, 208
job market flexibility, 42
listening skills, 158, 160, 166
as metaphorical rudder, 2, 6, 14
overwhelmed feelings, 166
perspective, 77
professional expertise, 200
self-awareness, 192, 194, 204
self-care, 6, 7, 8, 34–35, 43, 46, 217–33
    fundamental lessons/strategies, 225–26
special group-counseling training, 79
theoretical framework, 13–24
working within area of own competence, 174
See also counselor-client connection
metaphors
counselor's guidance, 2, 6, 14
grief experience, 169
layers of crisis, 49, 50
MI. *See* motivational interviewing

Michigan Alcohol Screening Test, 104–6
mindfulness, 224, 226, 228
minority clients. *See* multicultural counseling
miracle question, 156, 157
Mobile Crisis Unit, 46, 47
mood disorders, 51, 127
   trauma screening, 111
   See also depression
moral decisions, 85–86
motivation
   client level of, 161–62
   presenting vs. actual, 76–77
Motivational Enhancement Therapy, 157
motivational interviewing, 32, 76, 77, 149,
     157–61, 162, 176
   case study, 177
   exercise, 179
   four general principles, 158
   in grief therapy, 166
   main concepts, 158–60
   myths about, 157–58
   techniques, 160–61
   traps to avoid, 159–60
mourning, tasks of, 167–68
multicultural counseling, 191–210
   communication breakdown, 197
   in context of crisis counseling, 201–2
   cross-cultural competence, 197–98, 202
   cultural awareness, 201
   definition of multicultural, 192
   dialogue-friendly atmosphere, 198–200, 201
   history of, 193, 196
   influencing factors, 202–10
      age, 202–5
      gender, 205–6
      race/ethnicity, 208–10
      sexual orientation, 207–8
   overview, 193–94
   social-environmental aspects, 194–96, 200
   specific suggestions, 200–201
multimodal therapy, 19, 21–22, 75

9/11 attacks (2001), 1, 5, 6, 225
   children's group counseling, 79
   disaster mental health counseling, 30, 31
narrative truth, 168, 169
National Eating Disorders Screening Program
     (1998), 117
National Health and Nutrition Examination
     Survey III, 121
Native Americans. *See* race/ethnicity
natural disasters, 28, 44
   assessment tools, 96

natural healers, 154–55
negative coping, 33, 34
negative countertransference, 221
negative emotionality, 86
negative-positive balance, 165
negative thought patterns, 155–56
negative transference, 154
NHANES (National Health and Nutrition
     Examination Survey III), 121
nightmares, 99
normalcy, cycle of, 74
normative behavior, 194, 196
NOS (eating disorder not otherwise specified),
     51, 113

OARS+ strategies, 160
ODARA (Ontario Domestic Assault Risk
     Assessment), 109–10
older adults, 195, 202–5
   case study, 204
   exercise, 205
   general approaches, 203–4
   specific issues, 203
ongoing treatment (Stage 3), 33–34
Ontario Domestic Assault Risk Assessment,
     109–10
open questions, 160, 161
oppressed groups, 195, 196, 197, 206, 207

palliative action, 76
PAR™, 99
patriarchal terrorism, 108–11
personality
   factors in shaping, 153
   homicidal tendency, 129
   modules of, 4, 21–22, 76, 97–98
   positive traits, 163, 164, 165, 171, 172
personal needs. *See* self-care
PFA. *See* psychological first aid
phone therapy. *See* telephone setting
physical abuse, 44, 108
physical exercise, 76, 220, 228, 229
   excessive, 113
physical impairment, 44, 203, 204
physical sensations, grief-related, 167
planned short-term psychotherapy. *See* brief
     therapy
planning, 4, 172, 175
play (counselor self-care), 226, 228, 229
play therapy, 166
pleasure, loss of, 167
positive outlook, 172
positive psychology, 32, 149, 163–65, 176

case study, 178
exercise, 179
limits of, 164
techniques, 164–65
positive regard, 199
positive self-view, 172, 175
posttraumatic stress disorder, 32, 34, 89, 96, 98
assessment, 99–101
compassion fatigue comparison, 222
grief therapy, 166
rape survivors, 111
sexual abuse victims, 50–51
specific treatment techniques, 75
substance abusers, 173
symptom inventory, 101
three symptom types, 99–100
poverty, 194, 195, 208
powerlessness, 51, 113
precontemplation (change stage), 76, 77, 162
prejudice, 194, 195
preoccupation, 51, 113
preparation (change stage), 76, 77, 162, 163
prescription drug abuse, 50, 111
private practice setting, 42, 47
helpful responses, 47
privileged communication laws, 86
exceptions, 87
problem exploration
cognitive-behavioral therapy, 155–56
couples therapy, 83, 156, 157
psychological first aid, 4
solution-based brief therapy, 156–57
problem-solving skills, 171, 172, 176
professional conduct principles, 86
professional relationship. *See* counselor-client
connection
professional self-care. *See* self-care
Project Match, 157
PsychCorp, 99
psychiatric emergencies, 85
psychoanalytic theory, 16, 16(t)
psychodynamic brief therapy, 153–55
psychoeducational information, 33
psychological first aid, 19–21, 97
case study, 21
critical incident stress debriefing, 33
definition of, 3
eight core actions, 20
exercise, 21
five components, 4, 20
goal of, 4, 20
psychosocial/transition crisis intervention model,
23, 23(t)

PTSD. *See* posttraumatic stress disorder
public health perspective, 77
purging, 113

questions. *See* open questions; scaling questions

race/ethnicity, 196, 197–98, 202, 208–10
case study, 209
counseling suggestions, 209
exercise, 210
racism, 194, 195
rape. *See* sexual abuse
rating. *See* scaling questions
rational emotive therapy, 155
reconstruction phase (disaster), 32
record-keeping log, 156
recovery phase (disaster), 28
referral networks, 5
reflective listening, 158, 160
reinforcement, 163
relational self, 168–69
relationships. *See* interpersonal relationships
relaxation techniques, 224
reliability, assessment instrument, 98–99
religious solace. *See* spirituality
remedy phase (disaster), 28
rescue phase (disaster), 28
reserve capacity, 170, 174
resilience, 32, 149, 170–77
10 ways to build, 171–72, 175–76, 223
counselor, 6, 7, 218, 223, 224, 226
exercise, 231
definition of, 170
resistance, 29, 34, 154
resistance (brief therapy FRAMES component),
152, 153
resistance (motivational interviewing
component), 158, 159
responsibility (brief therapy FRAMES
component), 152, 153
RET (rational emotive therapy), 155
revolutionary epistemology, 168
rhetoric, 168
"righting reflex," 158
rituals, 169, 226
role-playing, 162, 168, 169
Russian doll metaphor, 49, 50

scaling questions, 157, 159, 161
scapegroup, 196
schemata
definition of, 197
distorted, 155

schizophrenia, 127
school crisis response team (SCRT), 44
school setting, 5, 42, 44–45, 85
  helpful responses, 44–45
  typical crises/issues, 44
secondary traumatic stress disorder, 221, 222
Seeking Safety, 34
self-actualization, 163
self-assessment, 3, 227
self-awareness (client), 86
self-awareness (counselor), 192, 194, 201, 217,
    223, 228, 229
self-care (client), 176
self-care (counselor), 6, 7, 8, 34–35, 43, 46,
    217–33
  case studies, 228–29, 230, 231
  exercises, 229–33
  fundamental lessons/strategies, 225–26
  general techniques, 222–24
  holistic plan, 50
  reasons for practicing, 218
  resources, 219, 220, 226–28
  specific techniques, 224–25, 228–29
  tips, 220
  top 10 practical suggestions, 226, 227
self-compassion (counselor), 221
  components, 224
self-concept, 171
self-disclosure, 170, 175
self-efficacy (brief therapy FRAMES
    component), 152–53
self-efficacy (motivational interviewing
    component), 158, 159
self-efficacy (stages of change), 76, 162
self-efficacy development, 76, 155
self-forgiveness (counselor), 220–21
self-help groups, 227
self-identity, 168–69
self-integration, 164
self-liberation, 163
self-medication, 107, 108, 111, 172–73
self-observation skills, 156
self-perception. See self-view
self-reevaluation, 162
self-reproach, 167
self-talk, 171, 220
  self-view, 18, 170
    change in, 174–75
    positive, 172, 175
    women's relationships, 205, 206
self-vulnerability, 174
sensations, 21, 22
sexism, 206

sex therapy, 166
sexual abuse, 42, 44, 50–51, 111–12
  assessment, 31
  case study, 51, 112
  eating disorder crossover, 113
  exercise, 51, 112
  rape crisis programs, 5
  rape hotlines, 43
  substance use/abuse crossover, 50, 111
sexual orientation, 207–8
  case study, 207
  exercise, 206, 208
  general approaches, 207
shock, 167
Short Michigan Alcoholism Screening Test,
    105–6(t)
short portable mental status questionnaire, 100
short-term psychotherapy. See brief therapy
signature strengths, identifying/using in new way
    (positive psychology technique), 165
single-session therapy, 153
situational crisis
  definition of, 28
  school setting, 44
situational theory, 18, 19(t)
sleep problems, 99, 204
SMAST (Short Mast), 105–6(t)
social-environmental factors, 77, 194–96, 200
  disaster context, 202, 203, 205
  racial/ethnic groups, 208, 209
  suicide risk, 127
social support. See support network
solution-based brief therapy, 156–57
somatic profile (BASIC personality), 4
special populations, 73–85
  case study, 88, 89–90
  couple/family counseling, 82–85, 89
  ethical/legal issues, 85–90
  group counseling, 78–82, 89
  individual counseling, 75–78, 89
specific populations. See multicultural counseling
spirituality, 32, 150, 155, 172–76, 177, 202,
    207, 226
  barriers, 174
  bridges, 174–75
  definition of, 173
  exercise, 179
  techniques, 175–76
stages of change model, 76–77, 149, 161–63, 176
  readiness to change, 77
  specific stages, 76, 162–63
  techniques, 162–63
stereotypes, 194, 197, 198, 203, 205, 206

stimulus control techniques, 163
strategic retreat, 222
strengths
  identifying, 169
  playing to, 171
  See also resilience
stress management (client), 8, 77
  critical incident debriefing, 33, 34, 80
  post-disaster, 29, 31
  psychological first aid, 3
  techniques, 222–25
  See also resilience
stress management (counselor), 217–28
STSD (secondary traumatic stress disorder),
  22, 221
substance use/abuse/dependence, 32, 33, 34, 44,
  47–52, 96
  addiction assessment, 101–6
  burnout-related, 221
  case study, 106
  co-occurring disorders, 49–52, 107
  eating disorder crossover, 113
  exercise, 106
  older adults, 203
  patriarchal terrorism, 108
  racial/ethnic minorities, 208
  sexual abuse offenders, 51, 111
  sexual abuse victims, 50, 111
  specific populations, 207
  specific treatment techniques, 75
  suicide overlap, 126, 127
  trauma-related, 172–73
suicide risk, 4, 44, 85, 126–28
  case study, 128
  exercise, 128
  factors and clues, 127
  older adults, 203
  prevention, 5, 43
summary statements, 160
Summit on Spirituality (1996), 173
supervision, mental health professionals, 227
support networks, 3, 171, 172, 202, 209
  mental health professionals, 226–27, 228
systems theory, 16, 16(t)

Tarasoff v. Regents of the University of California
  (Cal. 1976), 130
telephone setting, 42, 43–44, 85
  helpful responses, 43–44
  typical crisis/issues, 43
termination (change stage), 76, 162
terrorist acts, 1, 5, 6, 44. *See also* 9/11 attacks
test-retest (reliability), 98

theoretical framework, 14, 15
theoretical/philosophical assessment approach,
  96–97
therapeutic relationship, 33, 151, 152, 192, 208, 219
  mindfulness in, 224
therapy types and techniques, 32, 75–86, 149–78
  brief therapy, 149, 150–57
  client resilience, 149, 170–72
  couples/family therapy, 82–85
  grief therapy, 165–70
  group counseling, 78–82
  individual counseling, 75–78
  motivational interviewing, 76, 77, 149, 157–61,
    162, 176–79
  positive psychology, 149, 163–65
  spirituality, 150, 172–76
  stage of change model, 76–77, 149, 161–63
  See also assessment
thoughts
  feelings interaction, 155–56
  identification of, 33
three good things in life (positive psychology
  technique), 165
thriving
  definition of, 170
  improving as, 174
transference, 151, 154, 208
transgender individuals, 195, 207–8
transtheoretical model, 157, 161–62
trauma
  assessment, 31, 99–101, 111
  case study, 101
  children's specific treatment techniques, 76
  community responses, 44–46
  exercise, 101
  grief overlap, 166
  group members' exposure to, 80
  growth following, 174–75
  impact on mental health of, 29, 111, 172–73
  recent/specific treatment techniques, 34
  suicide risk, 127
  symptom inventory, 101
  triggers, 100
  vicarious, 221
  See also posttraumatic stress disorder
triangle of conflict/triangle of person, endpoints
  on, 154
trust, 76, 195, 200
TTM (transtheoretical model), 157, 161–62
24-hour hotlines, 5, 41, 43–44

vicarious traumatization, 221
victim blaming, 196

Vietnam veterans, 5
violence, 207
    duty to warn/report, 87–89
    patriarchal terrorism, 108–10
    rape crisis programs, 5
    school crises, 5, 44
    victim 24-hour hotlines, 43
    See also homicide; intimate partner violence;
        suicide risk
Virginia Tech shooting, 5

"warm lines" (phone), 43
warn, duty to, 87, 88–89
WEB scale, 109, 109–10(t)
well-being, 164
wellness center, 176
Western Psychological Services, 99
wisdom, 163

women
    childhood sexual abuse/adult alcohol problem,
        50, 111
    crisis counseling, 205–6
    eating disorders, 52, 112–13
    intimate partner violence, 108–10
    rape victims, 111
    as special population, 195
Women's Experience with Battering (WEB)
        scale, 109, 109–10(t)
women's movement, 5
workshops, 224
World Health Organization, 102
worldview. *See* schemata

yoga, 224
you are at your best (positive psychology
        technique), 165